An Intensively Compiled Practical English-Chinese Library of Traditional Chinese Medicine

(英汉对照)精编实用中医文库

Chief General Compilers CHEN Kaixian LI Qizhong(Executive) HE Xinghai

总主编 陈凯先 李其忠(执行) 何星海

Chief General Translators SHI Jianrong HU Hongyi XU Yao(Executive)

总主译 施建蓉 胡鸿毅 徐 瑶(执行)

Chinese Massage Therapy (Tuina)

中 国 推 拿

Chief Compiler ZHAO Yi LU Ping

Chief Translator HUANG Guoqi

主编 赵 毅 陆 萍

主译 黄国琪

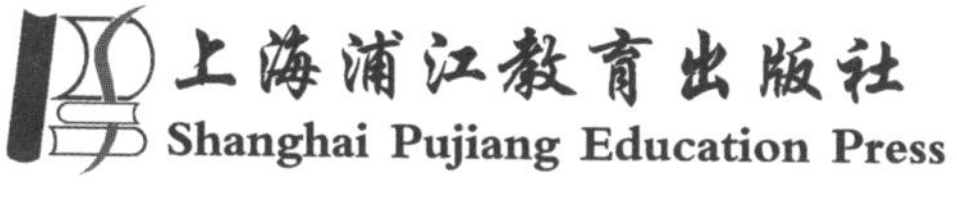

(Former Shanghai University of TCM Press)

An Intensively Compiled Practical English-Chinese Library of Traditional Chinese Medicine

Compilation Board of the Library

Chief General Compilers CHEN Kaixian LI Qizhong(Executive) HE Xinghai

Members(Listed in the order of the number of strokes in the Chinese names)

MA Lieguang	He Jiancheng	YU Xiaoping	SHEN Xueyong
ZHANG Tingting	CHEN Hongfeng	CHEN Dexing	ZHAO Yi
GUO Xin	HUANG Ping	YU Jian'er	ZHAN Hongsheng
MIAO Wanhong			

Compilation and Translation Committee of the Library

Chief General Translators SHI Jianrong HU Hongyi XU Yao(Executive)

Translations(Listed in the order of the number of strokes in the Chinese names)

ZHU Aixiu	YANG Yu	XIAO Yuanchun	ZHANG Yiping
ZHU Jianmin	HUANG Guoqi	DONG Jing	HAN Chouping

Chinese Massage Therapy (Tuina)

Chief Compiler ZHAO Yi LU Ping

Chief Translator HUANG Guoqi

《(英汉对照)精编实用中医文库》

编纂委员会

总　主　编　陈凯先　李其忠(执行)　何星海
编　　　委(按姓氏笔画为序)
马烈光　何建成　余小萍　沈雪勇
张婷婷　陈红风　陈德兴　赵　毅
郭　忻　黄　平　虞坚尔　詹红生
缪晚虹

编译委员会

总　主　译　施建蓉　胡鸿毅　徐　瑶(执行)
编　译　者(按姓氏笔画为序)
朱爱秀　杨　渝　肖元春　张亿萍
诸建民　黄国琪　董　晶　韩丑萍

《中国推拿》

主　　编　赵　毅　陆　萍
主　　译　黄国琪

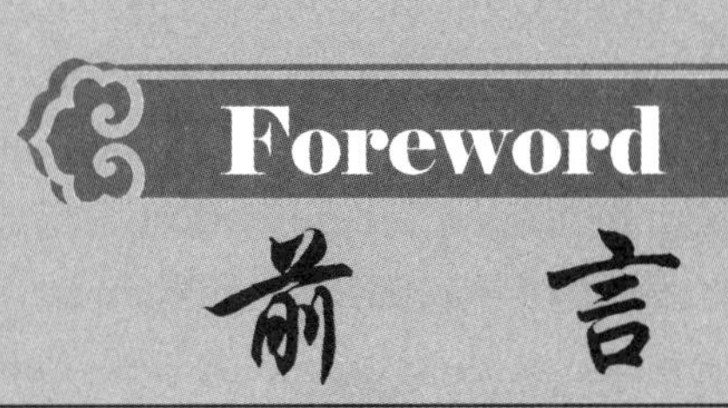

Foreword
前　言

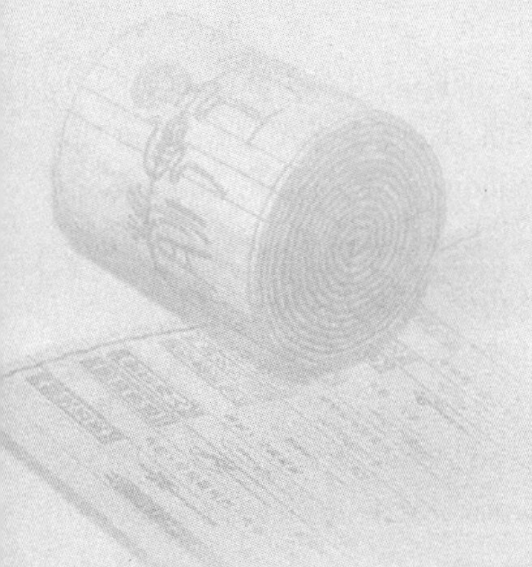

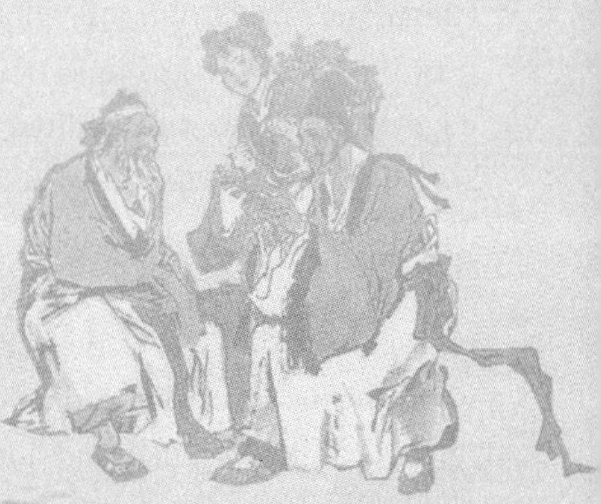

With the traditional medical philosophy and clinical experience as the principal body, the science of Traditional Chinese Medicine (TCM) is a comprehensive subject to study the rules of life activities and the disease prevention, diagnosis, treatment, rehabilitation as well as healthcare. The science of TCM has a long history of development and belongs to a summary of experiences that Chinese nation has fought against diseases for over several thousand years, is also an important component part of Chinese outstanding traditional culture and has contributed greatly to the healthcare undertaking and development of Chinese nation.

By increasing enhancement of modern living standard, change of living modes and acceleration of ageing process, the chronic diseases represented by tumors, cardiovascular diseases and diabetes become gradually the important factors in impacting the health of mankind, but TCM presents the better therapeutic effects. Nowadays, the modern medical mode of "society-psychology-biology" has been advocated in medical science, changing from the medical idea of "disease treatment" to "health promotion". The more and more patients in China and abroad have chosen natural and low side-effect Chinese herbal medicine for their problems. With the changes in medicine modes and in spectrum of diseases in the recent several dozens of years, TCM has increasingly been concerned by the medical experts and ordinary people in China and abroad, and the global " TCM upsurge" keeps rising. In order to meet the growing needs of the domestic and international professionals in learning the knowledge of TCM, we have edited particularly the series books of *An Intensively Compiled Practical English-Chinese Library of Traditional Chinese Medicine*.

The scientific, systematic and practical features have been emphasized in the series books. Based upon the full absorption of new progress in teaching and research achievements of TCM , the series books highlight the academic essentials of TCM, with precise exposition of medical philosophy and down-to-earth clinical practice, to introduce the "original and authentic" TCM to the readers. The series books introduce the commonly used therapeutic methods and clinical skills in Chinese medicine, by the clinically encountered and frequently seen diseases and the relevant ailments predominantly effective by Chinese medical therapies.By studying the series books, the readers can learn the knowledge and techniques of TCM on gradual progress and become proficient gradually in TCM.

The series books highlight"the precise features in three aspects"—capable in authors, refined in contents and accurate in translation. The majority of the authors of the series books are senior experts from the related faculties of Shanghai University of Traditional Chinese Medicine. The translator team is composed of the senior teachers with plentiful expertise in translation of TCM from international education college and foreign language center of Shanghai University of Traditional Chinese Medicine. In order to meet the needs of the readers in China and abroad, the basic and clinical core contents are selected and the latest research achievements are consulted based upon the principle "to seek its essentials but its completion" in the series books.

The series books can satisfy the beginners with certain knowledge of English language in studying TCM systematically and can also be used as the textbooks for education of TCM and pharmacy for foreign students. We sincerely hope the publication of the series books plays its promoting role for TCM going to the world.

Editors

June, 2017

中医学是以传统医学理论与实践经验为主体，研究人体生命活动规律和疾病预防、诊断、治疗、康复以及保健的一门综合性学科。中医学历史悠久，源远流长，是中华民族几千年来同疾病作斗争的经验总结，也是中国传统文化的重要组成部分，长期以来为中国人民的健康保健事业和民族繁衍作出了巨大的贡献。

随着现代生活水平的不断提高、生活方式的改变以及老龄化进程的加剧，以肿瘤、心血管疾病和糖尿病等为代表的慢性病日渐成为影响人类健康的重要因素，而中医药显示了良好的治疗效果。当今的医学倡导“社会—心理—生物”的现代医学模式，医学理念从“疾病治疗”向“健康促进”转变，国内外越来越多的患者选择天然、毒副作用低的中医药治疗疾病。近几十年来，随着医学模式的转变和疾病谱的改变，中医学日益引起越来越多的海内外医学专家和普通民众的关注，全球性的“中医热”正在持续升温。为了满足海内外人士日益高涨的学习中医学知识的需求，我们特地编撰了《(英汉对照)精编实用中医文库》丛书。

本丛书注重“三性”——科学性、系统性、实用性。丛书在充分吸取近年中医教学、科研进展的基础上，突出中医学术精华，理论阐述准确、临床切合实际，向读者介绍“原汁原味”的中医学；丛书介绍中医学常用的治疗方法和临床技能，所涉及的病证均为临床常见病、多发病和中医优势病种。丛书的 13 个分册涵盖了中医基础与临床的主干课程，通过阅读本丛书，读者可以由浅入深、循序渐进地学习中医药知识和技能。

本丛书突出“三精”——作者精干、内容精炼、翻译精准。丛书的中文作者绝大部分为上海中医药大学各相关教研室的资深专家，翻译团队由上海中医药大学国际教育学院和外语中心具有丰富的中医药学翻译经验的骨干教师组成。为了适合海内外读者的需求，丛书本着“求其精而不求其全”的原则，选取了基础和临床的核心内容，翻译上参考了最新的研究成果。

本丛书既可满足具有一定英语水平的初学中医者系统学习中医所用，也可供中医药留学生教育作为教材使用，衷心希望本丛书的出版在中医药走向海外进程中发挥应有的推动作用。

编者

2017 年 6 月

Note for compilation

编写说明

Chinese massage therapy (tuina) is an important component part in traditional Chinese medicine and is an important clinical subject in Chinese medicalpractice. This book introduces the basic knowledge, basic manual techniques and clinical applications of tuina therapy in seven chapters.

The first chapter introduces the basic knowledge, including the definition of tuina therapy, progressive learning method, and body postureof tuina therapy, and medical bed and instruments and commonly used media and ointments for clinical practice, and hot compress in combination with clinical practice. The second chapter introduces the development history of over 3000 years of tuina therapy. The third chapter introduces 20 types of the most commonly used basic manual techniques of tuina therapy. The fourth chapter introduces the clinical application of the manual techniques of tuina therapy on the different body parts. This is a bridge course of technique training for transiting to the clinical application after learning the basic manual techniques of tuina therapy. The fifth chapter is a general introduction about tuina treatment, including the therapeutic functions and therapeutic principles, and indications and contradictions of tuina therapy, and management of abnormal situations in clinical application. The sixth chapter gives the specific introduction of various diseases, introducing tuina treatments for 24 commonly encountered diseases, including 7 types of traumatic and orthopedic diseases, 13 types of internal and gynecological diseases and 4 types of pediatric diseases. Each disease is introduced briefly with its etiology, pathology and diagnostic essentials, and the basic therapeutic methods and pattern identification. The seventh chapter briefly introduces two kinds of training skills, "Tendon-Changing Exercises" and "Shaolin Internal Art".

The whole book is attached with over 100 drawings.

Specialacknowledgement goes to YAO Fei and ZHENG Juan who participate in part of the work during the compilation of this book.

Compiler

July, 2017

推拿是中国传统医学的重要组成部分，是中医的一门重要的临床学科。本书分七章介绍了中医推拿的基础知识、基本手法和临床应用。

第一章简要介绍推拿基本知识，包括推拿的定义，循序渐进学习推拿的方法，推拿的体位，推拿床与推拿器械，推拿常用介质与膏摩，以及配合推拿运用的热敷法。第二章介绍了中国推拿 3000 多年的发展历史。第三章介绍了 20 种最常用的推拿基本手法。第四章介绍推拿基本手法在人体不同部位的操作，这是学习了推拿基本手法后向推拿临床过渡的技能训练桥梁课程。第五章为推拿治疗总论，介绍了推拿的治疗作用和治疗原则，推拿的适应证和禁忌证，以及推拿异常情况的处理。第六章是推拿治疗各论，精选了 24 种常见病证的推拿治疗。包括 7 种骨伤科疾病，13 种内妇科疾病和 4 种儿科疾病。每一病证都简要介绍其病因、病理和诊断要点，重点介绍推拿基本治疗方法及辩证加减。第七章扼要介绍了“易筋经”和“少林内功”两种推拿练功法。

全书附图 100 余幅。

本书编写过程中，姚斐、郑娟娟参加了部分工作。谨此致谢。

编者

2017 年 7 月

Contents

目　录

Chapter 1 Basic knowledge of tuina therapy

第1章 推拿基本知识

Section 1 Brief introduction to tuina therapy

第1节 推拿概述

1 Tuina therapy and science of tuina therapy

In the ancient times, there were different Chinese characters for massage therapy. Respectively, Chinese characters for massage therapy were recorded in *Yellow Emperor's Inner Canon* (Huang Di Nei Jing) published over 2 000 years ago, and in *Medical Secrets* (Yi Men Mi Zhi) published in 1576 of the Ming Dynasty.

tuina therapy is an external therapy in Chinese medicine. Guided by the basic theory of traditional Chinese medicine, various standard manual techniques of tuina therapy are used as the therapeutic means to function on the acupoints or regions of the human body, to realize the goals to prevent and treat diseases.

With the guidance of traditional Chinese medicine and modern scientific theory, tuina therapy is a clinical subject of traditional Chinese medicine for explaining and studying the methods, rules and principles in order to prevent and treat diseases by

1 推拿与推拿学

推拿,古称按摩,还有按蹻等别名。"按摩"的名称记载于2 000多年前的《黄帝内经》,而"推拿"一词则首见于明代1576年的《医门秘旨》一书。

推拿疗法是中医学的一门外治法。它以中医学基本理论为指导,以各种规范性的推拿手法为治疗手段作用于人体的腧穴或部位,以达到防病治病的目的。

推拿学是在中医和现代科学理论的指导下,阐述和研究运用推拿手法防治疾病的方法、规律和原理的一门中医临床学科,以治疗的方

using the manual techniques of tuina therapy, with the therapeutic means as the distinctive feature.

2　How to learn tuina therapy

2.1　Learn both the basic knowledge of Chinese medicine and Western medicine

As a foundation to study tuina therapy, it is necessary to study and master the basic theory of traditional Chinese medicine, and the relevant theory of diagnostic technology of modern medicine, and to master the knowledgc of meridians, acupoints and anatomy of the human body.

2.2　Train the basic skills of manual techniques

It is necessary to study and train the manual techniques of tuina therapy painstakingly, and really master the commonly used basic manual techniques. Three phases should be established to learn the basic skills of the manual techniques.

Phase I: Learn and train the basic movements of the manual techniques, i.e. learn the "forms" of the manual techniques. The main learning method is supposed to imitate, in accordance with the explanation and demonstration of the teacher or in accordance with the demonstration in the video tapes, and in combination of the physiological feature of own hand, and repeatedly copy the teacher's movements and carefully experience their essentials, and have the teacher correct the mistakes during training, in order to gradually form the correct movements of the manual techniques and to obtain an "formed shape".

Phase II: Learn and train the penetrating power of the manual techniques, i.e. train the "spirit" and "effect" of the manual techniques. During this

法作为学科的标志性特征。

2　怎样学习中国推拿

2.1　学好中西医基础知识

作为学习中国推拿的基础，必须先学习和掌握中医学的基础理论，以及现代医学的相关理论和诊断技术，尤其应该掌握经络腧穴知识和人体解剖学知识。

2.2　练好推拿手法基本技能

必须认真刻苦地学习和训练推拿手法，真正地掌握常用基本手法。推拿手法基本技能的学习可以分为三个阶段。

第一阶段:手法基本动作的学习和训练，即学习手法之"形"。学习的方法主要是模拟，根据教师的讲解和示范，或根据视频资料的演示，结合自己手部的生理特点，反复临摹教师的动作并仔细体会其中的要领，并在练习中由教师纠正其错误的动作，逐渐形成正确的手法动作，达到"定型"。

第二阶段:手法渗透力的学习和训练，即练习手法之"神"，或"功力"。此阶段

phase, based upon the mastery of the basic movements of the manual techniques, it is necessary to train the power and persistence of the manual techniques. During the training, it is necessary to maintain identical coordination of the body, and use the force naturally and persistently with the nimble and consistent movements, and prevent local stiffness and over force from causing injury. Without changing the external forms, it is necessary to train the permeating ability of the manual techniques, in order to realize the "spirit" of the manual techniques after long-time training.

在掌握手法基本动作的基础上,再进行手法力量和持久性练习,练习过程中,注意保持身体协调一致,用力自然、持久,动作灵活、连贯;避免局部僵硬和过分用力,造成自我损伤,在不改变其外形的前提下,注重手法渗透力的训练,经过长时间的训练,达到手法"有神"。

Phase III: Train on the human body. In the previous two phases, the training is mainly processed on the rice bag. After the requirements are met, it is advisable to start training on the human body of the third phase. The training contents include the concrete practice of various basic manual techniques on different parts of the human body, and comprehensive practice of the commonly used associative techniques on every body parts. In the training, it is necessary to experience attentively the change of the movements and power of the hand, and continuously enhance the sense of the hand, and gradually adjust the movements and power in accordance with the anatomical structure of different tissues and the specificity of the muscular elasticity, in order to lay a good foundation for future clinical treatment.

第三阶段:人体操作训练。前面两个阶段主要在米袋上练习操作。达到要求后,可以开始第三阶段的人体操作训练。训练的内容是各种推拿基本手法在人体不同部位的具体操作实施,以及每个部位常用的组合性手法套路综合练习。练习时要时刻注意体会手下的动作和力量变化,不断提高自己的手感,逐步做到能根据不同组织解剖结构和肌肉弹性的特殊性及时调整动作和力量的大小,为过渡到推拿临床治疗打好基础。

2.3 Enhance the actual ability to treat diseases by tuina therapy

This period is mainly clinical probation in the department of tuina therapy, in order to learn the diagnostic methods and therapeutic skills and expe-

2.3 提高推拿治病的实际能力

这一阶段是在推拿科见习和实习。主要是向推拿医师学习推拿科常见疾病的诊

rience for the commonly encountered diseases from the clinicians of tuina therapy. This is the final transition period to apply the learnt theory of Chinese medicine and Western medicine and manual techniques of tuina therapy into the clinical service.

断方法以及推拿治疗技术和经验。这是将所学的中西医理论和推拿手法技能应用于临床的最后过渡阶段。

2.4 Train the internal works for tuina therapy

Being a qualified clinician of tuina therapy, it is necessary to master the theory and skills of tuina therapy but also to have a strong physique. The special training method for building up the physique is exactly a training of internal works. The traditional internal works for the students of tuina therapy mainly include tendon-changing exercises (Yi Jin Jing) and Shaolin internal art (Shao Lin Nei Gong). This training of internal works is supposed to train the physique and also train the mind and respiration. Only by the integration of the mind, energy and physique, can the internal works be built up enough for practice of tuina therapy. The training of internal works will be beneficial to guide and help the patients to process the training of internal works and functional rehabilitation in the future clinical workshop.

2.4 推拿功法的训练

要想成为一名合格的推拿临床医师,不仅要掌握中医推拿的理论和技能,还要有强健的体格。体格的专项锻炼方法,就是推拿功法训练。推拿专业医学生的传统功法主要有两种——易筋经和少林内功。推拿功法训练不仅是锻炼形体,还强调意念、呼吸的训练。意、气与形的结合,才能形成推拿操作的功力。推拿功法训练也有助于以后在临床上能指导和帮助病人进行功法训练和功能康复。

Section 2 Body position for tuina therapy

第2节 推拿的体位

In the treatment by tuina therapy, both the clinician and patient should choose a most appropriate body position, beneficial to the practice of tuina treatment. The principle to choose the body position is that the accepter is naturally relaxed in the limbs, with fully exposure of the body parts being

在推拿治疗过程中,医患双方都应选择一种最为合适的体位,以利于推拿治疗的实施。其体位的选择原则是:受术者肢体自然、放松,受术部位充分暴露,并且自

treated, and feels comfortable and safe subjectively. The practitioner is able to operate naturally and use the force conveniently, without any difficulty in shifting the left and right hand, and able to operate continuously without feeling tired.

觉舒适和安全。施术者操作自如,发力方便,左右手交替无障碍,并且能持久操作,不易疲劳。

1 Body position of the accepter

1 受术者的体位

1.1 Supine position

1.1 仰卧位

The accepter takes a supine position, with the two lower limbs extended naturally, and a pillow underneath the popliteal fossa. It is advisable to take this body position for applying massage therapy on the face, chest, abdomen, and anterior aspects of the four limbs.

受术者仰卧,两下肢自然伸直,腘窝下可垫枕而微屈。推拿面部、胸腹部、四肢前面时,常取此体位。

1.2 Prone position

1.2 俯卧位

The accepter takes a prone position, with the head resting in the hole at the head of a table, and a pillow underneath the ankle joint, with the two upper limbs naturally resting on the body side, or flexed and resting on the handles at the two sides of the table. It is advisable to take this body position for applying massage therapy on the nape, shoulder, lumbar region, back, buttocks, and posterior side of the lower limb.

受术者俯卧。头可置于床头的洞中,踝关节下面可垫枕。两上肢自然置于体侧,或前屈放在床头两侧的手托上。推拿项肩部、腰背部、臀部和下肢后部时,可取此体位。

1.3 Lateral recumbent position

1.3 侧卧位

This body position is not commonly taken. But, this body position can be taken in applying massage therapy on the shoulder, buttocks, and lateral aspects of the four limbs, and in doing obliquely pulling method of the lumbar vertebras. This body position is also advisable for those just after eating or unable to lie down prone because of fat body, or because of high age and weak constitution.

侧卧位不常用。但在推拿治疗肩、臀和四肢外侧部位时可用此体位,作腰椎斜扳法时也用到该体位。对于刚吃过饭或身体肥胖不能俯卧者,或年老体弱无法俯卧者,也可取此体位操作。

1.4 Standing position

This body position is seldom. It is advocated in the school of the internal-works massage therapy that the patient should train the standing exercises first before the treatment by tuina therapy, and should accept the chafing method and stick-hitting method in the standing position.

1.4 站立位

站立位推拿的情况较为少见。内功推拿流派主张患者在接受推拿手法治疗前，要先站桩练功，在站立体位下，接受擦法、棒击法等推拿手法治疗。

1.5 Upright sitting position

The accepter sits on a stool upright. This body position is advisable for applying the shaking method on the shoulder, and applying the pulling-extending method on the lumbar region.

1.5 端坐位

受术者正坐于凳子上。在作肩部摇法、坐位腰部拔伸法等操作时可用端坐位。

1.6 Bending sitting position

The accepter sits on a special tuina chair, with the face, chest, two forearms, buttocks, and anterior aspects of the two legs resting on the multiple force spots to support the body, in a very relaxed state in the whole body. This body position is advisable for applying one-finger pushing method on the nape, the rolling method on the shoulder and scapular region, the palm pushing method on the back, the chafing method on the back, and for patting the back and scapular region, and striking the nape and shoulder, and also for applying hot compression on the back.

1.6 伏坐位

受术者伏坐于一种特殊的伏坐式推拿椅上，面部、胸部、两手前臂、两臀、两小腿前部等多点分散受力支撑身体，全身处于一种非常放松的状态。可在此体位下作一指禅推颈项部、㨰肩部、滚肩胛、掌推背部、横擦背部、拍背部、掌振肩胛间区、叩击项肩部等操作，也适合作背部的湿热敷操作。

1.7 Semi-leaning position

This body position is mainly used for practice on the lower limb. This is a commonly used body position for treating the problems on the foot.

1.7 半靠位

主要用于下肢操作。半靠位是治疗足部病症的常用体位。

1.8 Hanging position or foot-up and head-down position

The hanging position means to hold the hanging pole with the two hands to suspend the body. The foot-up and head-down position means to hang the

1.8 悬吊位或倒悬位

悬吊位指双手抓住吊杆使身体悬垂，倒悬位是足高头低悬吊，这是一种比较特

foot higher than the head. This is a specific body position, beneficial to the extension of the spaces of the spinal joints in the lumbar vertebras. This body position is appropriate for treating lumbar intervertebral disc herniation, in the state of traction and extension.

殊的推拿操作体位。有助于腰椎等脊柱关节间隙的拉开。在牵引拔伸状态下推拿，适用于腰椎间盘突出症等病症的治疗。

2 Body position of the practitioner

The body position of the practitioner is usually decided by the body parts being treated. The sitting position is usually taken in massaging the head, face, chest and abdomen. The standing position is often taken in massaging the nape, shoulder, and back and lumbar region. Generally, it is not advisable to sit on the table of the accepter for doing tuina treatment.

2 施术者的体位

施术者的操作体位，主要取决于治疗部位。推拿头面部和胸腹部多取坐位；推拿颈项部、肩部、腰背部多取站立位。一般不要坐在受术者的床上操作。

Section 3 Table and equipment for tuina therapy

第3节 推拿床与推拿器械

1 Treatment table

The treatment table for tuina therapy is about 190 cm long and about 70 cm wide. The height of the treatment table is usually appropriate, if the practitioner stands up, with the two hands just touching the table surface, higher than Japanese treatment table, but lower than western tuina table. This is decided by the force direction of tuina therapy and the angle between the arm and the treatment table. If an electronic treatment table is selected, it is not necessary to consider about the height of the treatment table. An oval hole can be designed at the head of a treatment table, convenient for respiration, in order for the

1 推拿治疗床

中医推拿的治疗床，长约 190 厘米，宽约 70 厘米。床的高度一般以推拿医师站立位双手下垂，手指尖刚刚触碰到床面为宜。通常要高于日本式指压床，但低于西方的按摩床。这是由于中医推拿的用力方式的特点和手臂与床面的角度决定的。如能选用可电动升降的推拿床则不必考虑床的高度问题。床的头部可设计一个方便呼

head to rest on it. The surface of the treatment table should be comfortable. It is not advisable to offer a tuina treatment on a hard table.

吸的椭圆形的洞，以便头可放置其中。床面需软硬适中，不宜在硬板床上推拿。

2　Treatment chair for bending sitting position

This type of the treatment chair for bending sitting position (Figure 1-1) is designed for tuina on the upper body. The face, chest, two forearms, two buttocks and anterior aspects of the two legs can rest on the multiple spots to support the body. Therefore, the whole body is in a very relaxed state. This body position can be used for doing tuina on the nape, shoulder, upper arm, forearm, upper back and offering hot compression on the back.

2　伏坐式推拿椅

这种伏坐式推拿椅(图 1-1)专为推拿上半身的背部而设计。受术者的面部、胸部、两手前臂、两臀、两小腿前部等多点受力支撑身体，故全身处于一种非常放松的状态。可在伏坐位下推拿颈项部、肩部、上臂和前臂、上背部，也可以作背部的湿热敷。

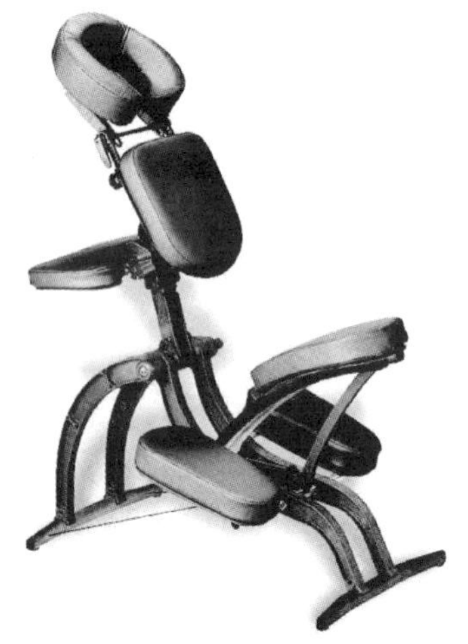

Figure 1-1　Treatment chair for bending sitting position

图 1-1　伏坐式推拿椅

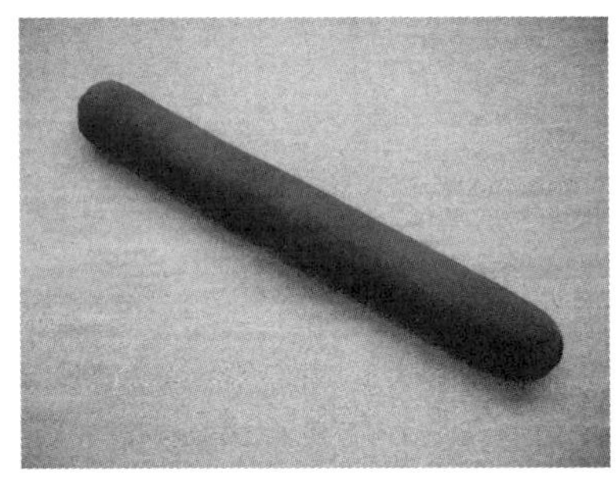

Figure 1-2　Mulberry-twig stick

图 1-2　桑枝棒

3　Mulberry-twig stick

Mulberry-twig stick is a tool used for stick-striking method in tuina therapy. In dog days in summer, 12 pieces of tender mulberry twigs in

3　桑枝棒

桑枝棒是推拿棒击法的工具。桑枝棒制作方法：在三伏天取长为 36～40 厘米、

length of 36～40 cm and in thickness of 0.5 cm are selected and peeled and dried in shadow. Firstly, each piece of mulberry twig is wrapped up with a piece of mulberry paper, and then encircled tensely with cotton threads. Afterwards, 12 pieces of mulberry twigs are tightened together, and wrapped up with mulberry paper and tied up with cotton threads and finally a cotton cover is sutured on it (Figure 1-2).

粗0.5厘米的嫩桑枝12根，去皮阴干。先用桑皮纸包裹每根桑枝，然后用棉线密密环绕一层，再将12根桑枝合并成一把，用桑皮纸包裹并用棉线扎紧，最后在外面缝上棉布套即可(图1-2)。

4 Other equipments

The equipments often used in the department of tuina therapy include acupoint-pressing stick, electronic vibrating massager, traction table, traction chair for cervical vertebras, and hot compression apparatus, etc.

4 其他推拿器械

推拿科常用的推拿器械还有点穴棒、电动振动式按摩器、牵引床、颈椎牵引架、热敷设备等。

Section 4 Media and pastes for tuina therapy

第4节 推拿介质与膏摩

1 Media for tuina therapy

It refers to the preparations with moistening effect and therapeutic effect, applied on the body surface of the accepter during tuina treatment. Those preparations are usually in forms of oil solution, water solution, tincture, paste or powder. The frequently used media for tuina therapy include green onion juice, ginger juice, green onion-ginger juice, talcum, sesame oil, olive oil, safflower oil, turpentine oil, and evergreen paste, etc.

1 推拿介质

推拿介质，指在推拿操作时涂于受术体表起润滑作用或兼有治疗作用的制剂。剂型一般有油剂、水剂、酊剂、膏剂或粉剂。推拿临床常用的介质有葱汁、姜汁、葱姜汁、滑石粉、麻油、橄榄油、红花油、松节油、冬青膏等。

1.1 Evergreen paste

Prepared of methyl salicylate, menthol, and Vaseline as excipient, one of the commonly used media in the clinic of tuina therapy, with the effects

1.1 冬青膏

由冬绿油(水杨酸甲酯)、薄荷脑和赋形剂凡士林等调配而成，是推拿临床最

to warm up the meridians, dredge the collaterals, stop inflammation and stop pain, appropriate for various types of pain due to soft tissue injury and diseases in deficient and cold pattern.

常用的介质之一。有温经通络、消炎止痛的作用，适用于各种软组织损害性疼痛和虚寒性疾病。

1.2 Sesame oil

It mainly gives a moistening effect, a commonly used medium in the rubbing and chafing method, also used for infantile tuina therapy at home, also for scraping method, cupping method or migrating cupping method.

1.2 麻油

主要起润滑作用。是摩擦类手法的常用介质，也用于家庭小儿推拿，亦可用于刮痧、拔罐和走罐。

1.3 Olive oil

It mainly gives a moistening effect.

1.3 橄榄油

主要起润滑作用。

1.4 Talcum powder

Mostly used in summer, also used for infantile tuina therapy to reduce friction between the hand and skin. Usually, it can be replaced by toilet powder at home.

1.4 滑石粉

多在夏季应用，也用于小儿推拿，可减少手与皮肤的摩擦。家庭一般可用婴儿爽身粉代替。

1.5 Turpentine oil

It is a kind of essential oil extracted from the pine tree, with the effects to activate blood, diminish swelling, circulate qi and stop pain, strong permeability through the skin, into the deep tissues, appropriate for obstructive pain in wind and damp pattern, aching pain in the joints and muscles. In the application, it is advisable to avoid contacting with the eyes and mucous membrane of the mouth and nose.

1.5 松节油

是一种从松树中提取的精油。有活血消肿、行气止痛作用，皮肤穿透力较强，能渗入深部组织，适用于风湿痹痛、关节肌肉酸痛等。使用时应避免接触眼睛和口鼻黏膜。

1.6 Safflower oil

It is prepared of safflower, methyl salicylate, and menthol, with the effects to activate blood, diminish swelling, circulate qi and stop pain, appropriate for various types of swelling and pain by soft tissue injury.

1.6 红花油

由红花、冬绿油、薄荷脑等配制而成。有活血消肿、行气止痛的作用，适用于各种软组织损伤肿痛。

1.7 Green onion juice or green onion-ginger juice

It is prepared by pounding fresh green onion

1.7 葱汁或葱姜汁

将新鲜葱白或加生姜捣

stalk or ginger and adding 75% alcohol, with the effects to expel wind, and relieve the exterior. Usually, green onion juice is used for common cold and fever. Green onion-ginger juice is often used in winter or for influenza in wind and cold pattern, in order to warm up the meridians and disperse cold.

烂,加入75%酒精,浸泡取汁备用。具有祛风解表的作用,用于感冒发热等症。通常用葱汁,冬季或风寒感冒用葱姜汁以温经散寒。

1.8 Massage lotion

It is an emulsion prepared of herbal drugs to expel wind, remove dampness, circulate qi and stop pain, appropriate for pain of soft tissue injury.

1.8 按摩乳

是由具有祛风胜湿、行气止痛等作用的中药配制而成的乳剂。适用于软组织损伤疼痛。

1.9 Massage cream

Many creams are available in the market, mostly used for facial massage, and beauty massage.

1.9 按摩霜

有多种市售商品。多用于面部按摩、美容按摩。

1.10 Medicated liquor

The herbal drugs are soaked into liquor for several days to get leach liquor. In accordance with the different pharmaceutical properties of herbal drugs, there are the different effects to circulate qi, activate blood, alleviate spasm, stop pain, and activate blood and disperse blood stasis, etc.

1.10 外用药酒

将中药浸泡于白酒中数日,取浸出液备用。根据所选中药的不同药性,而有行气活血、解痉镇痛、活血化瘀等不同作用。

1.11 Baby skin oil

Prepared of mineral oil, mostly used for infantile tuina therapy, skin care of infants, and also used for adults. It mainly gives a moistening effect. This type of oil is less in irritating the skin and is not easy to induce allergy. It can also be used for the scraping method, cupping method or migrating cupping method for lubrication.

1.11 婴儿润肤油

为矿物油。多用于小儿推拿、婴幼儿抚触,也可用于成人。主要起润滑作用。这种油对皮肤的刺激较小,不易引起过敏。也可用于刮痧、拔罐或走罐时的润滑。

1.12 Aromatic essential oil

It refers to the essential liquid extracted from the flower, leaves and fruit of the plants. Before the application, it needs to be diluted with vegetable oil. There are over 150 types of essential oil, and

1.12 芳香精油

精油是从植物的花、叶、果实等部位提取的精华液体,使用时需用植物油稀释。精油品种有150种以上,常

the commonly used ones are over dozens, such as lavender, rose, rosemary, black pepper, eucalyptus leaf, lemon, spearmint, neroli, ylang-ylang, pelargonium, jasmine and tea tree essential oil. Each essential oil has its specific major effects and can be used optionally. Several types of essential oil can also be combined based upon different recipes.

用的也有十几种，如薰衣草、玫瑰、迷迭香、黑胡椒、桉叶、柠檬、洋薄荷、橙花、香水树、天竺葵、茉莉、茶树精油等。每种精油各具其主要的功效特征，可选择性地应用，也可将多种精油按不同配方组合应用。

2　Paste massage therapy

It refers to an external therapy in Chinese medicine in which the manual techniques of the rubbing method and chafing method are given after herbal paste is applied on the patient's body surface. The herbal pastes belong to the component part of tuina therapy and also a channel for topical application of herbal products. The manual techniques can promote the permeation and absorption of active ingredients of the herbal drugs and the performance of pharmaceutical effect. The herbal drugs can assist the effects of the manual technique and also can moisten the muscles, beneficial to the practice of the manual techniques. Chinese characters for "massage pastes" were first seen in *Essential Prescriptions of the Golden Coffer* (Jin Kui Yao Lüe) by ZHANG Zhongjing of the Eastern Han Dynasty. The earliest paste massage method was recorded in *Herbal Formulas for Fifty Two Diseases* (Wu Shi Er Bing Fang).

2　膏摩

膏摩，是一种以中药膏摩剂（摩膏）涂于患者体表，并施以摩、擦等手法的中医外治法。膏摩是中医推拿疗法的重要组成部分，也是药物外用途径之一。手法可促进药物有效成分的渗透吸收和药理作用的发挥；药物可辅助手法起作用，并能润滑肌肤、有利于手法的操作。“膏摩”一词，首见于汉代张仲景的《金匮要略》。《五十二病方》记载了我国最早的膏摩法。

The massage pastes are paste-like ointment. The massage pastes used currently in the clinics are prepared based upon the ancient traditional herbal formulas by modern processing technology. In accordance with the different herbal formulas, there

膏摩剂，主要是一种糊状软膏。目前推拿临床使用的膏摩剂，是将我国古代传统的膏摩方，以现代制剂方法制备而成。根据所选膏摩

are respectively different effects to circulate qi and stop pain, activate blood and disperse blood stasis, benefit the kidney and strengthen yang, and strengthen the spleen and harmonize the stomach. The herbal formulas for massage pastes are mostly composed of the drugs to warm up the meridians and dredge and collaterals, expel wind and disperse cold, and circulate qi and stop pain, such as *Aconiti Praeparata Radix* (Fu Zi), *Chuanxiong Rhizoma* (Chuan Xiong), *Cinnamomi Cortex* (Rou Gui), *Asari Herba* (Xi Xin), *Pericarpium Zanthoxyli* (Hua Jiao), *Zingiberis Rhizoma* (Gan Jiang), and *Angelicae Dahuricae Radix* (Bai Zhi), etc, plus the herbal drugs selected upon pattern identification and aromatic products. The traditional processing technology of massage pastes is usually supposed to grind the herbal drugs into powder, soak with vinegar and fry with oil and filter and prepare into paste (or prepare with honey into pills, and melt with ginger juice before application). Because fatty pastes are much easier to be absorbed by the skin than hydrosoluble pastes, massage pastes are mostly in form of paste. Because animal oil is more beneficial to be absorbed by the skin than the vegetable oil, most pastes are prepared with animal oil. In the modern times, vaseline or lanolin is mostly used as the substrate. In order to be convenient for skin absorption, various types of skin permeation accelerators can be added, such as laurocapram, dimethyl ketone, etc.

方的不同,有行气止痛、活血化瘀、益肾壮阳、健脾和胃等不同作用。膏摩方的药物组成,以温经通络、祛风散寒、行气止痛类中药居多,如附子、川芎、肉桂、细辛、川椒、干姜、白芷等,再加上辨证用药和芳香药品。摩膏的传统制备方法,一般都是将药物研末,米醋浸泡,油煎过滤,炼为糊膏(或炼蜜为丸,使用时以姜汁化开)。因脂肪性糊剂比水溶性糊剂更易为皮肤吸收,所以摩膏以膏剂为多。又由于动物油比植物油更利于皮肤吸收,所以又以动物油制剂为多,现代多用凡士林或羊毛脂为基质。为便于皮肤吸收,还可加入各种皮肤渗透促进剂,如月桂氮䓬酮、二甲基亚酮等。

The famous ancient herbal formulas of massage pastes are Huanggao (Yellow Paste) (*Handbook of Prescriptions for Emergencies* (Zhou Hou Bei ji Fang)), Qinggao (Blue Paste) (*Thousand Golden*

知名的古代膏摩方有黄膏(《肘后备急方》)、青膏(《千金要方》)、白膏(《千金要方》)、陈元膏(《肘后备急

Prescriptions (Qian Jin Yao Fang)), Baigao (White Paste) Qian Jin Yao Fang), Old Element Paste (Chen Yuan Gao) (Zhou Hou Bei Ji Fang), Red Sage Paste (Dan Shen Gao) (Zhou Hou Bei Ji Fang), Shikimic Paste (Mang Cao Cao) (Zhou Hou Bei Ji Fang), Five-Ingredient and Licorice Massage Paste (Wu Wu Gan Cao Sheng Mo Gao) (Qian Jin Yao Fang), Aconitum Paste (Wu Tou Gao) (*Supplement to Thousand Golden Prescriptions* (Qian Jin Yi Fang), Deliberate Tumble Paste (Cuo Die Gao) (*The Medical Secrets of An Official* (Wai Tai Mi Yao)), Massage and Wind Paste (Mo Feng Gao) (*Ancient Literature from Dunhuang* (Dun Huang Yi Shu)), Stephania Tetrandra Paste (Han Fang Ji Gao) (*Peaceful Holy Benevolent Prescriptions* (Tai Ping Sheng Hui Fang)), Top Heliotrope Paste (Mo Ding Qing Lian Gao) (*Savior General Compendium* (Sheng Ji Zong Lu)), Great Tonic Massage Paste (Da Bu Yi Mo Gao) (Sheng Ji Zong Lu)), Deer Marrow Pills (Wai Lu Sui Wan) (*Han's Medical Rules* (Han Shi Yi Tong)), etc. The compatibility, efficacy and indications of those classic herbal formulas for tuina therapy are still valuable for reference.

方》)、丹参膏(《肘后备急方》)、莽草膏(《肘后备急方》)、五物甘草生摩膏(《千金要方》)、乌头膏(《千金翼方》)、蹉跌膏(《外台秘要》)、摩风膏(《敦煌遗书》)、汉防己膏(《太平圣惠方》)、摩顶青莲膏(《圣济总录》)、大补益摩膏(《圣济总录》)、外鹿髓丸(《韩氏医通》)等。这些经典膏摩方中的药物配伍和功效主治,至今仍有一定的参考价值。

Section 5　Hot compress

Hot compress therapy is a traditional external therapy with warming effect. Hot compress is often used together with tuina therapy. For instance, hot compress therapy is regarded as a common auxiliary method in the school of the internal tuina therapy. Based upon the treatment by the manual techniques, the heated towel is applied on the sick area, to

第5节　热敷

热敷疗法是一种具有温热效应的传统外治法。热敷常与推拿配合应用。如内功推拿流派就将热敷法作为常用的辅助治疗方法,在推拿手法治疗的基础上,将已加热的毛巾等敷于患部,借助

intensify the therapeutic effect of the manual techniques by its warming efficacy and herbal action. Hot compress can be divided into wet hot compress and dry hot compress. Hot compress can be given in the clinic or ward of the hospital, and can also be given at home by instructing the patient or family member.

其温热效应和药物作用以加强手法的治疗效果。热敷可以分成湿热敷与干热敷两大类。热敷可以在医院的门诊或病房进行,也可指导患者或其家属在家中自行操作。

1 Efficacy and indications of hot compress

1 热敷的功效与主治

Hot compress therapy is mainly supposed to realize the effects to warm up and dredge the meridians and collaterals, circulate qi and activate blood, relieve the exterior symptoms and disperse cold, dissipate blood stasis and stop pain, and regulate Zang-fu organs by its warming physical feature. The major efficacy of hot compress is "penetration of heat". According to different diseases, the drugs of different properties can be selected to produce the different effects to activate blood and disperse blood stasis, dredge the meridians and collaterals, and disperse cold and stop pain, etc.

热敷疗法主要凭借温热的物理特性而发挥温通经络、行气活血、解表散寒、祛瘀止痛、调整脏腑等治疗作用。热敷的主要效应是"透热",根据不同的疾病,选用不同性能的药物,可有活血祛瘀、疏经通络、散寒止痛等不同功效。

1.1 Warm up the meridians and stop pain

1.1 温经止痛

Hot compress applied on the meridians of the limbs has the effects to warm up the meridians, dredge the collaterals, and dissipate pathogenic cold from the meridians, appropriate for deficient cold pattern mainly manifested by extreme cold sensation in the hand and foot, and numbness and pain in the limbs.

热敷肢体经络,有温经通络、发散经脉寒邪的作用。适用于以手足厥冷、肢体麻木、疼痛为主症的经脉虚寒证。

1.2 Warm up cold and alleviate the exterior

1.2 温寒解表

Hot compress on Tianzhu (BL 10) (two sides of the nape), Dazhui (GV 14), Jianjing (GB 21), and bladder meridian of the back has the effects to warm up and disperse pathogenic cold, promote

热敷天柱(项部两侧)、大椎、肩井、背部膀胱经等部位,有温散寒邪、发汗解表之功。适用于外感风寒之邪束

perspiration and alleviate the exterior, appropriate for blockage of the muscles and body surface by exogenous wind and cold, manifested by superficial and tense pulse, no perspiration, aversion to cold, fever, stiffness and pain of the neck body ache, and lumbar pain. Liquid for wet hot compress can be added with green onion-ginger juice.

肌表，证见脉浮紧无汗，恶寒发热，头项强痛，身疼腰痛。湿热敷的液体，可加入葱姜汁。

1.3 Warm up the lung and dissolve phlegm

Hot compress on the chest and back has the effects to warm up the lung, dissolve phlegm, promote the lung in its distributing ability and stop cough. The flat pushing method (chafing) on the chest and back in the school of internal massage therapy, in combination of hot compress on the chest and back, is its typical application, mainly used for lingering cough, with thin and white sputum.

1.3 温肺化痰

热敷胸背部，有温肺化痰、宣肺止咳作用。内功推拿流派的平推（擦）前胸后背并配合胸背部热敷法为其典型应用。主治咳嗽不止，痰涎稀白者。

1.4 Warm up and dredge the heart yang

Hot compress on the upper back, Xinshu (BL 15) and sternum area has the effects to warm up and dredge the heart yang, used for arrhythmia, stuffy sensation in the chest and shortness of breath.

1.4 温通心阳

热敷上背部、心俞部和胸骨部，有温通心阳的作用。可用于心律不齐、胸闷气短者。

1.5 Warm up and promote the spleen and stomach

Hot compress on the epigastric region, Weishu (BL 21) and Pishu (BL 20) can warm up and excite yang qi of the spleen and stomach, and expel pathogenic cold from the Middle Energizer, appropriate for deficient cold of the spleen and stomach, gastric spasm due to cold, cold pain in the epigastric and abdominal region, vomiting, loose stool, and cold sensation in the four limbs, etc.

1.5 温运脾胃

热敷胃脘部和胃俞、脾俞部位，可温振脾胃阳气，祛除中焦寒邪。适用于脾胃虚寒，胃寒痉挛，脘腹冷痛，呕吐溏泻，四肢不温等。

1.6 Warm up and reinforce the kidney yang

Hot compress on Mingmen (GV 4), Shenshu (BL 23) and Shangliao (BL 31), Ciliao (BL 32),

1.6 温补肾阳

热敷腰骶部的命门、肾俞、八髎和小腹部的关元、丹

Zhongliao (BL 33) and Xialiao (BL 34) at woman's lumbar and sacral region, and Guanyuan (CV 4) and lower abdomen has the effects to warm up and reinforce the kidney yang, mainly used for prolapsed uterus, prolapsed bladder, impotence, seminal emission, soreness and weakness in the low back and knee, aversion to cold, cold sensation in the limbs, frigidity, tinnitus and deafness.

田，有温补肾阳作用。主治子宫下垂，膀胱下垂，阳痿遗精，腰膝酸软，畏寒肢冷，性欲冷淡，耳鸣耳聋者。

1.7 Warm up yang and regulate menstruation

Hot compress on Qihaishu (BL 24), Dachangshu (BL 25), and Shangliao (BL 31), Ciliao (BL 32), Zhongliao (BL 33) and Xialiao (BL 34) at woman's lumbar and sacral region, and Qihai (CV 6), Guanyuan (CV 4), Qugu (CV 2) and Henggu (KI 11) at the lower abdomen has the effects to warm up yang and regulate menstruation, mainly used for dysmenorrhea, irregular menstruation, amenorrhea, and cold pain in the lower abdomen.

1.7 温阳调经

热敷女性腰骶部的气海俞、大肠俞、八髎和小腹部的气海、关元、曲骨、横骨，有温阳调经作用，主治女子痛经、月经不调、闭经、小腹冷痛。

2 Wet hot compress

It refers to an external therapy by applying a heated wet towel on the body surface. It can be a simple wet hot compress by hot water, or can be given by soaking towel in the herbal liquid prepared of compound herbal formula. Ironing method by herbal decoction, herbal powder, or rice wine all belongs to wet hot compress.

2 湿热敷

湿热敷是一种以加温的湿布巾掩覆于体表的外治法。可以是单纯的热水湿热敷，也可以用中药复方的药汁浸泡布巾加温热敷。汤熨、药熨、酒熨，均属于湿热敷。

2.1 Herbal formula for wet hot compress

Besides the simplest hot compress by hot water, hot compress can be prepared with herbal decoction. Hereafter, several commonly used herbal formulas are introduced. The dose of the ingredients in the herbal formulas can be adjusted in accordance with the actual needs.

2.1 湿热敷方

除了最简单的热水热敷外，还可用中药煎汤热敷。这里仅介绍几种常用处方。方中中草药的剂量大小，可根据需要酌情调整。

2.1.1 Traditional herbal formula for hot compress

This is a commonly used herbal formula for hot compress in the school of internal massage therapy.

Composition: *Carthami Flos* (Hong Hua) 10 g, *Cinnamomi Ramulus* (Gui Zhi) 15 g, *Olibanum* (Ru Xiang) 10 g, *Myrrha* (Mo Yao) 10 g, *Lignum Sappan* (Su Mu) 50 g, *Cinnamonum camphora* (Xiang Zhang Mu) 50 g, *Chaenomelis Fructus* (Mu Gua) 10 g, *Arnebiae Radix* (Zi Cao) 15 g, *Lycopodii Herba* (Shen Jin Cao) 15 g, *Caulis Schizophragmae integriforlii seu Radix* (Zuan Di Feng) 10 g, *Liquidambaris Fructus* (Lu Lu Tong) 15 g, and *Homalomenae Rhizoma* (Qian Nian Jian) 15 g, mainly used for sprain, bruise, pain in pattern of wind and dampness, local aversion to cold, soreness in the joints, etc.

2.1.1 传统推拿热敷方

此方为内功推拿流派常用的热敷方。

组成：红花10克，桂枝15克，乳香10克，没药10克，苏木50克，香樟木50克，宣木瓜10克，老紫草15克，伸筋草15克，钻地风10克，路路通15克，千年健15克。主治扭伤、挫伤、风湿疼痛、局部怕冷、关节酸楚等。

2.1.2 Simple herbal formula for hot compress

Composition: *Cinnamonum camphora* (Xiang Zhang Mu) 50 g, *Siegesbeckiae Herba* (Xi Xian Cao) 30 g, *Mori Ramulus* (Sang Zhi) 50 g, and *Polygoni Cuspidati Rhizoma* (Hu Zhang Gen) 50 g, mainly used for pain and tumefaction caused by sprain and bruise, and soreness in the limbs, etc. It is advisable to combine with the fumigation and washing method in the local area.

2.1.2 简化推拿热敷方

组成：香樟木50克，豨莶草30克，桑枝50克，虎杖根50克。主治因扭挫伤而引起的疼痛肿胀，并治肢体酸楚等。可配合局部熏洗。

2.2 Operation of wet hot compress

2.2.1 Wet hot compress in the clinic

It is advisable to do it in the clinic or ward. Usually, by using "traditional herbal formula for hot compress", the practitioner of tuina therapy would give hot compress to the patient: ① Take a cloth bag, put in herbal drugs and tightly enclosed the bag. ② Get a stainless steel pot big enough and put the herbal drugs into the pot, and then pour in cold

2.2 湿热敷的操作

2.2.1 推拿临床湿热敷法

可在医院的推拿门诊或病房内进行，通常用“传统推拿热敷方”，由推拿医师为患者作热敷治疗：①取一个布袋，将中药置入布袋内，并将袋口扎好。②准备一个足够大的不锈钢锅，将药袋放入

water, about 3 cm below the level of top border. ③ Put the pot on a gas stove (or electromagnetic oven) and heat it, and after it boils, simmer it with low fire. ④ Get one or two face towels folded in half and then folded into four layers, with the transverse diameter larger than the longitudinal diameter. Hold the right upper angle and left upper angle respectively with the thumbs, index and middle fingers of the two hands, and soak the towel into the herbal liquid of the pot, and take it out from the herbal liquid after several seconds or a dozen of seconds, and then roll and dry up it. ⑤ Put the dried towel on the local area. If the patient feels too hot and cannot tolerate it, the practitioner should lift up the towel and put it down again after a while. ⑥ The towel for hot compress can be covered with a plastic film to keep warm. ⑦ When the towel is not too hot, change another towel taken from the pot and dried up. The towel should be thus changed for 2～4 times.

锅内，再往锅内注入冷水，使水平面离顶端边缘约 3 厘米。③将锅子放在煤气炉(或电磁炉)上加热，待其沸后，改用小火保温。④用一条或两条洗脸毛巾，将毛巾对折后再行对折成四层，毛巾的横径比纵径为大。用双手拇指和示、中二指，分别捏住毛巾的右上角和左上角，将毛巾浸入锅内药液中，数秒钟或十数秒钟后，将毛巾从药液中取出，卷拢、拧干。⑤将拧干的毛巾敷于局部，若患者感到毛巾过烫而难以忍受，医者应将毛巾取起，等待片刻后再敷。⑥热敷的毛巾外面可用塑料薄膜覆盖以保温。⑦等到毛巾不太热时，再换一条从锅内取出并拧干的毛巾。如此轮换 2～4 次。

2.2.2 Family simple wet hot compress

① Put one or two folded semi-wet towel in a plate. ② Put the towel plate into a microwave oven. ③ Heat the towel for about two minutes depending upon heat level of microwave oven. ④ Firstly, put a dry towel on the area to be applied with wet hot compress, then put the heated towel on it and wrap the heated towel with the dry towel underneath, and then put a piece of plastic film on it, and wrap it up with a quilt to prolong the warm time. ⑤ While the temperature comes down somewhat, take away the dry towel, and apply the hot towel directly on the body surface. ⑥ When the

2.2.2 家庭简易湿热敷法

①将一块或两块折叠好的半湿毛巾，放在碟子里。②把毛巾碟子放入微波炉内。③根据微波炉的火力大小加温 2 分钟左右后取出。④在需要湿热敷的体表部位先垫上一层干毛巾，然后把加温好的热毛巾置于其上，并用下面的干毛巾反包住湿热毛巾。上面可再用塑料薄膜覆盖，再用棉被包好，以延长保温时间。⑤在温度有所

temperature of the heated towel drops down (or after 3～5 minutes), take away the towel or change another hot towel. Usually, the treatment will be given for 20～30 minutes, once per day. ⑦ If necessary, it is advisable to heat the towel in microwave oven for several times.

下降时，去掉干毛巾，将里面的热毛巾直接敷于体表。⑥待热毛巾温度降低时(或3～5分钟后)，去掉或更换下一块热毛巾。一般治疗时间为20～30分钟，每日1次。⑦如有必要，可多次用微波炉加温毛巾并使用。

2.3 Precautions for wet hot compress

(1) Wet hot compress is mainly appropriate for upper back, lower back and four limbs.

(2) There must be no skin ulcer and skin lesion in the local body surface to be applied with hot compress.

(3) The temperature of wet hot compress should be within the patient's tolerance, usually 60～70℃. The time for hot compress is always 15～20 minutes.

(4) In the application of wet hot compress, the higher the temperature is the drier the towel should be twisted. Otherwise, it will easily burn the skin. If the temperature is not high, the towel can be a little bit wetter.

(5) In the application of wet hot compress, it is necessary to fully expose the limbs, and to maintain warm and breezeless in the room.

(6) The towel used for hot compress should be folded tidily. If it is a new towel, it is necessary to pat the towel after it is dried up, and then cover the local area for hot compress with this surface. Thus, it is easy to get close to the body surface, to transmit heat evenly and avoid burning the skin.

(7) Hot compress is a commonly used auxiliary means in the clinics of tuina therapy. The order of

2.3 湿热敷注意事项

(1) 湿热敷主要适用于腰背部和四肢。

(2) 热敷的体表局部必须没有皮肤溃疡和破损。

(3) 热敷温度以患者能忍受为度，一般为60～70℃，热敷时间以15～20分钟为宜。

(4) 湿热敷时，水温越高则毛巾应绞得越干，否则易烫伤皮肤；如果温度不高，可略带点湿。

(5) 热敷时需要充分裸露肢体，所以室内需保持温暖无风。

(6) 用于热敷的毛巾应折叠平整。若是新毛巾，在拧干后，可先将毛巾用手掌拍打一下，然后以此面敷贴于热敷局部，这样可以贴实受术体表，使热量能均匀传导，避免烫伤皮肤。

(7) 热敷是推拿科室常用的辅助治疗手段，某一部

hot compress and tuina treatment in one area should be tuina treatment before hot compress. In the application of hot compress, it is advisable to use the patting method through the towel, but without the pressing and kneading method. For the local area just after hot compress, it is not advisable to do any tuina treatment, in order to avoid inducing skin lesion.

位热敷与推拿的先后顺序，应该是先推拿再热敷。热敷时可隔着毛巾使用拍法，但不可按揉。刚刚热敷完后的局部，不宜再做推拿手法，以免造成破皮。

(8) During hot compress, the practitioner should always observe the patient attentively, in order to prevent the accidents of burns, etc.

(8) 热敷过程中，医者应自始至终观察患者，以防发生烫伤等意外。

(9) For the patients with low sensitivity in the local skin, it is advisable not to use hot compress. If it must be applied, it is necessary to observe more attentively, in order to avoid burns.

(9) 对于局部皮肤知觉迟钝者，应该慎用热敷法。必须使用时，应该加强观察，以免烫伤。

(10) Hot compress is prohibited for the patients with mental disorders.

(10) 神智不正常的患者禁用热敷法。

3 Dry hot compress

3 干热敷

Dry hot compress is mostly termed as "ironing method", in multiple forms. Traditionally, salt, sand, Kan-trigram and Li-trigram Sand (Kan Li Sha), Chinese herbal medicine are often heated and put into the cloth bag for ironing method. In modern times, many hot compress products by chemical heat production and electric heat production are available. Hereafter, several simple, easy and traditional dry hot compress methods are introduced.

干热敷多称为"熨法"，其形式很多，传统多将盐、沙、坎离砂、中草药等炒热后装在布袋内热熨，现代出现了很多化学产热和电子加热的热敷产品。这里仅介绍几种简单易行的传统干热敷法。

3.1 Ironing method for digesting food and removing food retention (self-designed herbal formula by ZHANG Zhenyun, author of *Improved Major Massage Techniques* (Li Zheng An Mo Yao Shu))

3.1 消食导滞熨法(《厘正按摩要术》作者张振鋆自制方)

Composition: *Aurantii Fructus* (Zhi Qiao) 30 g, *Raphani Semen* (Lai Fu Zi) 30 g, *Gleditsiae sinensis Fructus* (Da Zao Jiao) 1 piece and salt 15 g.

组成：枳壳 30 克，莱菔子 30 克，大皂角 1 条，食盐 15 克。上药共研为末，用白

After the above drugs are grinded into powder and fried hot with liquor, the herbal powder is put into a cloth bag and encircled tightly. While it is still hot, the bag is used to iron the epigastric region, in order to circulate qi, dissolve phlegm, digest food and remove food retention, for treating food retention and accumulation of phlegm in the epigastric region.

酒炒热，装入布袋内扎好。趁热敷胃脘部。有行气化痰，消食导滞作用，治疗食积痰滞，结于胃脘。

3.2 Phlegm-warming ironing method (from *Complete Work for Children's Diseases* (You You Ji Cheng))

One piece of Fu Zi and 30 g of Sheng Jiang are grinded and heated and wrapped up into a cloth bag. Firstly, the bag is used to iron the back of the child and then the chest. When the cloth bag is not so hot, it is advisable to open the bag and take out Fu Zi and Sheng Jiang and make them into a cake and put on the chest of the sick child. It has the effects to warm up phlegm and dilate the chest, mainly used for cold phlegm in the chest of sick child, and those with temporary coma, spitting out sputum like mung bean powder, in thick green color.

3.2 暖痰熨法(出自《幼幼集成》)

把一枚生附子和 30 克生姜，一起捣烂炒热。将炒热的附子和生姜用布包裹好。先将药包熨小儿背部，再熨小儿胸部。至药包不太热时，解开布包，将里面的附子和生姜取出，把它做成药饼，贴于患儿的胸口。有暖痰开胸之功，主治小儿胸有寒痰，一时昏迷，醒则吐痰如绿豆粉，浓厚而带青色者。

3.3 Soybean ironing method

One bowl of soybean is put into a cloth bag and encircled. Put the soybean bag into a microwave oven and heat it for about two minutes, depending upon the power of microwave oven. In accordance with the needs, soybean bag is used to iron pain of four limbs, or epigastric region and lower abdomen. After it cools down, soybean bag can be heated repeatedly. It has the effects to warm up the meridians, stop pain, warm up the center and strengthen the spleen, mainly used for cold sensation in the four limbs, cold pain in the joints, gastric spasm due to cold, and cold pain in the lower abdomen.

3.3 黄豆熨法

将干黄豆一碗，装入布袋内，缝好袋口。将黄豆包放入微波炉，根据微波炉的功率大小，加热约 2 分钟后取出。根据需要将热黄豆包敷于四肢疼痛处或胃脘、小腹等部位。冷却后黄豆包可反复加温使用。有温经止痛、温中健脾等作用，主治四肢畏寒、骨节冷痛、胃寒痉挛、小腹冷痛等。

Chapter 2 Brief history of tuina therapy

第 2 章 推拿发展简史

Since *Yellow Emperor's Inner Canon* (Huang Di Nei Jing), the manual technique therapy of Chinese medicine was termed by one phrase of Chinese characters for massage. In the Ming Dynasty, another phrase of Chinese characters for tuina appeared. Afterwards, two different phases of Chinese characters exist together for the same thing. Currently, this subject is officially termed as "Tuina" in Chinese language.

自《黄帝内经》起，中医手法疗法的学科名为"按摩"，明代开始有了"推拿"一称，此后两者并存通用。目前我国官方以"推拿"正式命名这一学科。

Section 1 Tuina therapy before Tang Dynasty

第 1 节 唐代以前的推拿

It is recorded in *Essential Questions* (Su Wen): "The central area is flat and humid, therefore, the heaven and earth exist and produce all things in numerous varieties. The people eat in large varieties but do not labor. Therefore, the diseases are mostly related to flaccidity, cold and heat, and should be treated by guiding technique and pressing technique. Therefore, the guiding technique and pressing technique come from the central area." The central area refers to the central China (nowadays, area of Henan Province), a birthplace of tuina therapy and

《素问 · 异法方宜论》记载："中央者，其地平以湿，天地所以生万物也众。其民食杂而不劳，故其病多痿厥寒热，其治宜导引按蹻。故导引按蹻者，亦从中央出也。"中央，指当时中国的中原地区（今河南省一带），是我国按摩疗法和导引疗法的发源地。河南出土的 3 000 多年前的甲骨文中，有"拊"等手

guiding therapy. In the oracle bone inscriptions of 3 000 years ago, unearthed in Henan Province, there were those records about the names of manual techniques and treatment of diseases by manual techniques. Massage therapy was then one of the major therapeutic methods.

法名称和以按摩手法治疗疾病的记载。按摩是当时主要的治病方法之一。

Guiding Book (Yin Shu) published in the book form before 186 BC was a monograph on guiding art. The basic contents in Yin Shu included the active movements of the limbs, and self-massage also including the passive suiding technique such as intraoral reduction method for dislocation of the temporo mandibular joint, pulling-stretching method of the cervical vertebras in the supine position for neck stiffness and pain, treading-stepping method of the lumbar region and backward stretching-pulling method for dysentery, and backward stretching-pulling method of the cervical vertebras for sore throat, etc. This was the first record on the spinal techniques in China.

成书于公元前 186 年以前的《引书》是一部导引术专著。引，指导引。《引书》中的基本内容为主动肢体运动和自我按摩，但也包括了被动导引手法。如记载了颞颌关节脱位的口内复位手法，治疗颈项强痛的仰卧位颈椎拔伸法，治疗痢疾的腰部踩踏法和腰部后伸扳法，治疗喉痹的颈椎后伸扳法等。这是我国脊柱手法的最早记载。

Herbal Formulas for Fifty Two Diseases (Wu Shier Bing Fang) published in the book form before 168 BC, there were over ten kinds of the massage techniques including the pressing, rubbing, scraping, pinching and caressing method, etc, and multi person massage therapy. In the book, there were also records about the pressing method to stop bleeding, therapy for infantile convulsion by using coin and therapy for skin itching and frostbite by medicated massage and medicated paste massage.

成书于公元前 168 年以前的《五十二病方》，涉及的按摩手法，有按、摩、刮、捏、抚等 10 余种，还出现了多人按摩法。该书记载了按压止血法，用钱匕推刮治疗小儿惊风抽搐，以及药摩和膏摩法治疗皮肤瘙痒、冻疮等。

Huang Di Nei Jing a classic of Chinese medicine, laid a foundation for the medical system of tuina therapy. In this book, the formal name for this subject, massage therapy, was mentioned for

中医经典著作《黄帝内经》为我国推拿医学体系的建立奠定了基础。在这本书中，第一次出现了手法疗法

the first time. The functional mechanism of tuina therapy was explained, such as to warm up the meridians and disperse cold, activate blood and reinforce blood, soothe the tendons and dredge the meridians. The contraindications and indications of tuina techniques were listed. In the book, there were also records about the specific manual techniques to press the abdominal aorta and press the carotid artery and their applications, and about paste massage therapy for facial paralysis by using "horse paste". In the book, the manual techniques were also used for making diagnosis and locating acupoints in acupuncture, having the palpation by the manual techniques to become an important component of tuina therapy. The theory of "using pain spot as a acupoint", mentioned in Huang Di Nei Jing, was mainly used to guide the treatment of pain in the soft tissues and has been used continuously up to the present.

的正式学科名——"按摩";阐述了按摩的作用机理,如温经散寒、活血补血、舒筋通脉等;提出了按摩手法的适应证和禁忌证;记载了按压腹主动脉法、按压颈动脉法等特殊手法及其运用;记载了用"马膏"膏摩法治疗面神经麻痹;还将手法用于诊断与针刺的定穴,使手法触诊成了推拿学的一个重要组成部分。《内经》提出的"以痛为输"理论,主要用于指导治疗经筋(软组织)病痛,一直沿用到现在。

It was recorded in *History of the Han Dynasty* (Han Shu) that there were ten volumes of *Yellow Emperor and Qi Bo on Massage* (Huang Di Qi Bo An Mo), which is publically acknowledged as earliest book on tuina therapy.

《汉书·艺文志》记载有一本《黄帝岐伯按摩》10 卷(已佚),公认是我国最早的推拿(按摩)专著。

Wuwei Medical Bamboo Slips of Han Dynasty (Wu Wei Han Dai Yi Jian) recorded a complete herbal formula for paste massage, "paste recipe for treating girls". The massage paste was composed of four ingredients of *Zanthoxyli Pericarpium* (Hua Jiao), *Chuanxiong Rhizoma* (Chuan Xiong), *Angelicae Dahuricae Radix* (Bai Zhi) and *Aconiti Lateralis Radix Praeparata* (Fu Zi), and used for massage, topical application and oral administration. The indications of paste massage method include

东汉的《武威汉代医简》记载了完整的膏摩方"治千金膏药方"。摩膏由川椒、川芎、白芷、附子 4 味中药组成,其用法可外摩、外敷和口服。膏摩的适应证有喉痹、血府痛、咽干,适合口服和外敷的病症,还有心腹痛、嗌痛、齿痛、金创、头痛和妇女产后诸病等。"三指摩"法成

pharyngitis, pain in the blood vessels, and dry throat. The oral administration and topical application are appropriate for pain in the chest and abdomen, pharyngalgia toothache, knife cuts, headache, and various postpartum diseases, etc. "Three-finger massage" method becomes one of the basic manual techniques in paste massage in the later generations.

了后世膏摩的基本操作手法之一。

In *Essential Prescriptions of the Golden Coffer* (Jin Kui Yao Lüe) by ZHANG Zhongjing of the Eastern Han Dynasty, the therapeutic methods were given mainly by herbal formulas, plus a little content about massage therapy. In the book, Chinese characters for "paste massage" were mentioned for the first time, together with acupuncture therapy and guiding therapy, for prevention and healthcare. This book gives a detailed explanation about the manual techniques to rescue the dying, such as external chest compression, artificial respiration by pressing the abdomen, traction of cervical vertebras, extension and flexion of four limbs, reflecting the highest level of tuina therapy in the Han Dynasty.

东汉张仲景的《金匮要略》,其治法以方药为主,也有少量按摩的内容。书中首次提到了"膏摩"一词,并将它与针灸、导引等疗法并列,用于预防保健。该书对手法抢救自缢死作了详细介绍,其急救手法包括胸外心脏按摩术、按腹人工呼吸法、颈椎牵引、四肢关节屈伸法等,体现了我国汉代推拿疗法的最高水平。

Up to *Handbook of Prescriptions for Emergencies* (Zhou Hou Bei Ji Fang) by GE Hong (284—364) of the Jin Dynasty, the manual techniques of tuina therapy have been developed from the simple to mature. There were the spine-pinching method by the opposite force of five fingers and coordinative operation of the two hands and the abdomen-upholding method by upward functional force. The spine-pinching method has been in the important position in infantile massage therapy. The manual techniques recorded in include the rubbing, finger-

推拿手法发展到晋代葛洪(284—364 年)的《肘后备急方》,已从简单趋于成熟,五指相对用力且双手协同操作的捏脊法和作用力向上的腹部抄举法已经出现。捏脊法后来在小儿推拿领域得到了重用。《肘后备急方》记载的推拿手法,还有摩、指按、按、抓、指弹、捻、摩捋、拍、指捏等。手法的适应证,包括

pressing, pressing, grasping, finger-plucking, twisting, palm-rolling, patting and finger-pinching method, etc. The indications of those manual techniques include various internal and external problems of sudden cardiac pain, sudden abdominal pain, cholera with muscular spasm, facial paralysis, headache, beriberi, regurgitation, and urticaria due to wind and heat. In Zhou Hou Bei Ji Fang, paste massage method was also systematically summarized. Paste massage method has been extensively applied for internal, external, gynecological and ENT problems.

卒心痛、卒腹痛、霍乱转筋、面瘫、头痛、脚气、胃反、风热隐疹等内外科诸疾。《肘后备急方》还对膏摩法作了系统总结，膏摩法已广泛应用于内、外、妇、五官科病证。

(*True Instructions* (Zhen Gao) compiled by TAO Hongjing (456—536) introduces a "Northern Emperor's Flexion" method, a Taoict-instructed technique for passive movement of the joints. mainly for treating apoplectic paralysis of the limbs. His famous book on life preservation, *Collections of Personality Cultivation and Life Prolonging* (Yang Xing Yan Ming Lu), discusses self massage method for life preservation in details.

陶弘景(456—536年)总结编撰的《真诰》介绍了一种道家传授的以关节被动运动手法为主的"北帝曲折"法，主要用以治疗中风肢体瘫痪。他的养生名著《养性延命录》详细论述了自我养生按摩法。

Taoist life preservation was prevailing in the Wei, Jin, Southern and Northern Dynasties (220—589). Self massage method for life preservation developed from a simple posture to the series of postures. The representative works is *Taoist Regimen of Supreme Purity* (Tai Qing Dao Lin She Sheng Lun). In its "section four of massage method", there were the famous eighteen posture of "self massage method" (termed massage methods from Indian in *Thousand Golden Prescriptions* (Qian Jin Yao Fang)) and Lao Tse massage method. Here, the so-called massage method mainly refers to the guiding method, i.e. the active movements of the limbs in

魏晋南北朝时期(220—589年)道家养生之风盛行，自我养生按摩法的操作，已从一招一式向套路化发展。代表性著作如道林的《太清道林摄生论》。其"按摩法第四"，有著名的"自按摩法"十八势(《千金要方》称之为天竺国按摩法)和老子按摩法。这里所谓的按摩法，主要是导引法，即结合自我按摩的肢体主动运动。但其中记载了大量自我按摩手法，如按、

combination of self massage. But, a large number of self massage techniques was recorded, such as pressing, pounding, twisting, plucking, touching, shaking, striking and extending method, etc. In addition to self massage, the passive and general health-care massage was also emphasized in Tai Qing Dao Lin She Sheng Lun, believing that it was necessary to massage promptly, as soon as you did not feel well. If general massage is given every day, the pathogenic factors would not be able to invade the body. This viewpoint to treat the unformed problem by massage therapy is influential to the later generations.

捶、捻、拔、摸、摇、打、伸等。《太清道林摄生论》除推崇自我按摩外，也重视被动性全身保健按摩的作用。认为稍微感觉不舒服，就应该及时按摩防治。如果能够每天接受全身按摩，外邪就不能侵犯人体。这种推拿治未病的观点，对后世影响很大。

Section 2　Tuina therapy in the Tang, Song and Yuan Dynasty

第 2 节　唐宋元时期的推拿

The period of the Sui and Tang Dynasties (581—907) was the most flourishing period in the history of China, in which the politics, economy, science and technology, and culture developed unprecedentedly and tuina medicine also entered the climax. In that moment, massage therapy was acknowledged officially and massage education was on the right tracks. The clinical and educational staffs were granted with series of professional titles. Massage therapy was clearly defined with the therapeutic scope. Paste massage therapy was extensively applied clinically.

隋唐时期（581—907 年），是中国历史上最强盛的时期，政治、经济、科技、文化都得到了空前的发展，推拿医学也进入了高潮。此期按摩疗法得到了政府的认可，按摩教育步入正轨，按摩临床和教学人员有了系列“职称”，按摩有了明确的治疗范围，膏摩得到了广泛的临床应用。

The Song and Yuan Dynasties (960—1368) lasted for over 400 years. By the records in *History of Song Dynasty* (Song Shi), there were massage prac-

宋元时期（960—1368 年）历时 400 余年。据《宋史 · 职官》记载，宋初太医署

titioners in the Imperial Medical Academy. But, in the medical reform in later period, the massage department was cancelled from the administration of imperial medical practitioners.

仍有按摩博士。但在后来的医疗改革中，太医局取消了按摩科。

In the period of Jin and Yuan Dynasties (1115—1368), the main achievements of tuina medicine were innovations of the manual techniques for bone injury.

金元时期（1115—1368年）推拿医学的主要成就是骨伤手法的创新。

1 The establishment of tuina medical education and medical system in Sui and Tang Dynasties

1 隋唐推拿医学教育和医疗体系的建立

The administration of the Sui and Tang Dynasties established the formal imperial medical college, "Imperial Medical Academy". By the records in *Six Law Codes of Tang Dynasty* (Tang Liu Dian), there were 20 massage doctors, 120 massage therapists, 100 massage students in the massage department in the Imperial Medical Academy. In the Sui Dynasty, there was no acupuncture department, but massage had been listed in parallel with herbal medicine, herbal drugs, and psychology-like healing art, because of its large scope.

隋代政府设立了正规的宫廷医学院"太医署"。据《唐六典》记载，隋代太医署按摩科有按摩博士 20 人，按摩师 120 人，按摩生 100 人。隋代尚无针灸科，而按摩已与医、药、祝禁并列，且规模庞大。

In the Tang Dynasty, oversized massage department was cut down, and acupuncture department was set up. By the records in Tang Liu Dian, in the massage department of the Tang Dynasty, there were 1 massage doctor, 4 massage therapists, key teaching staff members, and 15 massage students, studying in the school, and also 16 massage workers between massage therapists and massage students, belonging to medical staffs. The teaching contents in the massage department were massage therapy and guiding therapy. Then, the massage talents trained in the massage department

唐代对过于庞大的按摩科设置予以裁减，并增设了针灸科。据《唐六典》记载，唐代的按摩科配置按摩博士1人，按摩师 4 人，是教学核心人员；按摩生 15 人，为在校学生；在按摩师和按摩生之间增加了按摩工 16 人，属于治疗人员。按摩科的教学内容，主要是按摩和导引。当时按摩科培养的按摩人才，不仅承担治疗任务，还负

not only needed to undertake the medical mission but also to take the responsibility for imperial healthcare and for advising life preservation by guiding art, with their therapeutic scope in the eight types of diseases in relation with "wind, cold, summer-heat, dampness, hunger, over-eating, over-fatigue, and improper leisure". Then, diseases due to bone injury were also treated in the massage department.

有宫廷保健与指导导引养生的责任。其治疗范围为"风、寒、暑、湿、饥、饱、劳、逸"八疾。当时骨伤疾病的治疗也属于按摩科。

The establishment of massage department in the Sui and Tang Dynasties united the previous confused nomenclature for manual technique medicine, and massage therapy became the legal term for manual technique medicine.

隋唐时期按摩科的设立，统一了此前对手法医学的混乱命名，按摩成了手法医学的法定名称。

2 Massage therapy in *Origin and Outcome of Diseases* (Zhu Bing Yuan Hou Lun) and *Thousand Golden Prescriptions* (Qian Jin Yao Fang) of the Tang Dynasty

2 唐代《诸病源候论》和《千金方》中的推拿

Zhu Bing Yuan Hou Lun (published in form of book in 610) by CHAO Yuanfang, an imperial doctor in the Sui Dynasty, is a special book on pathogenic factors and symptom complex. In this book, there were no therapeutic herbal formulas for those listed diseases, but there were the detailed methods of guiding therapy for corresponding symptom complex, including large numbers of massage methods, mainly self-massage methods. In combination of the limb guiding techniques, those massage methods can be used to treat corresponding diseases, promote recovery, and also to maintain life preservation and prevent diseases.

隋太医博士巢元方的《诸病源候论》(成书于610年)，是一部病因证候学专著，该书所列的病证均无治疗方药，但却提供了详细的对症导引疗法。其中包括大量按摩法，主要是自我按摩法。这些按摩操作法结合肢体导引，既可对症施治和康复，又能养生防病。

In Qian Jin Yao Fang by Sun Simiao (581—682) of the Tang Dynasty, the massage therapy and

唐代孙思邈(581—682年)的《千金方》，除医药方面

regimen by massage at that time were summarized, in addition to its contribution to medicine and pharmacy.

的贡献外，对当时的按摩疗法与按摩养生法也作了总结。

In Qian Jin Yao Fang, massage therapy for pediatric diseases was discussed in a larger space, the application of paste massage therapy in particular. For instance, Five-Ingredient and Licorice Massage Paste (Wu Wu Gan Cao Sheng Mo Gao) was used to treat infantile common cold. For healthy children, it was also advised to massage the palm, sole and vertex of the child with the medicated paste, for avoiding invasion of pathogenic wind and cold.

《千金方》以较大篇幅论述了儿科疾病的推拿法，尤以膏摩法的应用为多。如用五物甘草生摩膏治疗小儿风寒感冒，对于健康的小儿，也提倡每天早起用以膏摩小儿手足心和头顶，用于预防风寒之邪的侵袭。

In Qian Jin Yao Fang, the records and discussions about paste massage method were another summary to paste massage method 300 years after *Handbook of Prescriptions for Emergencies* (Zhou Hou Bei Ji Fang).

《千金方》对膏摩法的记载和论述，是继《肘后备急方》300 年后对膏摩法的又一次总结。

In Qian Jin Yao Fang, many specific manual techniques and practicing methods were also recorded, such as midwifery by massaging the abdomen for difficult labor, reposition by manipulation for prolapsed uterus, continuous pressing method for ascarid epigastric pain, reposition by upward pressing method for prolapsed anus, shaking and rotating method for intoxication, pulling and guiding method by multiple people for acute lumbar pain, and neck-pulling method by stepping on the shoulder and pulling the air for sudden coma, etc.

《千金方》记载了不少有特色的推拿手法和操作法：如处理难产的摩腹助产法；子宫脱垂的推纳复位法；蛔心痛的持续按法；脱肛的仰按复位法；处理酒醉的摇转法；急性腰痛的多人牵引导引法；突然昏厥的踏肩捉发拔伸颈椎法等。

The manual techniques for making diagnosis and locating the acupoints belong to the component part of tuina medicine. There are a number of records in Qian Jin Yao Fang. For instance, in the treatment of pulmonary diseases by acupuncture, the needle would be inserted after the reaction ap-

手法用于诊断与定穴，是推拿医学的重要组成部分。《千金方》也有不少记载。如针刺治疗肺病前要先按压肺俞，有反应才可以针刺。特别是提出了寻找阿是

pears by pressing Feishu (BL 13). In particular, "Ashi method" was suggested to look for Ashi points. Namely, it is necessary to detect the tender spot or reactive spot on the body surface by the manual technique. No matter it is the acupoint or not, it is Ashi point if tenderness or painful reaction appears. This method is significant for the treatment of soft tissue pain by acupuncture and massage therapy.

穴的"阿是之法",即针对病痛,应该在体表用手法探寻压痛点或反应点,不论是不是腧穴所在,只要出现痛快或疼痛反应,就是阿是穴了。这种方法,对于软组织疼痛的针灸推拿治疗很有意义。

In drawing the experience on life preservation from the forefathers, SUN Simiao strongly advocated the methods for life preservation including self massage, proposing to remember the possibility of danger in peace, and to do massage and guiding art every day for preventing diseases. Two kinds of Taoist guiding regimens recorded in the book, Indian massage method and Lao Tse massage method, went around at home and abroad by SUN Simiao's strong advocate.

孙思邈汲取前人养生经验,极力倡导包括自我按摩在内的养生法。主张安不忘危,每天都应该按摩导引,预防疾病。书中记录的天竺国按摩法和老子按摩法这两种道家导引养生法,经过孙思邈的大力提倡已流传海内外。

3 tuina therapy in *Peaceful Holy Benevolent Prescriptions* (Tai Ping Sheng Hui Fang) and *Savior General Compendium* (Sheng Ji Zong Lu) of the Song Dynasty

3 宋代《太平圣惠方》和《圣济总录》中的推拿

In *History of the Song Dynasty* (Song Shi), *Massage Methods* (An Mo Fa) and *Essentials of Massage* (An Mo Yao Fa) were recorded, but all extinct unluckily.

《宋史》载有按摩专著《按摩法》和《按摩要法》,惜均亡而不传。

Tai Ping Sheng Hui Fang by WANG Huaiyin of the Northern Song Dynasty is a magnificent summarization on the medical achievements in the Tang and Song Dynasties. In this book, tuina medicine was mainly valued in the summary of paste massage method and herbal formulas for massage, in number of over one hundred, far beyond those in Qian Jin

北宋王怀隐的《太平圣惠方》,是对唐宋医药成就的一次大总结。其中推拿医学的价值主要体现在对膏摩、药摩方的整理。其数量近百首,远远超出了《千金方》和《外台秘要》。摩膏的制备较

Yao Fang and *The Medical Secrets of An Official* (Wai Tai Mi Yao). The preparation of massage pastes was improved than that in the Tang Dynasty. New understanding on the location appropriate for paste massage was formed, and massage on the vertex and lumbar region was emphasized. Massage tools like iron spoon appeared. The application of paste massage developed to the specific diseases. Paste massage for eye diseases was mentioned for the first time. Paste massage was operated more maturely.

唐代有了改进。对膏摩的部位也有了新的认识,摩顶、摩腰膏得到重视。出现了铁匙等膏摩工具。膏摩应用向专病发展,眼疾的膏摩首次提及,膏摩的操作趋向细腻。

In Sheng Ji Zong Lu, a large-scale officially compiled book of the herbal formulas, there was plentiful information about massage medicine. In the chapter of the therapeutic methods of the fourth volume, it was believed in the special topic on massage therapy that massage could not be mixed up with guiding art and could be distinguished as "pressing" and "rubbing". "Pressing" refers to singular application of the manual technique. "Rubbing" could be used together with medicinal stuffs. The manual technique is beneficial to the performance of herbal potency. The functions of massage are generalized as "removing obstruction and inhibiting hyperactivity". In Sheng Ji Zong Lu, "topical application of herbal drugs, and paste massage" are discussed in parallel with manual reduction and administration of herbal stuffs, as the standard of bone-setting therapy. Iron made of raw iron was invented as a tool for rubbing the vertex. The effect of herbal paste for correcting deficiency was confirmed. For instance, Great Tonic Massage Paste (Da Bu Yi Mo Gao) was used to rub the lower back and reinforce the kidney, used for treating various

北宋末年的大型官修方书《圣济总录》有较丰富的推拿医学资料。其第四卷治法篇,有按摩疗法专论。认为不可将按摩与导引混为一谈,更应该区别"按"与"摩"。按为单纯用手法,摩则可以结合药物。手法有助于药力的发挥。并以"开达抑遏"概括了按摩的功用。《圣济总录》将"封裹膏摩"与手法复位和用药并提,作为正骨疗法的常规。还发明了生铁熨斗子作为摩顶工具;并肯定了膏摩的补虚作用。如以大补益摩膏摩腰补肾,治疗男女各种肾虚病证。

types of kidney deficiency in males and females.

4 *Ten Types of Labors* (Shi Chan Lun) of the Song Dynasty and manual midwifery

In Shi Chan Lun by YANG Zijian of the Song Dynasty, various types of difficult labors due to abnormal fetal position were described for the first time, such as shoulder presentation, foot presentation, breech presentation, umbilical cord binding the shoulder, uterine prolapse during labor, and the manual correction of abnormal fetal position was systematically recorded. Although this book is extinct, its main contents were retained in *Complete Good Herbal Formulas for Women* (Fu Ren Da Quan Liang Fang) by CHEN Ziming of the Song Dynasty. The manual technique to correct the abnormal fetal position pioneered in Shi Chan Lun is the first innovation for manual midwifery and extends the therapeutic scope of tuina medicine.

4 宋代《十产论》与手法助产

宋人杨康候(字子建)的《十产论》(1098 年)最早描述了因异常胎位引起的各种难产,如横产(肩先露)、倒产(足先露)、偏产(臀先露)、碍产(脐带攀肩)、盘肠产(产时子宫脱垂),并系统记载了手法矫正异常胎位。此书虽已佚,但是其主要内容,被宋代陈自明的《妇人大全良方》保留了下来。《十产论》首创的矫正胎位异常的转胎手法,开手法助产之先河,扩大了推拿医学的应用范围。

5 Tuina therapy in *Confucians' Duties to Their Parents* (Ru Men Shi Qin) and *Effective Herbal Formulas of Practitioners in the Generations* (Shi Yi De Xiao Fang)

ZHANG Zihe, a medical practitioner of the Jin Dynasty, was a representative of "purgative school" from one of the four medical masters in the Jin and Yuan Dynasties. In Ru Men Shi Qin, he categorized various therapeutic methods into three types of "sweating, vomiting and purgation", and listed massage therapy and acupuncture therapy into the "sweating method". Massage therapeutic methods recorded in the book include massage on the breast by wood comb for mastitis in women, the pushing and kneading method in combination of purgative

5 《儒门事亲》和《世医得效方》中的推拿

金代医家张子和,是金元四大家之"攻下派"的代表。他在《儒门事亲》中将各种治法分成汗、吐、下三类,而将按摩与针灸等归入"汗法"。书中记载的按摩疗法应用有木梳梳乳治妇女乳痈,以推揉法配合泻下药治疗妇人腹中有块,自我揉腹催吐治疗伤食、伤酒,揉目并配合针刺治疗目上长瘤,按

drugs for abdominal lump in women, self massage on the abdomen to promote vomiting for improper food ingestion and improper alcohol drinking, massage on the eyes in combination of acupuncture for lump on the eye, massage on the abdomen for infantile abdominal lump, etc. "Pressing and Guiding" were first mentioned by Zhang Zihe.

摩腹部治疗小儿腹内痞块等。"按导"一词也是张子和首先提出的。

In Shi Yi De Xiao Fang by WEI Yilin of the Yuan Dynasty, the manual techniques for bone injury are somewhat innovated, such as two-person dynamic traction for lumbar pain, foot-up and head-down inverted hanging reposition for spinal fracture, foot-up and head-down inverted hanging reposition for dislocation of hip joint, i. e. "to set the bones by the hand" for reposition in the foot-up and head-down inverted hanging situation, and reposition by sitting stool and ladder for dislocation of the shoulder joint, etc.

元代危亦林的《世医得效方》在骨伤治疗手法上有所创新。如治疗腰痛的双人动态牵引法;治疗脊柱骨折的倒悬复位法;治疗髋关节脱位的倒悬复位法,即在倒悬的情况下"用手整骨节",使其复位;治疗肩关节脱位的坐凳、架梯复位法等。

Section 3 Tuina therapy in the Ming and Qing Dynasty

第3节 明清时期的推拿

The Ming Dynasty (1368—1644) is a reflourishing period of tuina medicine. In the early period of the Ming Dynasty, the massage department was once more legalized. The extant books on massage therapy started from the Ming Dynasty. Chinese characters for "tuina" appeared. The manual techniques of massage therapy were used in various clinics for adults and children. Infantile massage therapy was formed systematically. Healthcare massage and self massage for life preservation developed further. In the middle and later period of the Ming Dynasty, the massage depart-

明代(1368—1644年)是推拿医学再度兴盛的时期。明代初期按摩科重新合法化。现存的推拿专著始于明代。在此时期,"推拿"一词出现。推拿手法运用于成人和小儿各科临床。小儿推拿体系形成。保健按摩和自我养生按摩进一步发展。明代中后期按摩科被政府取消。

ment was cancelled by the authority.

Tuina medicine developed very slowly in the Qing Dynasty (1644—1911). The medical clinics were merged into nine clinics in the imperial hospital of the Qing Dynasty, without massage clinics. Except that the manual techniques were used in the bone setting and the manual technique of massage therapy were combined by fewer medical practitioners in their medical treatment, massage therapy basically existed and developed among the folk people. The bone-setting techniques represented by "eight bone setting methods" established its position in bone setting subject. Infantile massage therapy spread from the southern China to the whole, with its enlarged therapeutic scope and increasingly-growing manual techniques.

推拿医学在清代(1644—1911 年)发展缓慢。清代太医院将医学分科归并为九科,无按摩科。除了正骨科采用手法治疗和少数医家在医疗中结合运用推拿手法外,推拿基本上是在民间生存和发展的。以"正骨八法"为代表的正骨手法在正骨科中确立了地位。小儿推拿疗法从南方地区向全国辐射,治疗范围扩大,手法渐多。

1　The change of massage clinics in the Ming Dynasty

1　明代按摩科的变迁

In the early period of the Ming Dynasty, massage clinic was one of the thirteen medical clinics. But, after flourishing for two hundred years, up to 1571, medical institutions were reduced to eleven clinics, and massage clinic was cancelled by the authority since then. As for the reason that massage clinic declined once again, in addition to the limitation of hand touching massage due to feudal ethics, the negative influence of accidents on massage medicine could not be neglected.

Although massage developed for several thousand years, due to the limitation in the scientific levels then, the understanding of the human anatomy could not reach the height of the modern times. The manual techniques in massage therapy were not operated satisfactorily in delicacy and accuracy. The

明代初期,按摩科为医学 13 科之一。但在兴旺了 200 年后,至 1571 年,医学机构缩减为 11 科,按摩科从此被政府取消。按摩科再度由兴转衰的内在原因,除了封建礼教对以手法接触的按摩的限制以外,手法意外对按摩医学的负面影响也不可忽视。

尽管按摩已有几千年的发展,但受当时科学水平的局限,对人体解剖的认识还不可能达到现代的高度,按摩手法操作的精细度还不能尽如人意,对疾病的认识、诊

knowledge and diagnosis about diseases were limited by the levels of the medical science and medical education at that time. Moreover, the scholarly attainments of massage practitioners also impacted the efficacy of massage therapy. In this background, the therapeutic errors happened frequently, producing the negative social influence.

断也受到当时医学科学进步程度和医学教育水平的局限。其次，按摩人员本身的学识素养，也影响到按摩的疗效。在这一背景下，按摩误治现象时有发生，造成了负面的社会影响。

After massage clinic was cancelled, massage was forced to survive toward three directions: ① Keep it in the bone-setting clinic by name of "manual techniques". ② Treat children as the therapeutic targets, forming a system of infantile massage. ③ Survive in business of bath and hair dressing, as healthcare massage of folk people.

按摩科被取消后，按摩被迫朝三个方向分化：①以"手法"的名义保留在正骨科内；②治疗对象转向小儿，形成了小儿推拿体系；③在沐浴业和理发业求生存，转化为民间的保健按摩。

2 The establishment of infantile massage system in the Ming Dynasty

2 明代小儿推拿体系的建立

Based upon existing materials, Chinese characters for "tuina" were earliest recorded in *Medical Secrets* (Yi Men Mi Zhi) by ZHANG Siwei in 1574. Initially, it was only applied for children. Later, Chinese characters for "tuina" became the formal name.

据现有资料，"推拿"一词最早记载于1574年张四维的《医门秘旨》。最初仅应用于小儿，后来"推拿"成了正式的学科名。

In the later stage of the Ming Dynasty, infantile massage therapy started to prevail in the southern China. The earliest specific literature on infantile tuina was "Oral Instruction of Esoteric Tendon-Pinching Technique for Convulsion" in volume ten of *Complementation to Pocket Handbook of Herbal Formulas and Theory for Children* (Bu Yao Xiu Zhen Xiao Er Fang Lun) reedited by ZHUANG Yingqi in 1574, in which the locations, operation and indications of specific areas for infantile tuina, such as Pt. Sanguan, Pt. Liufu, were discussed for

明代后期，小儿推拿开始在中国南方地区流行。最早的小儿推拿专题文献是庄应琪于1574年补辑的《补要袖珍小儿方论》第10卷中的"秘传看惊掐筋口授手法论"，首次论述了三关、六腑等小儿推拿特定部位的定位、操作和主治，也有了手足推拿穴道图谱，手法以推擦为主而称为掐筋，主要的适

the first time, plus the acupoints chart for hand and foot tuina. The manual techniques were mainly the pushing method and chafing method, described as pinching the tendon, with infantile convulsion as the main indication.

应证是小儿惊风。

The symbol for the establishment of infantile tuina system was the publication of a group of books on infantile massage therapy, such as *Infantile Massage Canon* (Xiao Er An Mo Jing) (before 1601), *Complete Book on Secrets of Herbal Formulas and Pulses in Infantile Massage for Alive Infants* (Xiao Er Tui Na Fang Mai Huo Ying Mi Zhi Quan Shu) (1604), and *Secrets of Infantile tuina* (Xiao Er Tui Na Mi Jue) (1605). The operation charts of infantile massage therapy were published in *Secrets of Infantile tuina* (Xiao Er Tui Na Mi Jue).

小儿推拿体系建立的标志是《小儿按摩经》(1601 年以前)、《小儿推拿方脉活婴秘旨全书》(1604 年)、《小儿推拿秘诀》(1605 年)等一批小儿推拿专著的诞生。《小儿推拿秘诀》还出现了小儿推拿操作图谱。

The system of infantile massage therapy formed in the Ming Dynasty was unique in its operation, including the manual techniques and specific acupoints of infantile massage therapy. The format of the prescription in infantile massage therapy was written with the manual techniques and specific acupoints, plus number of the operation times, such as "push Pt. Pitu for three hundred times".

明代形成的小儿推拿体系有其独特的操作法。这种操作法包括了小儿推拿手法和小儿推拿特定穴。小儿推拿的处方格式是手法加特定穴,有的还加上操作次数,如"推脾土三百"。

3 Position of bone-setting techniques in the bone setting clinics in the Qing Dynasty

3 清代正骨手法在正骨科中的地位

It was believed in *The Golden Mirror of Medicine* (Yi Zong Jin Jian), a textbook of imperial hospital in the Qing Dynasty, that the manual techniques were the "priority mission for bone setting", confirming the position of the manual techniques in the bone setting clinics. In the book, the eight bone

清代的太医院教科书《医宗金鉴》认为手法为"正骨之首务",确立了手法在正骨科的地位。还论述了正骨八法——摸、接、端、提、推、拿、按、摩。其中摸法为诊断

setting methods—feeling, linking, holding, lifting, pushing, grasping, pressing and rubbing were discussed. Among them, the feeling method was a diagnostic technique. The theory of "bone dislocation", mentioned in Yi Zong Jin Jian , was of guiding significance for bone-setting massage and spinal massage, in which for the treatment of spinal bone dislocation (posterior articular dislocation, etc), it was suggested to relax the soft tissue by the manual technique first, and to do the reposition by pressing the spine afterward, in combination of oral administration and topical application of herbal drugs.

手法。《医宗金鉴》提出的"骨错缝"学说,对正骨推拿和脊柱推拿有指导意义。对脊柱错骨缝(后关节紊乱等)的治疗,主张先手法放松软组织,再行按脊复位手法,并配合药物内服外敷。

4 Prevalence of infantile massage therapy in the Qing Dynasty

Infantile massage therapy started in the later period of the Ming Dynasty and prevailed in the southern China. The number of the books on infantile massage therapy was obviously increased in the Qing Dynasty. The important ones are *Extensive Significance of Massage* (Tui Na Guang Yi) (about 1676), *Secret Book on Pediatric Massage* (You Ke Tui Na Mi Shu) (1691), *Iron Mirror of Pediatrics* (You Ke Tie Jing) (1695), and *Improved Major Massage Techniques*(Li Zheng An Mo Yao Shu)(1888). It was believed in You Ke Tie Jing that the practice of tuina was just equal to the application of herbal properties. The well-known "ode to substitution of tuina by drugs" in the book was exactly to generalize the functions of infantile massage by the efficacy of herbal drugs. Besides, "three-character scripture for tuina" published in *Complete Book of Infantile Massage* (Tui Na Xiao Er Quan Shu) (1877) was circulated extensively in the late Qing Dynasty.

4 清代小儿推拿的流行

小儿推拿兴起于明代后期,流行于中国的南方地区。清代小儿推拿著作的数量明显增加,重要者有《推拿广意》(约 1676 年)、《幼科推拿秘书》(1691 年)、《幼科铁镜》(1695 年)、《厘正按摩要术》(1888 年)等。其中《幼科铁镜》认为用推拿就是用药味,书中著名的"推拿代药赋",就用中药的功效来归纳小儿推拿操作法的作用。另外,《推拿小儿全书》(1877 年)记载的"推拿三字经",在清末以后流传很广。

Section 4　Tuina therapy in the Republican Period

第 4 节 民国时期的推拿

The development of massage therapy in the Republican Period (1911—1949) was characterized by the formation of regional folk tuina schools, introduction of western massage therapy and private practice of massage therapy.

民国时期(1911—1949年)推拿医学的发展特点，是地区性民间推拿流派的形成、西方按摩疗法的传入和推拿私人开业的普及。

1　Main massage schools in the modern times

1　近代主要推拿流派

1.1　One-finger massage school

1.1　一指禅推拿流派

The inheritance of one-finger tuina school could be traced back to LI Jianchen, a native of Henan province, in the Qing Dynasty. Around 1861, LI handed it down to DING Fengshan (1847—1920), a native of Yangzhou, Jiangsu. After 1921, DING migrated to Shanghai and started his practice, having over ten disciples of WANG Songshan, QIAN Fuqing, DING Shushan, etc. The representative books of this school are (*One Finger Meditation Skill* (Yi Zhi Ding Chan) (end of the Qing Dynasty), *Instruction to One-Finger Massage* (Yi Zhi Chan Tui Na Shuo Ming Shu) (Republican Period), and (*Huang's Medical Sayings* (Huang Shi Yi Hua) (Republican Period). The manual techniques of one-finger tuina school in the early period include the ten methods of pressing, rubbing, pushing, grasping, twisting, lifting, rolling, twiddling, entangling and kneading technique. Among them, one-finger pushing method by the shaking and rhythmical manipulation with the force point on the thumb is a symbolic technique. Based upon basic theory of Chinese medicine, clinically it is advocated to "push the acupoints and go through the me-

一指禅推拿流派的传承链可上溯到清代河南人李鉴臣。李氏于 1861 年前后传江苏扬州丁凤山(1847—1920)，丁氏于 1912 年后迁居上海并开业，弟子有王松山、钱福卿、丁树山等十余人。该派的代表著作有《一指定禅》(清末)、《一指禅推拿说明书》(民国)、《黄氏医话》(民国)。早期的一指禅推拿流派手法有按、摩、推、拿、搓、抄、滚、捻、缠、揉十法，其中以拇指为着力点并摆动式节律性操作的一指禅推法为标志性手法。临床上以中医基本理论为指导，主张"推穴道，走经络"。擅长治疗头痛、眩晕、失眠、胃脘痛、胃下垂、久泄、便秘、劳倦内伤、面瘫、月经不调、痛经、慢性鼻炎等内妇科杂病以及

ridians", specialized in treating miscellaneous internal and gynecological diseases of headache, vertigo, insomnia, epigastric pain, gastroptosis, long-term diarrhea, constipation, overstrain due to internal injury, facial paralysis, irregular menstruation, dysmenorrhea, and chronic rhinitis, etc, and cervical spondylopathy, shoulder pain, and joint pain, etc.

颈椎病、漏肩风、关节疼痛等症。

1.2 tuina school of rolling method

The tuina school of rolling method was initiated by DING Jifeng (1914—1998). His grandfather, DING Fengshan, and his father, DING Shushan, were the masters of one-finger tuina. In 1936, DING Jifeng opened his tuina clinic in Shanghai. In order to meet the needs of the increasing patients with apoplectic hemiplegia and soft tissue pain, he enlarged the flexion and extension of the wrist joint with the ulnar aspect of the hand dorsum as the touching surface, based upon the "rolling method" of one-finger tuina school, to increase the stimulation and enhance the effect of the manual technique. His rolling method was earliest recorded in his book published in 1945, *Brief Introduction to Massage Medical Principle* (Tui Na Yi Shu Yuan Li Jian Lun). Later, he integrated the rolling method with the passive movement of various joints, together with the kneading method and the pressing, grasping, twisting and rubbing method, forming the unique massage school of the rolling method. Based upon the theory of the meridians as its basic theory, the tuina school of rolling method was associated with the modern medical theory of physiology, anatomy, pathology and biomechanics as the guideline for clinical treatment. The manual techniques were appropriate for the body parts of nape, shoul-

1.2 㨰法推拿流派

㨰法推拿流派创始于丁季峰(1914—1998),其伯祖父丁凤山、父丁树山均为一指禅推拿大家。丁季峰1936年在上海开设推拿诊所,为适应日益增多的中风偏瘫和软组织疼痛患者的就诊需求,变法图新,在一指禅推拿流派"滚法"的基础上,将手背尺侧部作为接触面,并加大了腕关节的屈伸运动,既增加了刺激量,又提高了手法的效率,为与原来的"滚法"相区别,故取名㨰法。㨰法最早记载于他1945所著《推拿医术原理简论》。后来又将㨰法与各部关节被动运动相结合,并辅以揉法和按、拿、捻、搓等法,形成了风格独特的㨰法推拿流派。㨰法推拿流派以中医经络学说为基础理论,结合生理、解剖、病理、生物力学等现代医学理论,作为临床施治的指导。手法适用于颈、肩、腰、臀及四肢等部位,擅长治疗运动

der, low back, buttocks and four limbs and effective for diseases of the motor system and nervous system. The main indications included apoplectic hemiplegia, post polio syndrome, traumatic paraplegia, peripheral nerve paralysis, facial paralysis, headache, soft tissue injury in the nape, shoulder, lumbar region, back and four limbs, various chronic arthritis, intervertebral disc herniation, scapulohumeral periarthritis, neck pain, and cervical spondylopathy, etc.

系统、神经系统疾病。主要适应证有：中风偏瘫、脊髓灰质炎后遗症、外伤性截瘫、周围神经麻痹、面瘫、头痛、颈肩腰背及四肢软组织损伤、各种慢性关节炎、腰椎间盘突出症、肩周炎、落枕、颈椎病等。

1.3 School of internal-works tuina

This school of internal-works tuina is characterized by the chafing method of the strong effect in warming and dredging the meridians and warming up and replenishing the internal organs as the main therapeutic technique, and by instructing the patients to train "Shaolin internal works (Shao Lin Nei Gong)" to prevent and treat diseases. MA Wanqi (1884—1941), a native of Jining, Shandong, learnt this art from his hometown fellow, LI Shujia. In 1920s, MA Wanqi practiced his medicine in Shanghai with internal-works tuina, handed down this art to his brother, MA Wanlong, and his disciple, LI Xijiu. In practice of internal-works tuina, the holistic concept was stressed to support the constitution and expel pathogens. In the clinical application, there was a whole set of routine techniques for whole body tuina. The main indications included internal injury due to deficiency and depletion, pulmonary tuberculosis, asthma, pulmonary emphysema, hypertension, gastric and duodenal ulcer, chronic gastritis, gastroptosis, epigastric pain, diarrhea, constipation, insomnia, dysmenorrhea, amenorrhea, injury of chest and hypochondria, and soft tissue

1.3 内功推拿流派

内功推拿的特点是以温通经络和温补脏腑作用较强的擦法为主治手法，并指导病人锻炼“少林内功”，以防治疾病。由山东济宁的马万起(1884—1941)受之于同乡李树嘉。马氏于 20 年代以内功推拿行医于上海，传胞弟马万龙、弟子李锡九。内功推拿强调整体观念，重视扶正祛邪。临床应用时，有一套全身操作常规手法。主要适应证有虚劳内伤、肺结核、哮喘、肺气肿、高血压、胃和十二指肠溃疡、慢性胃炎、胃下垂、胃脘痛、泄泻、便秘、失眠、痛经、闭经、胸胁屏伤，以及软组织损伤等。

injury, etc.

In terms of tuina schools formed in the Republican Period, there were also the Zangfu organ pushing-pressing method by WANG Yaru of Hebei province, the pressing-guiding method by YUAN Zhenglun and YUAN Zhengdao brothers influential in Shanghai, abdominal tuina method by LUO Junchang in Chongqing region, bone-setting massage in various regions, and infantile massage therapy, etc.

民国时期形成的推拿流派还有河北王雅儒的脏腑推按法，在上海颇有影响的袁正伦、袁正道兄弟的按导术，重庆地区骆俊昌的腹诊推拿法，以及分布多地的正骨推拿法、小儿推拿法等。

2 Introduction of western massage therapy

2 西方按摩疗法的传入

The introduction of western massage therapy into China was symbolized by the publication of western massage books in Chinese language. The books were mostly translated or edited from Japanese works into Chinese language or directly translated from the original works of English language.

西方按摩疗法传入中国的标志，是中文西方按摩著作的刊行。其书多从日文著作翻译或编译成中文，或直接从英文原著翻译。

Teaching Materials on Massage Art from Western Countries (Xi Yang An Mo Shu Jiang Yi) edited and translated by DING Fubao in 1910 was the earliest-introduced works on western massage art. The author of the original book was Kawai Kyouhei. A group of books on western massage was published by compilation and translation in the Republican Period, such as *Health Massage* (Wei Sheng An Mo Fa) (1917), *Western Massage* (Xi Yang An Mo Shu) (1928), *Practical Massage Art and Revised Exercises* (Shi Yong An Mo Shu Yu Gai Zheng Ti Cao) (1932), *Special Issue of Spinal Massage Art* (An Ji Shu Zhuang Kan) (1935), *Latest Teaching Materials on Western Massage* (Zui Xin An Mo Shu Jiang Yi) (1936), and *Introduction to Massage* (Tui Na Fa Yin Yan) (1947), etc.

1910 年丁福保编译的《西洋按摩术讲义》，是最早介绍西方按摩术的著作。原著者是日本的河合杏平。民国时期编译或翻译出版了一批西方按摩著作，如《卫生按摩法》(1917 年)、《西洋按摩术》(1928 年)、《实用按摩术与改正体操》(1932 年)、《按脊术专刊》(1935 年)、《最新按摩术讲义》(1936 年)、《推拿法引言》(1947 年)等。

tuina therapy did not reject western massage

中医推拿对西洋按摩术

and could learn from the other's strong points and overcome own shortcomings for intensifying the research on anatomy, physiology and pathology of the human body, making the diagnosis by consulting the terms of diseases in western medicine, doing tuina by the combination of the meridians and acupoints with the anatomical parts, and integrating the manual techniques of the joint movement into the massage system of Chinese medicine, and stressing the contraindications in massage treatment, etc. *Hua's massage Art* (Hua Shi An Mo Shu) published by YANG Huating (1934), *Examples of massage Science* (An Mo Shu Xue Ju Yu) by ZHONG Jiqian (1935) *Practical Guideline for Massage Art* (An Mo Shu Shi Yong Zhi Nan) (1933) is exactly a special book on the integration between Chinese medicine and western medicine and between Chinese techniques and western techniques. Western massage therapy is positively significant to enhance the exchange between tuina medicine and western massage medicine.

并不排斥，并能取长补短，加强了对人体解剖、生理病理的研究，诊断参考西医病名，推拿操作采取经络腧穴与解剖部位相结合，将关节运动类手法融入了中医推拿体系，重视推拿治疗的禁忌证，等等。此期出版的杨华亭的《华氏按摩术》(1934年)、钟吉倩的《按摩学举隅》(1935年)、《按摩术实用指南》(1933年)，就是中西医结合、东西方手法会通的推拿专著。西洋按摩疗法对中西推拿医学的交流提高有积极意义。

3 Population of private practice

In the Republican Period, tuina practitioners mostly engaged in their practice in the form of private clinic.

In the column of Chinese medicine practitioners in *Shanghai Guideline* (Shang Hai Zhi Nan) published by Commercial Press in 1914, there were DING Fengshan, a founder of one-finger tuina school, and ZHANG Jinglian, a famous practitioner of infantile tuina.

After base for one-finger tuina school moved from Yangzhou to Shanghai at the end of the Qing

3 推拿私人开业的普及

民国时期推拿医生主要以私人诊所形式执业。

1914年商务印书馆《上海指南》的中医师栏目中，就有一指禅推拿流派创始人丁凤山和小儿推拿名家张静莲。

一指禅推拿流派的基地自清末民初从扬州迁往上海

Dynasty and beginning of the Republican Period, his disciples spread in various regions of Shanghai in the form of private clinics. For instance, QIAN Fuqing, a disciple of DING Fengshan, his private practice was listed in "*The Total Practitioner List of Western Medicine and Chinese Medicine in China*" of 1915, Shang Hai Zhi Nan from 1916 to 1930, and in the "*List of Medical and Pharmaceutical Business of Shanghai and China*" of 1943, and in "*The Member List of Shanghai Chinese Medical Practitioners Association*" of 1948, etc.

以后，其弟子们以私人开业的形式遍布上海各地。如丁凤山的弟子钱福卿，其开业记载可见于 1915 年《全国中西医士总览表》、1916 到 1930 年的《上海指南》，以及 1943 年《上海暨全国国医药界名录》、1948 年《上海市中医师公会会员录》等。

With the increasing standardization of the medical management, the tuina practitioners also had themselves engaged positively into the health management system of the government. In the first registration of the practitioners of western medicine and Chinese medicine, organized by Shanghai Health Bureau in 1928, 27 tuina practitioners were listed. In the ninth registration examination for Chinese medical practitioners, organized by Shanghai Health Bureau in 1934, there were more than eleven qualified tuina practitioners. The massage practitioners also positively joined Chinese medicine associations of Chinese medicine and of Chinese medical practitioners in various regions in China. In the "*List of Chinese Medicine*" in 1932 by the Shanghai Association of Chinese Medicine, there were 21 tuina staffs. In "*Member List of Shanghai Association of Chinese Medicine*" of 1934, there were 29 tuina practitioners. Tuina staffs and tuina-related staffs recorded in the "member list of Shanghai Association of Chinese Medicine Practitioners" of 1948 accounted for 83. By incomplete statistics, from 1920s to 1940s, the total number of the listed formal tuina practitioners in

随着医疗管理的不断规范，推拿从业人员也积极将自己纳入政府卫生管理体系之中。1928 年上海市卫生局组织第一次西医、中医登记，就有 27 个推拿医师（医士）名列其中。1934 上海市卫生局第 9 届国医登记考试，合格的推拿医生至少有 11 人。推拿医生还积极加入了各地的国医公会、中医师公会等中医社团。1932 年上海市国医学会《国医名录》中有推拿人员 21 人。1934 年的《上海市国医公会会员录》，有推拿医生 29 人。1948 年《上海市中医师公会会员录》记载的推拿和推拿相关会员达到 83 人。据不完全统计，上世纪 20 年代到 40 年代，上海有名可查的正规推拿医生总数超过了 160 人。由此可见民国时期推拿医疗的发展规模和

Shanghai was over 160. Therefore, the development scale and track of tuina medicine in the Republican Period could be seen.

轨迹。

Section 5　Modern development of tuina therapy

第 5 节 推拿的现代发展

1　Recovery and popularization (1950—1976)

From 1950s to 1976, tuina medicine was in a period of recovery and popularization. This period was characterized by the development of academic education of tuina medicine, and engagement of tuina practitioners in the hospital and clinical treatment.

In 1954, Tianjin United Clinic of Chinese Medicine opened the massage clinic. In 1955, Beijing Guanganmen Hospital opened the massage clinic, and Beijing Association of Chinese Medicine organized a massage course. In 1956, Beijing set up a massage hospital. Shanghai Medical School organized a tuina training course. In 1958, it was renamed massage school affiliated to Shanghai College of Traditional Chinese Medicine, in 3 year-schooling system, starting the formal academic education of tuina. In the same year, tuina clinic was established in Shanghai. In 1959, Wuhan Chinese Medicine Hospital and Chinese Medicine Clinic of Hebei Province respectively established massage clinic. In 1960, entrusted by the health ministry, Shanghai Tuina School organized the first national seminar of tuina practitioners. In the same year, No. 7 Military Medical University organized two-year tuina professional course. In 1965,

1　复苏与普及(1950—1976 年)

从 1950 年代至 1976 年，推拿处于复苏和普及期。这一时期的特点是推拿学历教育的开展，推拿医生进入医院和推拿临床治疗的普及。

1954 年，天津中医联合门诊部开设按摩科。1955 年，北京广安门医院开设按摩科，北京中医学会开设按摩研究班。1956 年，北京成立了按摩医院。上海卫生学校于 1956 年开办推拿训练班，1958 年更名上海中医学院附属推拿学校，学制 3 年，从此开展了正规的推拿学历教育。1958 年，上海成立推拿门诊部。1959 年武汉市中医院和河北省中医门诊部分别设立按摩科。1960 年，卫生部委托上海推拿学校举办了第一期全国推拿医师进修班。同年，第七军医大学开办两年制推拿专业班。1965

Shandong College of Traditional Chinese Medicine organized advanced tuina course. In 1973, Shanghai College of Traditional Chinese Medicine organized the second national training course of tuina teachers. In 1974, Shanghai College of Traditional Chinese Medicine established the three-year discipline of acupuncture, tuina and traumatology.

年山东中医学院举办推拿进修班。1973 年，上海中医学院举办了第二期全国推拿师资训练班。1974 年，上海中医学院设立三年制针灸、推拿、伤科专业。

In this period, the clinical study on massage therapy gradually started in various regions. In addition to orthopedic and traumatic diseases, massage therapy was also applied in the treatment of cholelithiasis, biliary ascariasis, infantile ascaris intestinal obstruction, diphtheria, malaria, mastitis, electric ophthalmia, and hordeolum, etc. Tuina anesthesia was also successfully applied in thyroidectomy, herniorrhaphy, subtotal gastrectomy, and Cesarean section.

这一时期推拿临床研究在各地逐渐展开。除骨伤科疾病外，推拿还应用于胆结石、胆道蛔虫症、小儿蛔虫性肠梗阻、白喉、疟疾、乳腺炎、电光性眼炎、麦粒肿等。推拿麻醉也成功地应用于甲状腺摘除、疝修补、胃大部切除、剖宫产等手术。

2 Development and prosperity (since 1977)

2 发展与繁荣(1977 年以来)

Since the end of "cultural revolution" in 1976, tuina clinical service, education and scientific research have been developing comprehensively. tuina therapy became the formal state nomenclature for manual technique medicine and manual technique clinics. The departments of massage therapy were set up in Chinese medicine hospitals. Tuina major was established in the colleges and schools of Chinese medicine. The academic activities of massage therapy have been unprecedentedly active. The main events are as follows:

1976 年“文化大革命”结束以后，推拿的临床、教学、科研全面展开。推拿成为国家对手法医学和手法临床分科的正式命名。中医医院设有推拿科，中医院校开设推拿专业。推拿学术活动空前活跃，主要大事有：

In the spring of 1978, Shanghai College of Traditional Chinese Medicine started to enroll the five-year students in the major of acupuncture, tuina and

1978 年春，上海中医学院招收五年制针灸、推拿、伤科专业学生。1979 年上海中

traumatology. In 1979, Shanghai College of Traditional Chinese Medicine set up the faculty of acupuncture therapy and faculty of massage therapy for discipline of acupuncture and tuina. In 1979, first national conference on tuina academic experience opened in Shanghai College of Traditional Chinese Medicine. In 1982, Shanghai College of Traditional Chinese Medicine set up a five-year undergraduate program of tuina discipline. In 1983, massage association was established in the Fujian Province. National conference of massage and guiding was held in Wuhan. Guangdong seminar on massage and qigong was held in Guangzhou. In 1984, Association of Tuina Medicine was set up in Chongqing, and *Journal of tueina Medicine* was initiated at the same time. The third national training course for tuina teachers was held in Shanghai College of Traditional Chinese Medicine. In 1985, *Journal of Massage and Daoyin* was initiated by Guangdong Provincial Institute of Chinese Medicine. Three-year tuina program was set up in the faculty of acupuncture in Nanjing College of Traditional Chinese Medicine. The Majors of tuina or acupuncture and tuina were also successively established in some colleges of Chinese medicine. In 1986, the faculty of massage therapy was set up in Shanghai College of Traditional Chinese Medicine and started to enroll the postgraduate students for massage discipline. In 1987, tuina volume edited by DING Jifeng of *Chinese Medical Encyclopedia* (Zhong Guo Yi Xue Bai Ke Quan Shu) was published. In 1987, the national academic organization of tuina therapy—Tuina Society of Chinese National Association of Chinese Medicine (later named Tuina Society of China Asso-

医学院成立针灸推拿系，设针灸、推拿专业。1979 年，首届全国推拿学术经验交流会在上海中医学院召开。1982 年，上海中医学院设立五年制本科推拿专业。1983 年，福建省成立按摩学会，武汉召开全国按摩与导引学术会议。广州召开广东省按摩气功学术交流会。1984 年，重庆市成立推拿医学研究会，并创办《推拿医学》杂志；上海中医学院举办第三期全国推拿师资培训班。1985 年，广东省中医研究所创办《按摩与导引》杂志，南京中医学院针灸系开设三年制推拿专业。一些中医学院也相继设立推拿专业或针灸推拿专业。1986 年，上海中医学院推拿系成立，开始招收推拿专业研究生。1987 年，丁季峰主编的《中国医学百科全书》推拿学分册出版。1987 年，全国性推拿学术团体——中华全国中医学会推拿学会（后改称中华中医药学会推拿分会）在上海成立。1988 年，中华中医药学会推拿分会的首次全国推拿学术交流会在上海举行，至 2014 年已举办了 15 次全国学术会议。1989 年，上海市中医药研究院推拿研究所成立。

ciation of Chinese Medicine) was established in Shanghai. In 1988, the first national academic conference of massage medicine organized by Tuina Society of China Association of Chinese Medicine was held in Shanghai. Up to 2014, 15 national academic conferences had been held already. In 1989, the Research Institute of Massage was set up in Shanghai Academy of Traditional Chinese Medicine and Pharmacy. In 1991, first international seminar on "massage and daoyin" was held in Wuhan by Wuhan Massage Association. In 1996, the faculty of acupuncture and massage therapy was established in Nanjing University of Traditional Chinese Medicine. Tuina discipline developed from professional training program to undergraduate program in many colleges and universities of Chinese medicine. In 1997, Shanghai University of Traditional Chinese Medicine started to enroll doctoral students of tuina discipline for the first time. In 1999, the national medical center of massage therapy in Shanghai Yueyang Hospital was approved by the State Administration of Traditional Chinese Medicine. In 2001, the national academic seminar on tuina literature and academic schools was held in Shanghai.

1991 年，武汉按摩学会在武汉举办"按摩与导引"首届国际学术研讨会。1996 年，南京中医药大学成立针灸推拿学院。不少中医院校的推拿专业也从专科发展到本科。1997 年，上海中医药大学首次招收推拿博士生。1999 年，上海岳阳医院的全国推拿专科医疗中心获国家中医药管理局批准。2001 年，全国推拿文献与学术流派学术交流会在上海召开。

The development of tuina medicine in this period was pioneered by the initiation of scientific research and experiments. Some researchers from other subjects also joined the study on tuina science. The research on massage therapy by multiple subjects was created. From the various angles of physiology, biochemistry, and neurotic electrophysiology, the research personals initiated the study on the tuina techniques and their efficacy and obtained a group of quality achievements. The researching tar-

这一时期的推拿医学的发展以科研实验的开展为先导。一些其他学科的科学研究者也加入了推拿科学研究的行列，多学科渗透研究推拿的局面已经形成。研究人员从生理、生化、神经电生理等各个角度，对推拿手法及其效应开展了研究，取得了一批有质量的成果。研究方

gets included mechanics study on manual techniques, study on tuina analgesia, and study on tuina biological effectiveness, etc. The scientific research projects were "dynamic analysis of swinging techniques in Chinese medical tuina", "study on collection and management of data from tuina techniques determination apparatus", "study on permeability of tuina techniques and functional mechanism of biological tissues", "analgesic mechanism study on stimulation of manual techniques in different forces to nociceptive pain", "dynamic study on swinging manual techniques", etc. "Study on theoretic foundation of TCM specific therapies" and its subsidiary projects of "TCM specific manual techniques for spinal diseases" and "study on theoretic foundation of 'meridian tendons' and 'bone dislocation'" were scheduled into the "developing plan of state key basic study" ("973" plan).

向主要有推拿手法动力学研究、推拿镇痛研究、推拿生物效应研究等。科研课题有"中医推拿摆动类手法动力学分析""推拿手法测定仪数据采集处理研究""推拿手法深透性与生物组织作用机制研究""轻重不同手法对伤害性疼痛刺激的镇痛机理研究""中医摆动类手法的动力学研究"等。"基于中医特色疗法的理论基础研究"及其子课题"中医特异性手法治疗脊柱病""'经筋'和'骨错缝'理论基础研究",列入国家科技部"国家重点基础研究发展计划"("973"计划)。

Tuina education also developed to the high level. Shandong College of Traditional Chinese Medicine and Shanghai College of Traditional Chinese Medicine successfully designed and manufactured the dynamic determination apparatus of tuina manual techniques successively and have already applied it in the teaching and research. Tuina education is developing toward the digitalization, multimedia and network. A group of the works had been published in the relation with the classification, and reinforcing and reducing effect of the manual techniques, accidents, school of manual techniques, and introduction of specific manual techniques. The communication on massage therapy increased progressively at home and abroad. The international education and communication of tuina medicine de-

推拿的教育工作也向高层次发展。山东中医学院和上海中医学院在 80 年代相继研制成功的推拿手法力学测定仪,已应用于推拿教学和科研。推拿教学正向数字化、多媒体化、网络化发展。发表了一批有关推拿手法的分类、补泻、手法意外、流派手法和独特手法介绍等论文。国内外推拿的交流日益增加。推拿的对外教学与交流已广泛开展。按脊、指压、反射区按摩法等国外"推拿"法也被介绍进了中国内地。2012 年和 2013 年上海中医

veloped extensively. The foreign massage methods of chiropractic, acupressure and reflex massage were also introduced into the mainland of China. In 2012 and 2013, two teacher training courses of "Science of Tuina Techniques", a project of state continuous education, were held in Shanghai University of Traditional Chinese Medicine.

药大学举办了两期国家继续教育项目"推拿手法学"师资培训班。

The clinical study of tuina medicine also developed extensively and profoundly. In addition to orthopedic and traumatic diseases, the clinical treatment and study had been initiated and the encouraging achievements had been obtained in diabetes, schizophrenia, coronary heart disease, angina pectoris, asthma, pulmonary emphysema, neurodermatitis, chronic fatigue syndrome, acute mastitis, and tumors. Since 2011, tuina clinics have been successively upgraded to be the state key specific clinics in the hospitals in Changchun, Yunnan, Shanghai, Tianjin, Zhejiang, and Fujian. The diagnostic and therapeutic plans have been ruled and optimized to design the clinical channel for some most appropriate diseases in tuina clinics. The research missions for classification and systematization of tuina technology of skin regions and channel tendons, tuina technology of Zangfu organs, tuina technology of joint movement, tuina technology of joint regulation, tuina technology of acupoints, guiding technology, infantile tuina technology, tuina technology and paste massage technology by auxiliary equipment, stepping technology and spine-pinching technology are in process.

推拿的临床研究也向广度和深度发展。除骨伤科疾病外，开展了对诸如糖尿病、精神分裂症、冠心病、心绞痛、哮喘、肺气肿、神经性皮炎、慢性疲劳综合征、急性乳腺炎、肿瘤的临床治疗与研究，并取得了可喜的成果。2011 年以来，长春、云南、上海、天津、浙江、福建等地多所医院的推拿科相继成为国家临床重点专科。对推拿科一些优势病种的诊疗方案作了梳理、优化，制定了临床路径。对中医推拿有特色的皮部经筋推拿技术、脏腑推拿技术、关节运动推拿技术、关节调整推拿技术、经穴推拿技术、导引技术、小儿推拿技术、器械辅助推拿技术和膏摩技术、踩蹻技术和捏脊技术的分类整理研究工作正在开展。

The specific manual techniques and academic schools of massage medicine, such as one-finger tuina, had been successively and successfully de-

一指禅推拿等特色推拿手法及流派在多地相继申报非物质文化遗产成功。各级

clared as intangible cultural heritage in many regions. The inheritance of famous TCM practitioners in tuina medicine in various levels and academic schools has been initiated.

推拿名老中医和学术流派的传承工作已经展开。

In this period, the published important books on tuina are: *Practical tuina of Chinese Medicine* (Shi Yong Zhong Yi Tui Na Xue) (LUO Jinghong, 1982), *Science of Massage* (Tui Na Xue) (YU Dafang, 1985), *Science of Massage-Chinese Medical Encyclopedia* (Zhong Guo Yi Xue Bai Ke Quan Shu-Tui Na Xue) (DING Jifeng, 1987), *Shandong Massage Medical Art* (Qi Lu Tuina Yi Shu) (SUN Chengnan, 1987), *Science of Massage Manual Techniques* (Tui Na Shou Fa Xue) (CAO Renfa, 1987), *Annals of Chinese Massage Medicine-Origin of Manual Techniques* (Zhong Hua Tui Na Yi Xue Zhi-Shou Fa Yuan Liu) (LUO Jinghong, 1987), *Science of Chinese Medical Massage* (Zhong Yi Tui Na Xue) (Edited by CAO Renfa, 1992, second edition in 2006), *Chinese Massage* (Zhong Guo Tui Na) (JIN Yicheng, PENG Jian, 1992), *Compendium of Chinese Massage* (Zhong Guo Tui Na Da Cheng) (WANG Zhihong, YAN Juntao, 1993), *Compendium of Massage* (Tui Na Da Cheng) (DING Jifeng, 1994), *Atlas of Massage Manual Techniques* (Tui Na Shou Fa Tu Pu) (SHEN Guoquan, YAN Juntao, 1994, second edition in 2004), *Research Compendium of Modern Chinese Medicine and Pharmacy-Massage Volume* (Xian Dai Zhong Yi Yao Yan Jiu Da Xi-Tui Na Fen Ce) (YAN Juntao, ZHAO Yi, 1998), *Li Zumo on Chinese Traditional Manual Technique Medicine* (Li Zu Mo Lun Zhong Guo Chuan Tong Shou Fa Yin Xue) (LI Zumo, 1998), *Compendium of Chinese Massage* (Zhong Guo Tui

此期出版的重要的推拿著作有:《实用中医推拿学》(骆竞洪,1982)、《推拿学》(俞大方,1985)、《中国医学百科全书·推拿学》(丁季峰,1987)、《齐鲁推拿医术》(孙承南,1987)、《推拿手法学》(曹仁发,1987)、《中华推拿医学志·手法源流》(骆竞洪,1987)、《中医推拿学》(曹仁发主编,1992,2006二版)、《中国推拿》(金义成、彭坚,1992)、《中国推拿大成》(王之虹、严隽陶,1993)、《推拿大成》(丁季峰,1994)、《推拿手法图谱》(沈国权、严隽陶,1994,2004二版)、《现代中医药研究大系·推拿分册》(严隽陶、赵毅,1998)、《李祖谟论中国传统手法医学》(李祖谟,1998)、《中国推拿全书》(夏治平,2000)、《推拿手法学》(周信文,2000)、《推拿手法学》(王之虹,2001)、《推拿学》(严隽陶,2003)、《推拿手法学》(王国才,2003)、《中国脊柱推拿手法全书》(李义凯,2005)、《推拿学》(范炳华,2008)、《推拿手法学》(赵毅、季远,2013)等。

Na Quan Shu) (XIA Zhiping, 2000), *Science of Massage Manual Techniques* (Tui Na Shou Fa Xue) (WANG Zhihong, 2001), *Massage Science* (Tui Na Xue) (YAN Juntao, 2003), *Science of Massage Manual Techniques* (Tui Na Shou Fa Xue) (WANG Guocai, 2003), *Chinese Compendium of Spinal Massage Manual Techniques* (Zhong Guo Ji Zhu Tui Na Shou Fa Quan Shu) (LI Yikai, 2005), *Massage Science* (Tui Na Xue) (FAN Binghua, 2008), *Science of Massage Manual Techniques* (Tui Na Shou Fa Xue) (ZHAO Yi, JI Yuan, 2013), etc.

Twelve Regular Meridians 十二正经

1. Lung Meridian of Hand-Taiyin	手太阴肺经
2. Large Intestine Meridian of hand-Yangming	手阳明大肠经
3. Stomach Meridian of Foot-Yangming	足阳明胃经
4. Spleen Meridian of Foot-taiyin	足太阴脾经
5. Heart Meridian of Hand-Shaoyin	手少阴心经
6. Small Intestine Meridian of Hand-Taiyang	手太阳小肠经
7. Bladder Meridian of Foot-Taiyang	足太阳膀胱经
8. Kidney Meridian of Foot-Shaoyin	足少阴肾经
9. Pericardium Meridian of Hand-Jueyin	手厥阴心包经
10. Triple Energizer Meridian of Hand-Shaoyang	手少阳三焦经
11. Gallbladder Meridian of Foot-Shaoyang	足少阳胆经
12. Liver Meridian of Foot-Jueyin	足厥阴肝经

Chapter 3 Manual techniques of tuina therapy

第3章 推拿手法

Section 1 Classification of manual techniques

第1节 推拿手法的分类

During the development of tuina medicine for several thousand years, the medical practitioners in the successive dynasties created and invented many effective manual techniques. It can be seen in the literature of the ancient and modern times that there are three or four hundred types of the written manual techniques. These manual techniques are respectively characteristic in the structures, operating skills, force forms and medical efficacy. The manual techniques are numerous in types. In order to learn, research and use the manual techniques conveniently, the scholars generalize, summarize and classify the manual techniques from different angles. The commonly used manual techniques can be divided into the following types.

在推拿医学几千年的发展过程中,历代医家创造、发明了许多行之有效的推拿手法。在古今文献中可见之于文字记载的手法就有三四百种之多。这些手法在术式结构、操作技巧、发力方式、医疗效果等方面都各具特点。手法的分类方法很多,为了便于学习、研究、应用推拿手法,学者们分别从不同角度将手法加以归纳总结、分门别类。常用的推拿手法分类有以下几种。

1 Classification by motion mode of the manual techniques

1 根据手法的动作形态分类

This is the classification in the classic textbook of massage therapy and is seen earliest in *Science of*

这是经典的推拿教科书分类法。最早见于上海中医

tuina (Tui Na Xue) edited in 1975 by Shanghai College of Traditional Chinese Medicine, in which the manual techniques are divided into six major types, i.e. winging type, rubbing and chafing type, vibrating type, pressing type, striking type, and joint-moving type. This kind of classification is helpful to study the structures and scientific principles by modern sports biomechanics.

学院 1975 年主编的《推拿学》，将推拿手法分成六大类，即摆动类、摩擦类、振动类、挤压类、叩击类和运动关节类手法。这一分类方法有利于从现代运动生物力学着手，来学习与研究手法的术式结构及其科学原理。

2 Classification by motion shape of the manual techniques

In accordance with the condition of the manual techniques, this classification is supposed to divide the manual techniques into three types of singular manual techniques, complex manual techniques and compound manual techniques.

2 根据手法术式结构的简繁分类

本分类法根据手法术式结构的简繁，可将推拿手法分成单式手法、复合手法与复式手法三类。

2.1 Singular manual techniques

Also termed basic manual techniques, it refers to the type of the manual techniques with singular element in the structure, such as pushing method, grasping method, pressing method, rubbing method, pinching method, patting method, etc.

2.1 单式手法

又称基本手法，是指手法的术式结构为单一成分的一类手法，如推法、拿法、按法、摩法、捏法、点法、拍法等。

2.2 Complex manual techniques

It refers to the type of the manual techniques composed of two or over structure of the simple manual techniques, such as pressing-kneading method, grasping-kneading method, and pulling-shaking method, etc.

2.2 复合手法

是指由两种或两种以上单式手法术式结构成分相结合而形成的一类手法，如按揉法、拿揉法、牵抖法等。

2.3 Compound manual techniques

The manual techniques were specially used for children in the ancient times. It refers to the assembled manual techniques operated with the stipulated procedure by the several kinds of singular manual techniques on a group of the acupoints or specific

2.3 复式手法

古代专门用于小儿的手法，是指由几种单式手法在一组特定穴或特定部位上以规定程序操作的组合型手法。这类手法往往根据操作

areas. This type of the manual techniques is termed with the specific names in accordance with the operating mode and feature, such as horse swimming across the heaven river, picking up bright moon from bottom of water, hornet entering the cave, etc.

方式和特点，冠以特定的名称，如打马过天河、水底捞明月、黄蜂入洞等。

3 Classification by force direction of the manual techniques

The manual techniques can be divided into two major types.

3 根据手法的作用力方式分类

可将所有手法分成两大类。

3.1 Manual techniques for soft tissue

By the direct functional force, they function on the soft tissues, i.e. directly transmit the force to the operated areas by the touch of the hand, to induce the distortion and fluctuation of internal pressure in the local soft tissues. Most manual techniques belong to this type of the manual techniques for soft tissues.

3.1 软组织类手法

通过直接作用力作用于软组织，即通过手的接触而直接传递到受术部位，引起局部软组织变形和内压波动，大多数推拿手法都属于软组织类手法。

3.2 Manual techniques for joints

By the indirect functional force, they function on the joints, i.e. function on the remote articular ligament by the bone lever and tension of soft tissues, to induce the change of joint motion, such as the shaking method, pulling method, pulling-extending method, and flexing-extending method for the spine and joints.

The functions of manual techniques are overlapping in the two types of the manual techniques. For instance, if the pressing method is used for reposition of the thoracic vertebras and lumbar vertebras, it belongs to the manual technique for joint. The shaking method can also function on the muscles and ligaments around the joint. If the pulling

3.2 骨关节类手法

通过间接作用力作用于骨关节，即手法力通过骨骼杠杆及软组织的张力作用于远隔的关节韧带，引起关节运动状态的改变。包括摇法、扳法、拔伸法、屈伸法等脊柱或关节手法。

这两大类手法的作用有所交叉，比如按压法如果用于胸椎、腰椎复位，即属于骨关节类手法；摇法也可作用于关节周围的肌肉、韧带等软组织；扳法如果缓慢操作不用“寸劲”发力，也可用于

method is operated slowly without release of "inch force", it can also be used to prolong the muscles and relax the soft tissues.

拉长肌肉放松软组织。

5 Classification by the targets of the manual techniques

They are divided into the adult manual techniques and infantile manual techniques, etc.

5 根据手法的应用对象分类

分为成人推拿手法、小儿推拿手法等。

6 Classification by the academic schools

They are divided into the one-finger manual technique, internal-works manual techniques, and bone-setting manual techniques, etc.

6 根据推拿流派分类

分为一指禅推拿手法、内功推拿手法、正骨推拿手法等。

Section 2 Basic requirements of manual techniques

第2节 推拿手法的基本要求

The basic requirements of the manual techniques are the basic standard abstracted from the various manual techniques for guiding all manual techniques.

The basic requirements of the manual techniques were defined in *Science of Tuina* (Tui Na Xue) published by Shanghai College of Traditional Chinese Medicine in 1975 to "be persistent, forceful, even and gentle for obtaining deep penetration", acknowledged by the academic circles.

推拿手法的基本要求是从各种手法中抽象出来的适用于指导所有手法的基本准则。

1975 年上海中医学院《推拿学》将推拿手法基本要求确定为"持久、有力、均匀、柔和,从而达到深透",得到了学术界的认可。

1 Basic requirements of the manual techniques for soft tissues

1.1 Persistent

It means that during the operation of the manual techniques, the movement and force should be maintained consistently in the period of enough time, without interruption, without distortion and

1 软组织手法的基本要求

1.1 持久

持久,是指手法在操作过程中,能够严格地按照规定的技术要求和操作规范持续地运用,在足够的时间内

without lack of force, strictly based upon the stipulated technical requirements and continuous application of the operating standard, in order to ensure the stimulation of the manual techniques to the human body to be accumulated to the critical point, so as to realize the effects to regulate the functions of Zangfu organs and change the pathological state.

保持动作和力量的连贯性，不间断、不变形、不乏力，以保证手法对人体的刺激能够积累到临界点，以起到调整脏腑功能、改变病理状态的作用。

1.2 Forceful

It means that this type of force is not a brute force or violent force, and it is a kind of technical force. Any kind of the manual techniques is based upon this force.

1.2 有力

有力，即有力量，且这种力量不可以是蛮力和暴力，而是一种含有技巧的力量。无论何种手法总是以力为基础的。

1.3 Even

It means that the force, frequency and amplitude of the manual techniques must be maintained even. The force must not be strong sometimes or weak sometimes. The frequency should not be fast sometimes or slow sometimes. The amplitude should not be large sometimes or small sometimes. The manual techniques should be operated stably and rhythmically.

1.3 均匀

均匀是指手法操作的力量、频率和幅度都必须保持均衡。力量不可忽强忽弱，频率不宜时快时慢，幅度不要时大时小，应使手法操作既平稳而又有节奏。

1.4 Gentle

It means that during the operation of the manual techniques, the movements should be stable and gentle. In the change of the manual techniques, it is necessary to natural, coordinative, light without floating tendency and heavy without stagnant tendency. Gentle does not mean weak and feeble. It implies firmness should be contained in gentleness, in order to avoid stiff and rude force and avoid adding suffering to the patient. It is exactly as what is said in "general introduction to manual techniques" of *The Golden Mirror of Medicine* (Yi Zong Jin Jian)

1.4 柔和

柔和是指手法操作时，动作平稳缓和，手法变换时自然、协调，轻而不浮，重而不滞。柔和并不是软弱无力，而是柔中有刚，不可生硬粗暴，增加患者的痛苦。正如《医宗金鉴·正骨心法要旨》"手法总论"所说："法之所施，使患者不知其苦，方称为手法也。"

that only if the patient does not feel suffering, can the manual techniques be termed so.

1.5 Deep penetration

It means that after the above four requirements of persistent, forceful, even and gentle state arc ensured in the manual techniques, a kind of penetrating force can be formed, to permeate into the skin and directly reach the deep tissues and internal organs by the stimulation of the manual techniques on the body surface, or indirectly have the biological effect of the manual techniques to reach the target organ via various channels, so as to realize the effect to regulate Zangfu organs. Deep penetration refers mainly to deep penetration of the force, also includes the deep penetration of heat at the same time.

1.5 深透

深透是指手法具备了持久、有力、均匀、柔和这四项要求后,形成了一种渗透力。这种渗透力,可透皮入内,直接深达手法刺激部位的深层组织和内脏器官,或间接地通过各种途径使手法的生物效应到达目标脏器,起到调整脏腑虚实的作用。深透,主要是指力的深透,但也同时包括了热的深透。

2 Basic requirements of the manual techniques for joints

It refers to the manual techniques for the movement of the joints. They are specific in the operation. But the basic requirements can be generalized as "stable, accurate, ingenious, and fast".

2 骨关节手法的基本要求

骨关节手法是指运动关节类手法,在操作上有其特殊性,其基本要求可概括为"稳、准、巧、快"四个字。

2.1 Stable

It is needed to be stable and natural, and to move within the scope of the rules and permission according to the actual situation, and avoid brute and rude action. It is also necessary to reflect the safety principle of the manual techniques, not to do any uncertain manual techniques for the movement of the joints, and not to abuse the manual techniques and use the manual techniques blindly.

2.1 稳

"稳"即稳重。要求操作时要平稳自然,因势利导,要在规定与允许的范围内动作,避免生硬粗暴。"稳",还体现了手法的安全性原则,不做无把握的运动关节类手法,不滥用手法,不盲目施术。

2.2 Accurate

It includes the accuracy in the manual tech-

2.2 准

包括手法术式的准确和

niques and in the functional area. Namely, it is necessary to select the manual techniques purposefully and locate the area accurately, to have the selected manual technique accurately function on the targeted joint.

作用部位的准确。即选择手法要有针对性，定位要准。要求选用手法的时候要能够精确地作用到目标关节。

2.3 Ingenious

It means ingenious and nimble. It is necessary to use the ingenious force during the operation of the manual techniques, to overcome the hardness by gentleness and to win the victory by nimbleness, and not to use the force absurdly. Only by using the ingenious force, can it be possible to "achieve great goal by doing little" and to save the force for self protection. To be "ingenious" is the basic requirement for the manual techniques for the movement of the joints. Only by painstaking study and training, can it be possible to really reach the realm of "seizing the opportunity externally and having ingeniousness internally" requested by the predecessors.

2.3 巧

就是技巧、灵巧的意思。手法操作时要用巧力，以柔克刚，以巧制胜，不用蛮力。运用巧力才能"四两拨千斤"，才能省力并自护。用好"巧"是运动关节类手法的基本功，只有经过刻苦学习和艰苦训练，才能真正达到前人要求的"机触于外，巧生于内"的境界。

2.4 Fast

In using the force, it is necessary to release and withdraw the force quickly, i.e. "inch force", and not necessary to release the force too far and too long.

2.4 快

手法用力时要疾发疾收，即用所谓的"寸劲"，发力不可过长，发力时间不可过久。

Section 3 Basic manual techniques

第3节 基本手法

1 Rolling method

It refers to the manual technique to roll back and forth by the ulnar aspect of the hand back on the massage area, with the dorsum of the fifth

1 㨰法

以第五掌指关节背面吸定，用手背近尺侧部分在受术部位作来回滚动的手法，

metacarpophalangeal joint adhering on the skin. The rolling method was created by Mr. DING Jifeng around 1940 and is a representative technique in rolling tuina school.

称为㨰法。㨰法是丁季峰先生于 1940 年前后始创,是㨰法推拿流派的代表性手法。

Form

It is necessary for the practitioner to be naturally relaxed in the fingers, to adhere to the massage area with the dorsum of the fifth metacarpophalangeal joint or ulnar aspect of the hypothenar, to drop the shoulder and have the elbow joint as the fulcrum, to roll the ulnar aspect of the hand back on the massage area back and forth continuously, with the active swinging motion in the forearm to take the extension and flexion of the wrist joint and rotating motion of the forearm (Figure 3-1)

术式

术者手指自然放松,以第五掌指关节背面或小鱼际尺侧缘吸定于受术部位,沉肩,以肘关节为支点,前臂作主动摆动,带动腕关节的伸屈和前臂的旋转运动,使手背近尺侧部在受术部位作持续不断的来回滚动(图 3-1)。

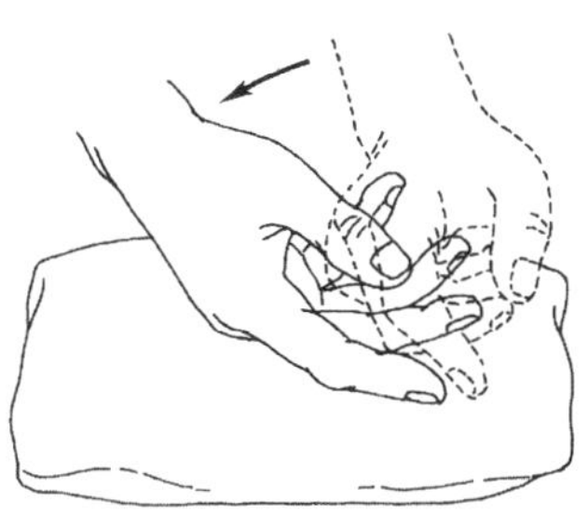

Figure 3-1 Rolling method

图 3-1 㨰法

Explanation

(1) Frequency is 120～160 times per minute.

(2) It is needed to relax and drop the shoulder, flex and abduct the shoulder joint forward a little bit, keep a distance of 1～2 fists between the elbow and chest, and to maintain the stability relatively and not to move forward, backward, leftward and rightward in large amplitude.

说明

(1) 频率为每分钟120～160 次。

(2) 肩部放松下垂,肩关节略前屈、外展,肘部与胸壁相距 1～2 拳,在操作中肘部应相对稳定,不宜大幅度前后左右运动。

(3) The included angle in the flexion of the elbow joint is 130°～150°. It is advisable to adjust the force by changing the included angle.

(3) 肘关节屈曲的夹角为130°～150°。可通过夹角的变化来调整施术压力。

(4) It is needed to be big in the amplitude in the flexion and extension of the wrist joint, and to roll forward in maximum by flexing the wrist joint in 60°～80°, and roll backward in maximum by extending the wrist joint in 30°～40°.

(4) 腕关节伸屈幅度要大，前滚至极限时屈腕达60°～80°，回滚至极限时伸腕达30°～40°。

(5) It is needed to be natural in all fingers and not to flex or extend the fingers too much.

(5) 各手指任其自然，不可过度屈曲或伸直。

(6) It is needed to use force in rolling back and forth, and to have the force ratio in forward rolling and backward rolling in about 3∶1.

(6) 来回都要用力，前滚和回滚的用力比例约为3∶1。

(7) It is needed to be even in pressure, frequency and amplitude in the operation and to be coordinative and rhythmical in the movement.

(7) 㨰法操作的全程，其压力、频率、幅度要均匀，动作要协调而有节律性。

(8) It is needed for the practitioner to stand with the two feet apart naturally and to bend the body forward a little bit. It is advisable to increase the pressure by increasing the forward-bending angle of the upper body.

(8) 术者站立操作时，两脚自然分开，上身略前倾。可通过加大上身前倾角度来增加施术压力。

(9) It is needed not to drag, flip up, twist and throw out. Dragging is usually induced by releasing the force with the shoulder joint wrongly, or by too fast motion to change the rolling friction to the sliding friction. Flipping up is caused by too small force in rolling back or no rolling back, forming a one-way impact force. Twisting is related to move the adhering spot upward to the hypothenar, and too large amplitude in the flexion and extension of the wrist joint, and too small in the amplitude in the rotation of the forearm. Throwing out is caused by releasing the force with the flexion and extension of the wrist joint, not the active flexion and extension

(9) 不可拖动、跳动、拧动和甩动。拖动通常是错误地以肩关节开合发力，或移动速度过快，将滚动摩擦变成了滑动摩擦；跳动是回滚力过小或没有回滚而形成单向冲击用力；拧动是将吸定点上移到了小鱼际，且腕关节屈伸幅度过大而前臂旋转幅度过小；甩动是没有肘关节的主动屈伸而以腕关节的屈伸发力。

of the elbow joint.

(10) It is needed to cooperate with the passive movement of the corresponding joint in the clinical practice.

(10) 㨰法临床操作中常配合相应关节的被动运动。

Application

The contact surface of the rolling method is comparatively larger and moderate and comfortable in stimulation, appropriate for nape, shoulder, back, lumbar region and buttocks, and four limbs with thick muscles. The rolling method is often used to roll the trapezius muscle, deltoid muscle, lumbar region and posterior aspect of the thigh, etc.

应用

㨰法接触面较大，刺激平和舒适，适用于颈项部、肩背部、腰臀部以及四肢等肌肉较丰厚的部位。常用的操作法有㨰斜方肌、㨰三角肌、㨰腰背部、㨰股后部等。

2 One-finger pushing method

2 一指禅推法

It refers to the manual technique to adhere to the body surface with the tip or cushion of the thumb, to lead the flexion and extension of the thumb by swinging the forearm, and to have the produced power to function on the massage area continuously. One-finger pushing method is a representative manual technique in one-finger tuina school.

用拇指的指端或指纹面着力，通过前臂的摆动带动拇指作屈伸运动，使产生的功力持续不断地作用于施术部位，称为一指禅推法。一指禅推法是一指禅推拿流派的代表性手法。

Form

It is necessary for the practitioner to have a loose fist, extend the thumb naturally to cover the fist eye and focus the force on the tip or cushion of the thumb on the massage area, with the elbow joint as a fulcrum, by the active swinging motion of the forearm, to lead the swinging motion of the wrist joint, and the flexing and extending movement of the metacarpophalangeal joint or the interphalangeal joint of the thumb, so as to have the produced power to function on the massage area rhythmically (Figure 3-2). This manual technique can be operated by the two hands.

术式

术者手握空拳，拇指自然伸直并盖住拳眼，用拇指指端或指纹面着力于受术部位，以肘关节为支点，前臂作主动摆动，带动腕关节摆动以及拇指掌指关节或指骨间关节的屈伸运动，使产生的功力节律性地作用于受术部位(图 3-2)。本法也可双手操作。

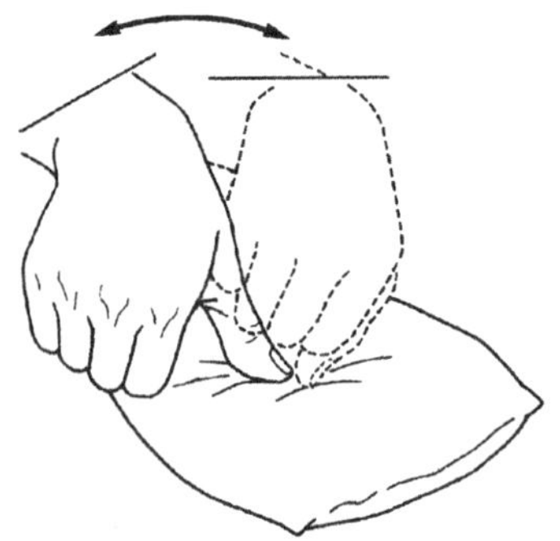

Figure 3-2　One-finger pushing method by finger tip
图 3-2　一指禅指端推法

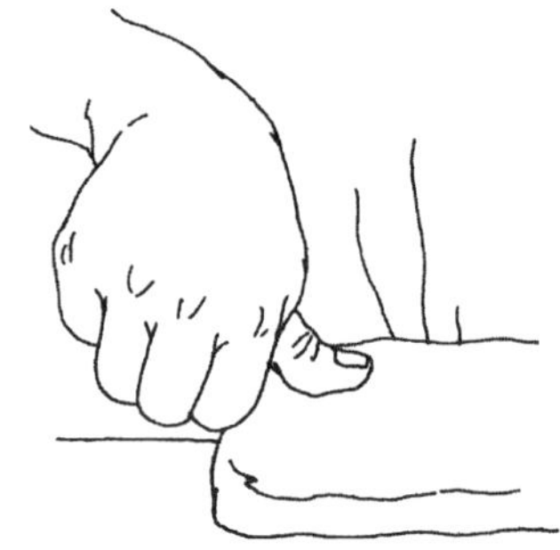

Figure 3-3　One-finger pushing method by finger cushion
图 3-3　一指禅指腹推法

Explanation

(1) In accordance with the different force spots of the thumb, one-finger pushing method can be divided into the pushing method by the finger tip or by the finger cushion. It is necessary for the practitioner with straight thumb to adopt the one-finger pushing method by the finger tip, and for the practitioner with the large extending amplitude in the interphalangeal joint of the thumb to focus the force on the finger cushion (Figure 3-3) (force by finger tip optional). The contact surface is smaller and local pressure in larger in the finger tip. The contact surface is larger and gentler in the finger cushion. In training and application, it is necessary to select the appropriate mode in accordance with the physiological condition of the individual's thumb and different massage areas.

(2) In the operation of the one-finger pushing method by the finger tip, there are two ways: by flexion and extension of the interphalangeal joint of the thumb, or by no flexion and extension of the interphalangeal joint of the thumb. In the operation

说明

(1) 根据拇指着力部位的不同，一指禅推法可分为指端推和指腹推两类。拇指较挺直者一般采用指端着力式一指禅推法，而拇指指骨间关节背伸幅度较大者，多采用指腹着力(图 3-3)(也可指端着力)。指端推者接触面积较小，局部压强较大。指腹推者接触面积较大，因而较为柔和。练习和应用时可根据个人拇指生理条件及不同的受术部位而选择相宜的操作。

(2) 一指禅指端推法操作时拇指指骨间关节有屈伸和不屈伸两种术式。屈伸拇指式一指禅推法操作时，拇指指骨间关节须跟随腕部的

of the one-finger pushing method by flexing and extending the thumb, it is necessary for the interphalangeal joint of the thumb to follow the swing motion of the wrist joint to have the rhythmical flexion and extension. For those with larger extension in the interphalangeal joint in the operation of the pushing method by the finger tip, it is only possible to adopt the flexing-extending mode of the interphalangeal joint. For those with comparatively straight interphalangeal joint of the thumb, it is advisable to decide the mode according to the situation.

(3) Frequency is about 120～160 times per minute.

(4) In the operation of the one-finger pushing method, it is needed to sink the shoulder, drop the elbow, hang the wrist, and to be loose in the palm and firm in the finger.

Application

One-finger pushing method is smaller in the contact surface, focused in power and strong in the permeability. Therefore, it can be used on the head, face, nape, chest, abdomen, four limbs and various parts of the whole body, especially appropriate for dot-like acupoints or lineal migration on the meridians. The commonly used methods are one-finger pushing method on Baihui (GV 20), on the nape, on Jugu (LI 16), and on the bladder meridian of the back, etc.

3 One-finger pushing method by finger side

It refers to the manual technique to adhere to the body surface with the radial side of the last knuckle of the thumb. It is named so in Chinese lan-

摆动而作节律性的屈伸活动。拇指指骨间关节背伸度较大者欲作指端着力推法时，只能采用指骨间关节屈伸术式。而拇指指骨间关节较挺直者，可根据情况决定屈伸与否。

(3) 频率为每分钟120～160 次。

(4) 一指禅推法操作时，要求沉肩、垂肘、悬腕、掌虚、指实。

应用

一指禅推法接触面小，功力集中，渗透性强，故可应用于头面部、颈项部、胸腹部及四肢等全身各部，尤其适合于点状的腧穴并沿着经络线状移动。常用操作法有一指禅推百会穴、一指禅推项部、一指禅推巨骨穴、一指禅推背部膀胱经等。

3 一指禅偏锋推法

用拇指末节桡侧缘着力作一指禅推法的手法，称为一指禅偏锋推法。由于是用

guage, because it is operated with the side of the thumb, similar to writing style by the side of the wirting brush in Chinese calligraphy.

拇指的侧面操作，类似于中国毛笔书法的偏锋行笔，故名。

Form

It is needed for the practitioner to straighten the metacarpophalangeal part, focus the radial side of the last knuckle of the thumb on the massage area, with the wrist joint naturally relaxed, slightly flexed or straightened naturally, sink the shoulder and drop the elbow, and by the elbow joint as a fulcrum and the active swinging motion of the forearm, lead the leftward and rightward swinging motion of the wrist joint and lead flexion and extension of the metacarpophalangeal joint or internphalangeal joint of the thumb, so as to have the produced power to function on the massage area. (Figure 3-4)

术式

术者掌指部自然伸直，以拇指末节桡侧偏锋着力于受术部位，腕关节自然放松，呈微屈或自然伸直状态。沉肩、垂肘，以肘关节为支点，前臂作主动摆动，带动腕关节左右摆动和拇指掌指关节或拇指的指骨间关节的屈伸活动，使所产生的功力作用于受术部位（图 3-4）。

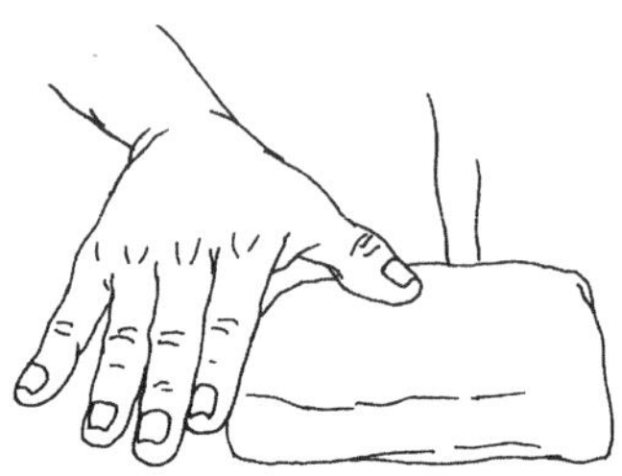

Figure 3-4　One-finger pushing method by finger side

图 3-4　一指禅偏锋推法

Explanation

(1) Frequency is 120～160 times per minute.

(2) The movement should be light, fast, and stable in rhythm.

(3) The wrist joint is naturally relaxed and not be bend.

说明

(1) 频率为每分钟120～160 次。

(2) 动作要轻快、平稳而有节奏感。

(3) 着力点要吸定，不可来回摩擦。

(4) The middle finger and forearm should be on a straight line, beneficial to lateral flexion of the wrist joint.

(4) 中指与前臂成一直线，有利于腕关节的左右侧屈摆动。

(5) It is needed for those with large amplitude in the extension of the interphalangeal joint of the thumb to flex the interphalangeal joint of the thumb properly and slightly, in order to avoid too large in the contact surface of the radial side of the thumb.

(5) 部分拇指指骨间关节背伸幅度较大者，应适当微屈指骨间关节，以保证拇指末节桡侧接触面不至于过大。

(6) In terms of the training steps of the one-finger pushing method by the finger side, it is needed to start from the kneading method by the hyperthenar, and then train on the palm or rice bag, and finally train on the head and face of the human body.

(6) 一指禅偏锋推法的训练步骤，可以先从摆动式鱼际揉法开始，然后在掌心或米袋上练习，最后过渡到在人体头面部练习。

Application

The one-finger pushing method by the finger side is light, fast, gentle and comfortable in the movement and can be applied on the head, face, chest, abdomen and hypochondriac region, especially on the head and face most commonly. The one-finger pushing method by the finger side is usually applied to push the forehead, the orbit, and the anterior midline of the chest, etc.

应用

一指禅偏锋推法动作轻快、柔和、舒适，应用于头面部、胸腹部和胁肋部等，尤以头面部最为常用。常用的操作法有一指禅偏锋推前额、偏锋推眼眶、偏锋推胸部前正中线等。

4 Pressing method

It refers to the manual technique to press the body surface by the finger cushion, or palm vertically, including the finger-pressing method, palm-pressing method, and elbow-pressing method.

4 按法

按法是指用指腹、手掌等垂直按压体表的手法。主要包括指按法、掌按法和肘按法。

Form

1. Finger-pressing method

It is needed to focus the force on the massage area with the thumb cushion, and press vertically downward by increasing force, with the rest four

术式

1. 指按法

以拇指指腹(指纹面)着力于受术部位，由轻而重垂直向下按压，其余四指握拳，

fingers in fist or opened, to assist the force (Figure 3-5). When the patient feels sore, numb, heavy and distending, it is needed to keep pressing for several seconds, and then relax gradually. Thus, it is repeated. The finger-pressing method can be operated with one finger or several fingers, also by the two hands or the piled fingers of the two hands (Figure 3-6). Usually, it is applied on the acupoints.

或张开支撑,以协同助力(图3-5);待受术者产生酸、麻、重、胀等感觉时持续数秒,然后逐渐减压放松。如此反复操作。指按法可单指操作或多指操作,也可双手操作或双手叠指操作(图3-6)。一般在腧穴上施术。

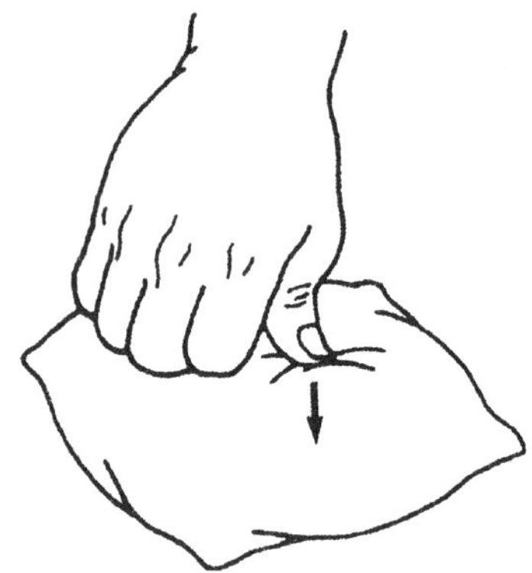

Figure 3-5　Finger-pressing method
图3-5　指按法

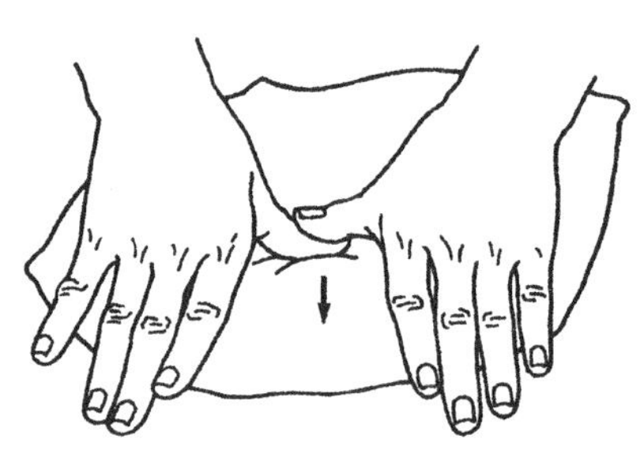

Figure 3-6　Pressing method by piled fingers
图3-6　叠指按法

2. Palm-pressing method

(1) Pressing method by the single palm　It is needed for the practitioner to bend the wrist joint, press the body surface with the palm root or whole palm vertically downward by the force of the upper arm increasingly, and then decreasingly to reduce pressure gradually (Figure 3-7).

(2) Pressing method by the piled palms　It is needed to put one palm on the back of another hand, by leaning forward with the body and force from the body trunk for transmitting the force along the vertical axis of the upper arm to the massage area, and press vertically downward, and then reduce pressure gradually (Figure 3-8).

2. 掌按法

(1) 单掌按法　术者腕关节背伸,用掌根或全掌着力于体表,上臂发力,由轻而重垂直向下按压,再逐渐减压(图3-7)。

(2) 叠掌按法　将一手掌心叠置于另一手手背,上身前倾,以躯干发力,使力沿上肢纵轴传导到受术部位,垂直向下按压,再逐渐减压(图3-8)。

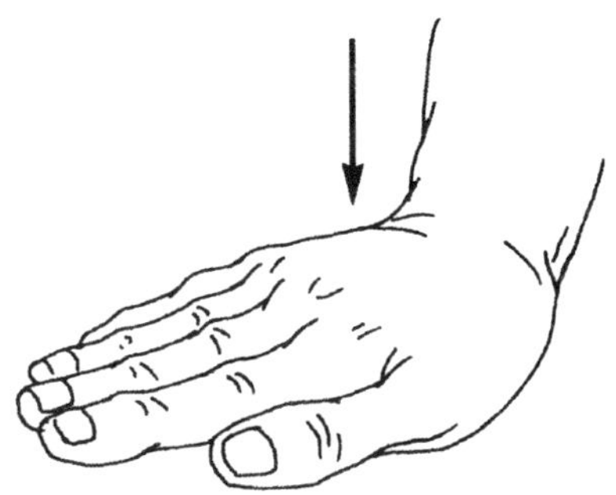

Figure 3-7 Palm-pressing method
图 3-7 掌按法

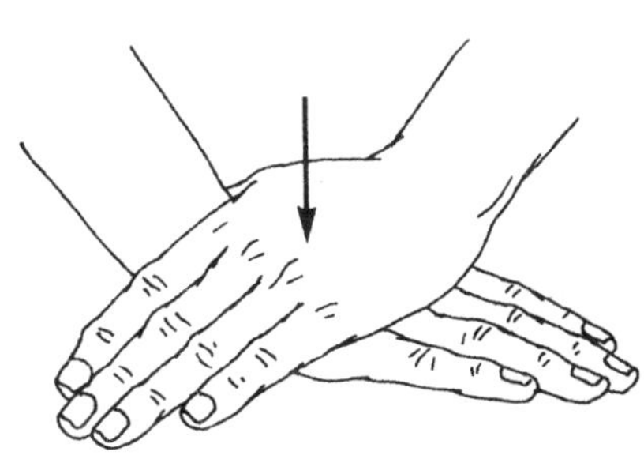

Figure 3-8 Pressing method by the piled palms
图 3-8 叠掌按法

3. Elbow-pressing method

It is needed to focus the force from the upper part of the ulna proximal to the elbow on the body surface of the massage area, lean forward in the upper body, and press stably and vertically downward (Figure 3-9).

3. 肘按法

以前臂尺侧上端近肘部着力于受术体表，上身前倾，平稳向下垂直按压(图 3-9)。

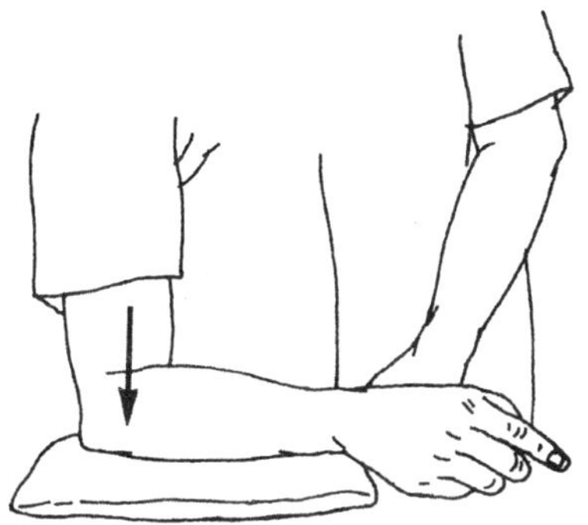

Figure 3-9 Elbow-pressing method
图 3-9 肘按法

Explanation

(1) It is needed to keep the pressing direction vertically to the body surface.

(2) It is needed to increase the force stably and decrease the force gradually, and not to use the impact force.

说明

(1) 按压的方向应与受术体表垂直。

(2) 用力要由轻到重平稳加压，再由重而轻逐渐减压，不可冲击式用力。

(3) It is needed to regulate the pressing powder by piling the fingers, piling the palms, extending the elbow, and lean forward in the upper body.

(3) 可用叠指、叠掌、伸肘、上身前倾等姿势来调整按压的力量。

(4) It is needed not to do the elbow-pressing method with the olecroanon.

(4) 肘按法不要用尺骨鹰嘴操作。

Application

应用

The finger-pressing method is smaller in the contact surface, appropriate for acupoints or Ashi points of the whole body, appropriate for various parts or acupoints of the whole body. Frequently, this method is applied to press the vertex, Taiyang (Extra), Jianjing (GB 21), Tianzong (SI 11), Zusanli (ST 36), Ashi points, and press the temple with index and middle finger, press the abdomen with three fingers, and press Huantiao (GB 30) with the piled fingers.

指按法接触面积较小，适用于全身各部位或腧穴。常用操作法有指按头顶，指按太阳，指按肩井，指按天宗，指按足三里，指按阿是穴，示、中二指按颞部，三指按腹部，叠指按环跳等。

The palm-pressing method is larger in the contact surface, with strong pressure but moderate stimulation, appropriate for large and flat areas of the low back, abdomen, and lower limb. Frequently, this method is applied to press the posterior aspect of the thigh by the palm, press the back by the symmetrical palms, and press the spine by the piled palms, etc.

掌按法接触面积大，压力虽大但刺激缓和，适用于面积大而又较为平坦的腰背部、腹部、下肢等部位。常用操作法有掌按股后部，对称掌按背部，叠掌按脊柱等。

The elbow-pressing method is strong in stimulation, usually used for the upper part of the scapula, buttocks, posterior part of the thigh, and lumbar and sacral region with thick muscles. For example, press Huantiao (GB 30) at the buttocks by the elbow.

肘按法刺激较强，一般用于肩胛上部、臀部、股后部、腰骶部等肌肉丰厚处。如肘按臀部环跳穴等。

[Appendix 1]　Pointing method　It refers to the manual technique to press the body surface vertically with the finger tip, the knuckle of the interphalangeal joint or elbow tip. This method is evolved

[附1] *点法*　*以指端、指骨间关节骨突或肘尖垂直按压体表，称为点法。点法由按法演化而来。以拇指或*

from the pressing method. If press with the finger tip of the thumb or middle finger, it is termed the finger tip-pointing method. If press with the flexed finger, or knuckle of the interphalangeal joint of the thumb, it is termed the knuckle-pointing method. If press with the elbow tip, it is termed the elbow-pointing method. In comparison with the pressing method, the contact surface is smaller and the stimulation is stronger, appropriate for acupoints or tender spots of various body parts. The pointing method is often used to poke Fengchi (GB 20), Fengfu (GV 16), Yifeng (TE 17), Dingchuan (Extra), Feishu (BL 13), Tianzong (SI 11), Hegu (LI 4), Huantiao (GB 30), Biguan (ST 31), Zusanli (ST 36), Qiuxu (GB 40), and Yongquan (KI 1), etc.

中指指端着力者称为指端点法，以屈曲的示指或拇指指骨间关节骨突着力者称为指节点法，以肘尖部着力者称为肘点法。点法与按法相比，接触面积较小，刺激强度较大，适用于全身各部位腧穴或压痛点（以痛为腧）。常用操作法有点风池、点风府、点翳风、点定喘、点肺俞、点天宗、点合谷、点环跳、点髀关、点足三里、点丘墟、点涌泉等。

[Appendix 2] Nipping method It refers to the manual technique to press the therapeutic spots stably with the nail of the thumb. In order to avoid piercing the skin, it is advisable to put a piece of thin cloth on the massage area. This method is the manual technique with strong stimulation and is often used for emergency by nipping Renzhong (GB 26), Laolong (Extra), and Shiwang (Extra). The light nipping method is appropriate for infantile tuina, for instance, nip Pt. Sihengwen, Pt. Banmen, etc.

［附 2］掐法　用拇指指甲端，在治疗点上平稳按压的手法，称为掐法。为避免刺破皮肤，可在受术部位上先铺一薄布。掐法是重刺激手法，常用于急救，有掐水沟、老龙、十王等操作法。较轻的掐法适用于小儿推拿，如掐四横纹、板门等。

5 Kneading method

It refers to the manual technique to adhere to the body surface with the finger or palm forcefully, including the finger-kneading method, palm-kneading method, and forearm-kneading method, etc.

5 揉法

以指、掌等部位着力于体表，并带动皮下组织作环旋运动的手法称为揉法。包括指揉法、掌揉法、前臂揉法等。

5.1 Finger-kneading method

It means to adhere to the massage area with the finger cushion and knead with a light, gentle and

5.1 指揉法

用指腹着力于受术部位上，作轻柔缓和的环旋揉动，

circular motion to lead a kneading motion with the subcutaneous tissues. The commonly used ones are the thumb-kneading method and middle finger-kneading method (Figure 3-10), and two finger-kneading method by the index and middle finger (Figure 3-11). The finger-kneading method is smaller in the contact surface and is focused in power, appropriate for the meridians and acupoints, and also for infantile tuina.

并带动皮下组织一起揉动。常用的有拇指揉法和中指揉法(图3-10),以及用示、中指着力的二指揉法(图3-11)。指揉法施术面积小,功力较集中,适用于在经络腧穴上操作,也用于小儿推拿。

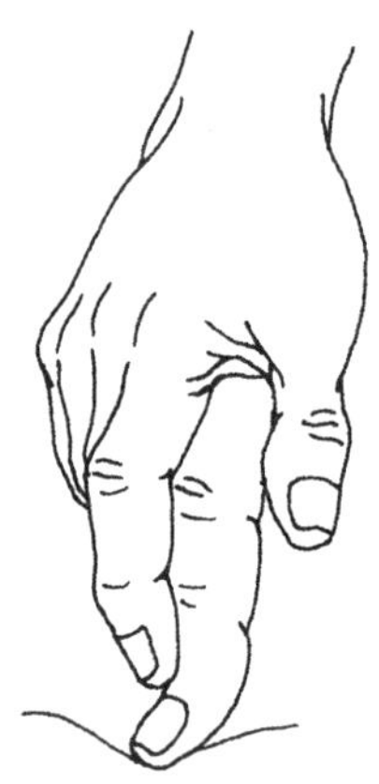

Figure 3-10 Middle finger-kneading method
图3-10 中指揉法

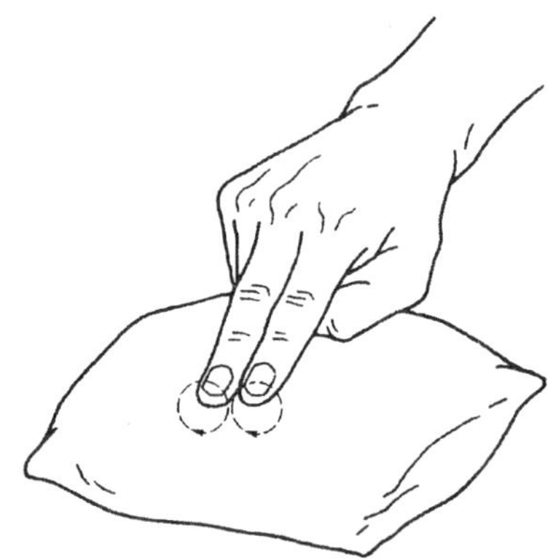

Figure 3-11 Two finger-kneading method
图3-11 二指揉法

5.2 Palm-kneading method

It means to adhere to the massage area with the palm, palm root or thenar, with the elbow joint as a fulcrum, to knead with a stable circular motion and lead a kneading motion of the subcutaneous tissues. In doing the palm root-kneading method (Figure 3-12), it is needed to flex the metacarpophalangeal joint of the palm slightly and knead stably with the palm root. If the palm-kneading method is done by one palm on the dorsum of the other hand, it is termed the kneading method by the piled palms (Figure 3-13).

5.2 掌揉法

用手掌、掌根或鱼际着力于受术部位上,以肘关节为支点,作平稳的环旋揉动,并带动皮下组织一起揉动。作掌根揉(图3-12)时,要求手掌的掌指关节略屈曲,以掌根部平稳下压并揉动。如以一手掌心叠加于另一手手背之上作掌揉法,称为叠掌揉法(图3-13)。

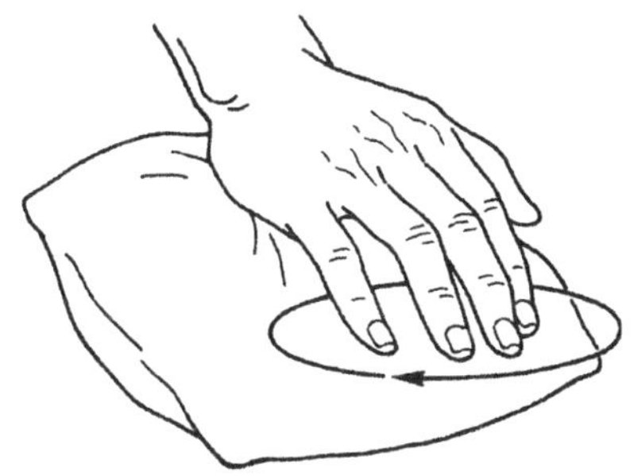

Figure 3-12 Palm root-kneading method
图 3-12 掌根揉法

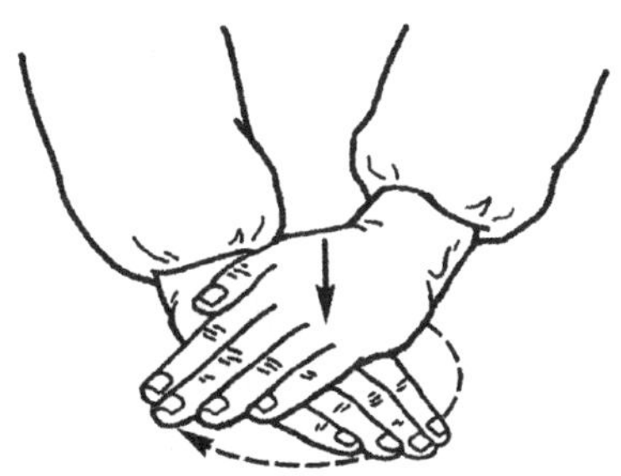

Figure 3-13 Kneading method of piled palms
图 3-13 叠掌揉法

5.3 Thenar-kneading method

This is the thenar-kneading method of swinging mode. It is requested for the practitioner to sink the shoulder, drop the elbow, relax and flex or straighten the wrist joint, with the thumb adducted slightly and the rest four fingers relaxed naturally, and adhere to the body surface with the thenar, with the elbow joint as a fulcrum, and make a active swing with the forearm, so as to lead the wrist joint for a lateral flexing motion, and take the subcutaneous tissues of the massage area to knead by the adhered thenar (Figure 3-14).

5.4 Forearm-kneading method

It means to adhere to the massage area with the upper 1/3 part of the ulnar side of the forearm, with the shoulder joint as a fulcrum, to knead with a circular motion by the upper arm taking the forearm (Figure 3-15), and lead the subcutaneous tissues to knead together.

Explanation

(1) In various kneading methods, it is necessary to lead the subcutaneous tissues to knead together, and not to make friction on the body surface.

(2) The frequency of the ordinary circular

5.3 鱼际揉法

这是一种摆动式的鱼际揉法。术者沉肩、垂肘，腕关节放松微屈或自然伸直，拇指略内收，其余四指自然放松，用鱼际吸定于受术体表，以肘关节为支点，前臂作主动摆动，带动腕关节作左右侧屈运动，并通过吸定的鱼际部带动受术部位的皮下组织一起揉动(图 3-14)。

5.4 前臂揉法

用前臂尺侧的上 1/3 部位着力于受术部位，以肩关节为支点，连同上臂带动前臂作环旋揉动(图 3-15)，并带动皮下组织一起揉动。

说明

(1) 各种揉法必须带动皮下组织一起揉动，不要在体表摩擦。

(2) 普通环旋式揉法的

kneading method is 100～120 times per minute. But the frequency of the thenar-kneading method of swinging mode is similar that in the pushing method by the thumb side, in 120～160 times per minute.

(3) The thenar-kneading method of swinging mode is a basic training method for the beginners of the manual techniques, helpful to enhance the elasticity and flexibility of the wrist joint. It is necessary to train it before learning the one-finger pushing method by the finger side.

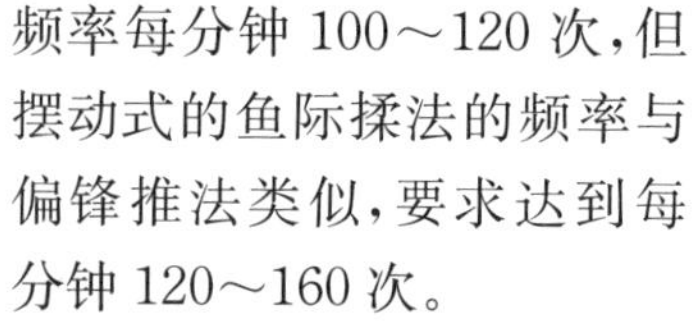

频率每分钟 100～120 次，但摆动式的鱼际揉法的频率与偏锋推法类似，要求达到每分钟 120～160 次。

（3）摆动式的鱼际揉法是推拿手法初学者的基础练习法，有助于提高腕关节的灵活性和柔韧性，应该在学习一指禅偏锋推法之前练习。

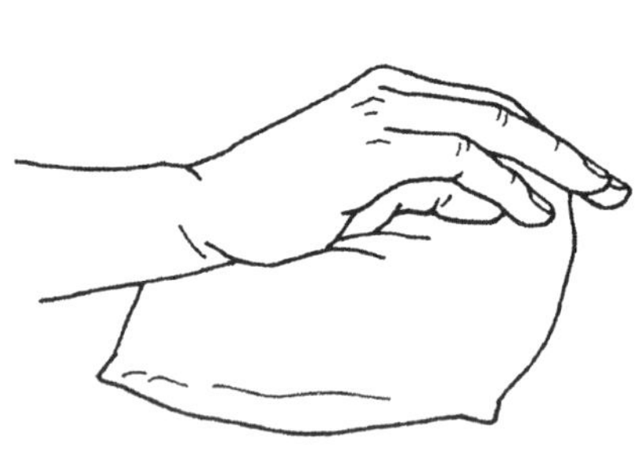

Figure 3-14　Thenar-kneading method of swinging mode

图 3-14　摆动式鱼际揉法

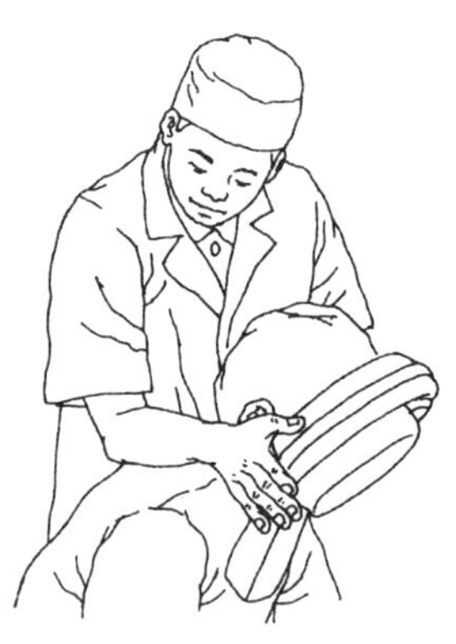

Figure 3-15　Forearm-kneading method

图 3-15　前臂揉法

Application

The finger-kneading method is extensively applied for the acupoints and Ashi points of various body parts. The palm-kneading method is mostly used on the back. The thenar-kneading method of swinging mode is often used on the forehead and temple. The elbow-kneading method is mostly used on the nape, shoulder, back and buttocks with thick muscles. The methods are commonly used to knead Baihui (GV 20), Quchi (LI 11), Hegu (LI 4), Taichong (LR 3) and Jiexi (ST 41) by the thumb,

应用

指揉法广泛用于全身各部腧穴和阿是穴。掌揉法多用于背部。摆动式鱼际揉法常用于前额部、颞部。前臂揉法多用于项肩部、背部、臀部等肌肉丰厚处。常用的操作法有拇指揉百会、曲池、合谷、太冲、解溪；中指揉印堂；二指揉上睛明、迎香；三指揉腹部；鱼际揉前额；叠掌揉腰

knead Yintang (Extra) by the middle finger, knead Shangjingming (Extra) and Yingxiang (LI 20) by the two fingers, knead the abdomen by the three fingers, knead the forehead by the thenar, knead the low back by the piled palms, and knead Jianjing (GB 20) and buttocks by the elbow, etc.

背部;前臂揉肩井、臀部等。

6 Pinching method

It refers to the manual technique to press the massage area forcefully with the thumb and rest four fingers.

Form

The practitioner squeezes and presses the skin and muscles forcefully with the thumb and rest four fingers. There are the pinching method by the two fingers, pinching method by the three fingers, and pinching method by the five fingers, etc. The pinching method by the two fingers means to use the force with the radial sides of the thumb and index or cushion of the index finger oppositely. The pinching method by the three fingers means to use the force with thumb and two fingers of the index and middle finger oppositely (Figure 3-16). The pinching method by the five fingers means to use the force with the thumb and rest four fingers oppositely (Figure 3-17).

6 捏法

拇指与其他手指相对用力挤压受术部位的手法,称为捏法。

术式

术者以拇指与其他手指指腹相对用力挤压肌肤。有二指捏法、三指捏法、五指捏法等。二指捏法为拇指与示指中节桡侧或示指末节指腹相对用力。三指捏法为拇指与示中二指相对用力(图 3-16)。五指捏法为拇指与其余四指相对用力(图 3-17)。

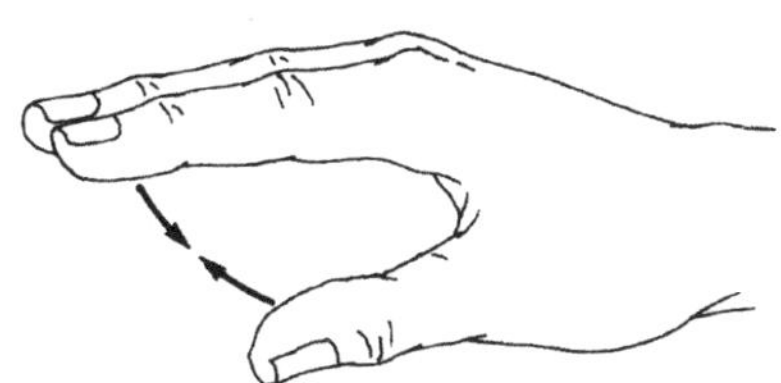

Figure 3-16 Pinching method by three fingers
图 3-16 三指捏法

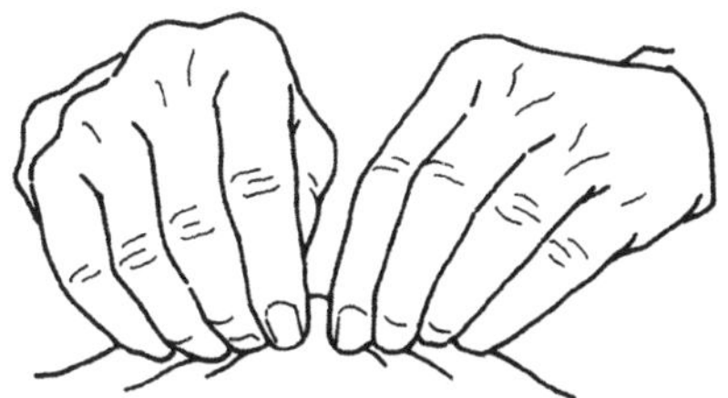

Figure 3-17 Pinching method by five fingers
图 3-17 五指捏法

Explanation

(1) The continuous operation should be rhythmical.

(2) In pinching the soft tissues, it is needed to straighten the interphalnageal joint as much as possible, to increase the contact area of the manual technique, and not to dig and grasp with the tip of the finger.

(3) It is advisable to pinch and migrate toward the vertical axis of the four limbs. If used to promote the reflux of venous blood and lymphatic fluid, it is advisable to migrate concentrically.

(4) If the uplifting movement is combined, it will be evolved into the grasping method.

(5) There is another palm-pinching method by squeezing and pinching the skin and muscles with the palm (palm root, thenar) and the four fingers, mostly used for the upper part of the scapula and four limbs.

(6) To pinch up the skin bilaterally along the spine, in combination of the uplifting movement, is termed "spine-pinching method" traditionally, mostly used for infantile massage therapy.

Application

By mutual assistance of toughness and gentleness, the pinching method can be used on the back, spine, four limbs and nape. It is commonly used to pinch Neiguan (PC 6) and Waiguan (TE 5), pinch Hegu (LI 4), pinch the spine, and sternocladomastoid muscle, and heel tendon, etc.

Appendix Grasping method

It refers to the manual technique to grasp and pinch forcefully with the tips of the five fingers.

The practitioner spreads the five fingers and

说明

(1) 连续操作时要有节律性。

(2) 指捏软组织时，指骨间关节尽量伸直，以增加手法的接触面积，不要用指端抠抓。

(3) 可边挤捏边沿四肢纵轴方向移动。如用于促进静脉血和淋巴液回流，一般向心性移动。

(4) 捏法如果配合上提动作，则演变成拿法。

(5) 还有一种以手掌（掌根、鱼际）与四指相对挤捏肌肤的掌捏法。多用于肩井部（肩胛上部）和四肢。

(6) 捏住脊柱两侧皮肤，并结合上提动作，属于拿法，但传统称为“捏脊法”，多用于小儿推拿。

应用

捏法刚柔相济，可用于背脊、四肢以及颈项部。常用的操作法有捏内外关、捏合谷、捏脊、捏胸锁乳突肌、捏跟腱等。

［附］抓法

以五指指端相对用力抓捏的手法称为抓法。

术者五指张开，指骨间

flexes the interphalangeal joints, contacts the massage area with the tips of the five fingers, and flexes the various interphalangeal joints forcefully to grasp and dig forcefully and oppositely (Figure 3-18). It is commonly used to grasp the five meridians (grasp the vertex).

关节屈曲,以五指指端接触受术部位,各指骨间关节用力屈曲,相对用力抓抠(图 3-18)。常用操作法有抓五经(抓头顶)。

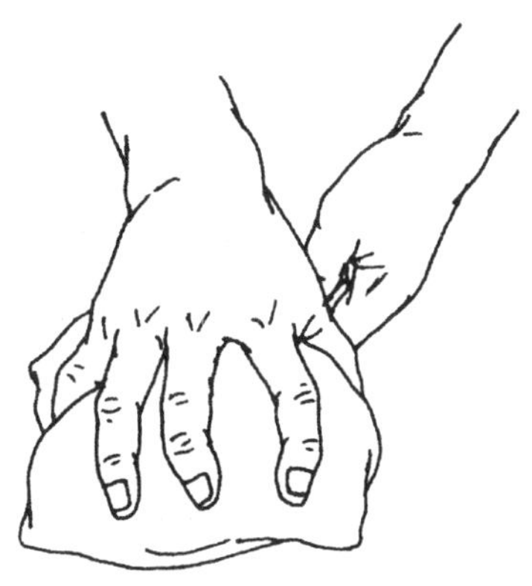

Figure 3-18 Train the grasping method on rice bag
图 3-18 抓法的米袋练习

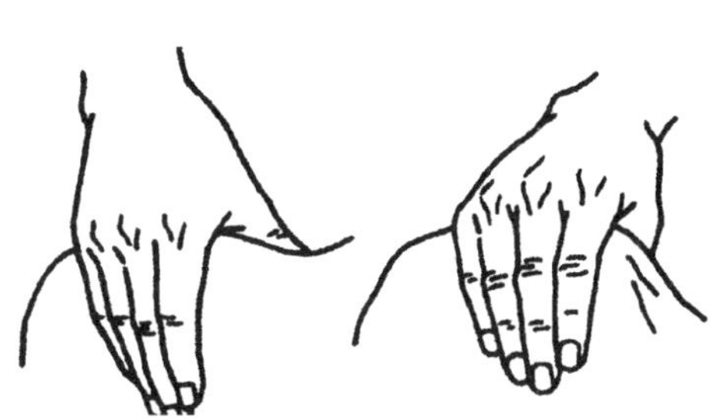

Figure 3-19 Seizing method
图 3-19 拿法

7 Seizing method

It means to pinch and lift up.

Form

With the thumb and cushions of the rest fingers in forceful opposition, the practitioner holds and uplifts the muscles and then slowly put them down repeatedly. The seizing method by the three fingers is supposed to have the thumb cooperated with the index and middle finger. The seizing method by the five fingers is supposed to have the thumb cooperated with the rest four fingers. (Figure 3-19).

Explanation

(1) It is needed to relax the wrist joint, and to be nimble and light in the movements.

7 拿法

捏而提起谓之拿。

术式

术者用拇指与其余手指的指纹面相对用力,夹住肌肉并将其垂直提起,再慢慢放下,反复操作。拇指与示中二指协同操作者称为三指拿法;拇指与其余四指协同操作者称为五指拿法(图 3-19)。

说明

(1) 腕关节要放松,动作灵活而轻巧。

(2) It is needed to straighten the interphalangeal joints to enlarge the contact area, and not to dig and nip with the finger tips and nails by flexing the fingers.

(2) 指骨间关节宜伸直，以加大接触面积。不可屈指用指端、指甲抠掐。

(3) It is needed to have a sending-back movement after uplifting movement, in order to be consistent and gentle in the movements.

(3) 提起后要有回送动作，以使动作连贯而柔和。

(4) It is needed to pinch and send back with increasing force and then decreasing force stably, and not to use the force suddenly or relax suddenly.

(4) 捏拿和回送的操作要由轻到重，再由重到轻，平稳过渡，不可突然用力或突然放松。

(5) It is needed to repeat the lifting and seizing movement for several times, forming a rhythmical operation.

(5) 提拿动作一般重复多次，形成节奏性操作。

(6) It is needed to avoid the protruded bones.

(6) 要避开骨突部位。

(7) It is advisable to operate with the single hand or two hands.

(7) 可单手操作也可双手操作。

Application

应用

The seizing method is a common manual technique clinically, often used on the nape, shoulder, back and four limbs. It is frequently used to seize the nape, sternocladomastoid muscle, the upper part of the trapezius muscle, four limbs, deltoid muscle, the extensor muscles of the forearm, and the poster aspect of the leg, etc.

拿法是推拿临床的常用手法，常用于颈项部、肩背部、四肢部。常用操作法有：拿项部、拿胸锁乳突肌、拿斜方肌上部、拿四肢、拿三角肌、拿前臂伸肌群、拿小腿后部等。

8 Rubbing method

8 搓法

It refers the manual technique to hold and rub the limb back and forth with the two hands.

用双手夹住肢体来回搓动，称为搓法。

Form

术式

The practitioner holds the limb with the palms of the two hands and rubs it back and forth (Figure 3-20)

术者用双手掌面相对夹住肢体，作方向相反的来回搓动(图3-20)。

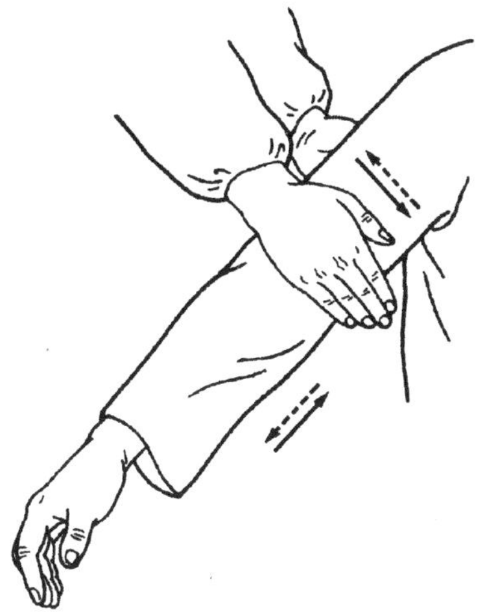

Figure 3-20 Rub the upper limb
图 3-20 搓上肢

Explanation

(1) The frequency is about 200 times per minute.

(2) In the rubbing movment, it is needed to take the subcutaneous tissues and not to make obvious friction with the skin.

(3) It is needed to be light and nimble, and not to hold the limb too tightly.

(4) In rubbing the back and four limbs, it is needed to move the two hands upward and downward along the vertical axis of the body trunk or limb.

(5) In rubbing the upper limb, it is needed to rub fast and migrate slowly, and rub lightly in the elbow joint.

(6) It is needed not to hold up breathing.

(7) If it is combined with the rotating movement, it is termed the rubbing-rotating method, for example, rub and knead the shoulder.

说明

(1) 频率约每分钟 200 次。

(2) 搓动时要求带动皮下组织,不要与皮肤有明显的摩擦。

(3) 动作要轻巧灵活,肢体不可夹得太紧。

(4) 搓背部、四肢时,双手可沿躯干或肢体的纵轴作上下移动。

(5) 搓上肢时,搓动要快,移动要慢,移动到肘关节时用力要轻。

(6) 不可屏气。

(7) 如带有旋转动作,称为搓揉法。如搓揉肩部。

Application

The rubbing method is mainly appropriate for the four limbs. Clinically, it is often used as the auxiliary method or finishing technique. It is commonly used to rub the upper limb, rub and knead the shoulder, rub the part of Jianjing (GB 21), the posterior aspect of the thigh, and rub the leg and hypochondriac part (Figure 3-21), and rub the low back, etc.

应用

搓法主要适用于四肢。临床上常作为辅助手法或结束手法。常用的操作法有搓上肢，搓揉肩部，搓肩井部，搓股后部，搓小腿，搓胁肋部（图 3-21），搓腰背部等。

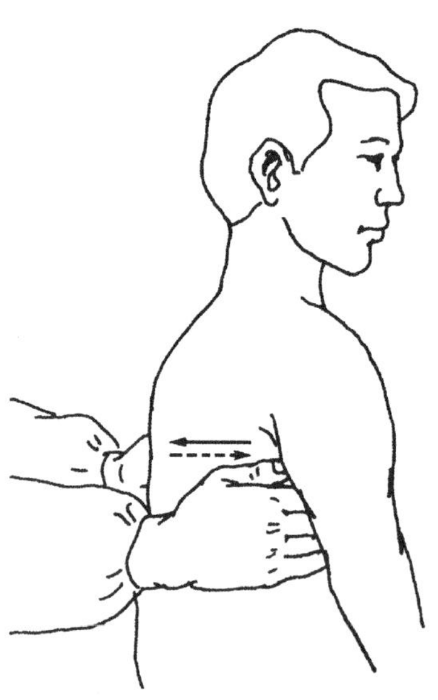

Figure 3-21　Rub the hypochondriac region

图 3-21　搓胁肋

9　Twisting method

It refers to the manual technique to hold and rub the finger or toe of the patient back and forth with the thumb and index finger.

Form

The practitioner holds the finger or toe with the cushion of the thumb and radial side (or cushion of the last finger section) of the middle section of the index finger and rubs back and forth in opposi-

9　捻法

用拇指与示指夹住受术者的手指或脚趾来回搓动，称为捻法。

术式

术者用拇指末节指纹面与示指中节桡侧（或末节指纹面）相对夹住受术者的手指或脚趾，作方向相反的搓

tion (Figure 3-22). It is also advisable to hold and twist the finger or toe with the ulnar side of the index and radial side of the middle finger.

动(图 3-22)。也可用示指尺侧和中指桡侧夹住手指或脚趾捻动。

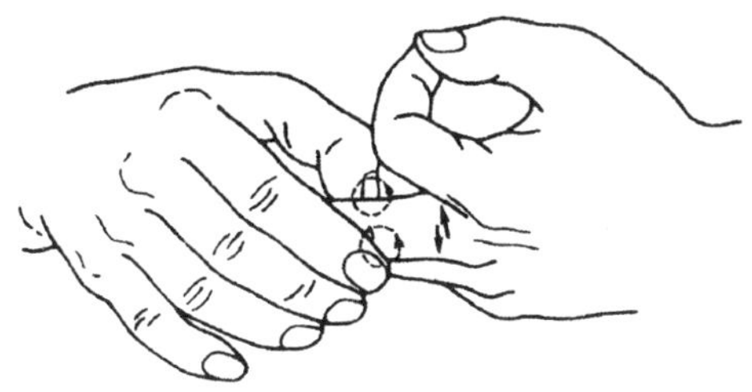

Figure 3-22 Twisting method

图 3-22 捻法

Explanation

(1) The frequency is about 200 times per minute.

(2) It is needed to take the subcutaneous tissues in the twisting method, and not to have obvious friction with the skin.

(3) It is needed to be light and nimble.

(4) In twisting the finger, it is needed to migrate slowly along the vertical axis of the finger to the remote part.

(5) After twisting the finger, it is needed to pull the fingers mostly.

说明

(1) 频率约每分钟 200 次。

(2) 捻法要求带动皮下组织,不要与皮肤有明显的摩擦。

(3) 动作要轻巧灵活。

(4) 捻手指时,可沿手指的纵轴向远端缓慢移动。

(5) 捻手指后,多配合拔伸手指。

Application

To twist the sides of the fingers is mainly to function on the nerve and meridians. To twist the upper and lower side of the fingers is mainly to function on the tendons. To twist the interphalangeal joint of the finger is mainly to function on the articular ligaments. It is often used to twist the finger and twist the toe.

应用

捻手指的侧面主要作用于神经、经络;捻手指的上下面主要作用于肌腱;捻指骨间关节主要作用于关节韧带。常用操作法有捻手指、捻脚趾。

10 Pushing method

It refers to the manual technique to make a

10 推法

在体表作单向直线推动

straight pushing motion in a singular direction. By the different force positions, it can be divided into the thumb-pushing method, palm-pushing method and elbow-pushing method.

的手法，称为推法。根据着力部位的不同可分为拇指推法、掌推法、肘推法等。

Form

术式

10.1 Finger-pushing method

10.1 指推法

(1) Pushing method by the thumb cushion　By spreading the thumb and closing the rest four fingers, make a pushing action of the palm motion on the straight line with the thumb toward the index finger (Figure 3-23).

（1）拇指指腹推法　虎口张开，四指并拢，拇指向示指方向作对掌运动式直线推动（图 3-23）。

(2) Pushing method by the thumb side　By the radial side of the thumb, make a pushing action on the straight line toward the tip of the index finger. It can be operated alternatively with the single hand or two hands.

（2）拇指侧推法　以拇指桡侧缘着力，向示指指尖方向作直线推动。可单手也可双手交替操作。

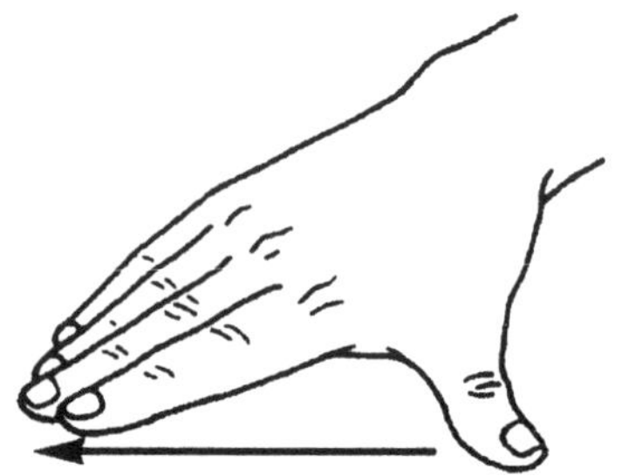

Figure 3-23　Pushing method by thumb cushion
图 3-23　拇指指腹推法

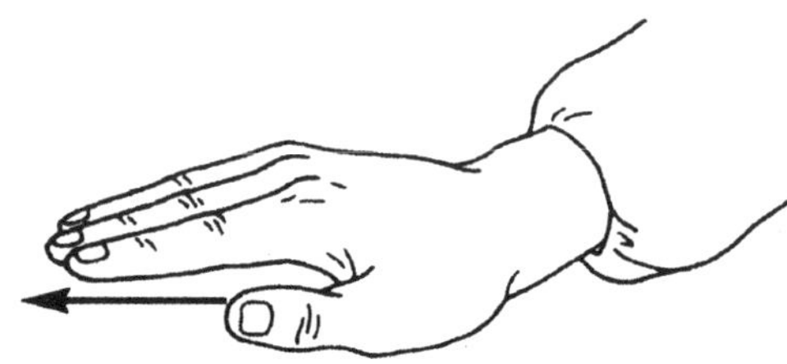

Figure 3-24　Palm-pushing method
图 3-24　掌推法

10.2 Palm-pushing method

10.2 掌推法

By force on the certain part with the palm or palm root, with the palm root as a key point, make a pushing action on the straight line by the extending the elbow (Figure 3-24). The pushing method only by the force from the palm root is termed the palm root-pushing method. The palm-pushing method can be operated with the two hands simultaneously.

术者用手掌或掌根着力于一定的部位上，以掌根为重点，以伸肘的力量为主作直线推动（图 3-24）。仅以掌根着力推动者称为掌根推法。掌推法可双手同时操作。

10.3 Elbow-pushing method

The practitioner flexes the elbow joint to make a pushing action on a straight line, by the force from the upper part of the forearm proximal to the elbow tip, with the movement of the shoulder joint (Figure 3-25).

10.4 Divergent pushing method

By the cushions of the two thumbs or thenar of the two hands, push divergently from the midpoint to the two sides of the massage area, like ← · → (Figure 3-26).

10.3 肘推法

术者肘关节屈曲，用前臂上段近肘尖处着力，以肩关节的运动为主，作直线推动(图 3-25)。

10.4 分推法

用双手拇指的指纹面或双手鱼际等部位，从受术部位的中点向两旁对称分开推动，形如← · →(图 3-26)。

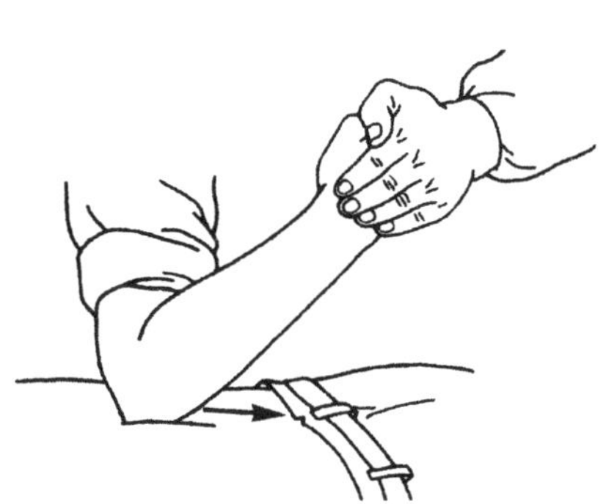

Figure 3-25 Elbow-pushing method
图 3-25 肘推法

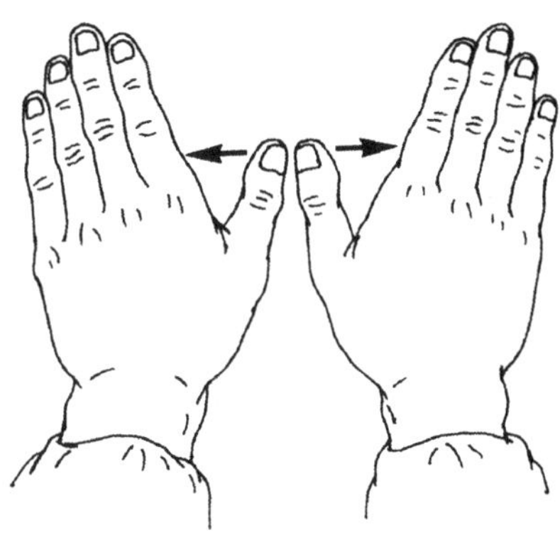

Figure 3-26 Divergent pushing method
图 3-26 分推法

Explanation

(1) It is needed to have a pushing action on a straight line, not tortuous and crooked.

(2) It is needed to adhere to the skin tightly in the whole operation, with even pressure.

(3) It is needed to be fast or slow in the speed of the pushing method. It is necessary to be slow and stable in the palm-pushing method and elbow-pushing method.

(4) The elbow-pushing method is comparatively strong in stimulation and should be selected in accordance with the pathological situation and tolerance of

说明

(1) 推法为直线运动，不可扭曲歪斜。

(2) 要求全程贴实皮肤，压力均匀。

(3) 指推法的速度快慢均可，掌推和肘推法宜慢而平稳。

(4) 肘推法刺激较强，应视病情需要和受术者的耐受性酌情选用，老弱瘦小者慎

the patient and must be used carefully in those with high age, weak constitution and thin body.

用。

(5) The palm-pushing method applied on the four limbs can be centrifugal and concentric, because of different effects. The centrifugal pushing method has the effect to promote the arterial blood to flow to the four limbs. The concentric pushing method has the effect to promote the reflux of venous blood and lymphatic fluid.

(5) 四肢的掌推法的方向可以是离心性的,也可以是向心性的,作用有所不同。离心性的推法有促进动脉血向四肢输送的作用,向心性的推法有促进静脉血和淋巴液回流的作用。

(6) In using powerful force, it is needed to apply a little oily medium on the massage area, in order to be beneficial to the manual operation and avoid skin lesion.

(6) 用力较重时,可在受术部位涂上少许油性介质,以利于手法操作,防止皮肤破损。

Application

应用

The finger-pushing method is appropriate for various parts of the whole body. The palm-pushing method is appropriate for the body parts of large area, such as low back, chest, abdomen and thigh, etc. The elbow-pushing method is mostly used for the low back and posterior aspect of the thigh with thick muscles. The method is commonly used to open Pt. Tianmen, push Pt. Qiaogong (push from Yifeng (TE 17) along the sternocladomatoid muscle to the superclavicular fossa downward with the cushion of the thumb), push the bladder meridian of the low back by the palm, push the four limbs by the palm, and push the bladder meridian of the upper back by the elbow, push the posterior aspect of the thigh by the elbow, and push the trapezius muscle, palm and abdomen divergently, etc.

指推法适用全身各部,掌推法适用于面积较大的部位,如腰背部、胸腹部及大腿部等。肘推法多用于腰背部、股后部等肌肉丰厚处。常用操作法有开天门,推桥弓(用拇指指腹从翳风穴沿着胸锁乳突肌由上而下推至锁骨上窝),掌推腰背部膀胱经,掌推四肢,肘推背部膀胱经,肘推股后部,分推斜方肌,分推掌心,分推腹部等。

11 Chafing method

11 擦法

It refers to the manual technique to make a chafing action on the body surface on a straight line

在体表作单向直线来回摩擦运动的手法,称为擦法。

back and forth in a singular direction. By the different force positions, it can be divided into the hypothenar-chafing method (side-chafing method), thenar-chafing method, palm-chafing method, and finger-chafing method, etc.

根据着力部位的不同，可分为小鱼际擦法（侧擦法）、鱼际擦法、掌擦法、指擦法等。

Form

The practitioner straightens the elbow joint and maintains certain tension, and adheres to the body surface with the force part and presses downward slightly, by the united flexion and extension of the shoulder joint and elbow joint, to take the finger or palm to make a chafing action on the body surface of the massage area on a straight line back and forth. To chafe with the hypothenar forcefully is termed the hypothenar-chafing method (Figure 3-27), also termed the side-chafing method. To chafe with the thenar forcefully is termed the thenar-chafing method (Figure 3-28). To chafe with the whole palm forcefully is termed the palm-chafing method. To chafe with the thumb, middle finger or finger cushions of the index, middle finger and ring finger forcefully is termed the finger-chafing method.

术式

术者腕关节伸直并保持一定的紧张度；着力部位贴附于体表，稍用力下压；以肩关节和肘关节的联合屈伸动作，带动手指或手掌在受术体表作均匀的直线往返摩擦运动。用小鱼际着力摩擦的，称为小鱼际擦法（图 3-27），又称为侧擦法。用鱼际着力摩擦的，称为鱼际擦法（图 3-28）。用全掌着力摩擦的，称为掌擦法。用拇指、中指或示、中、环三指指纹面着力摩擦的，称为指擦法。

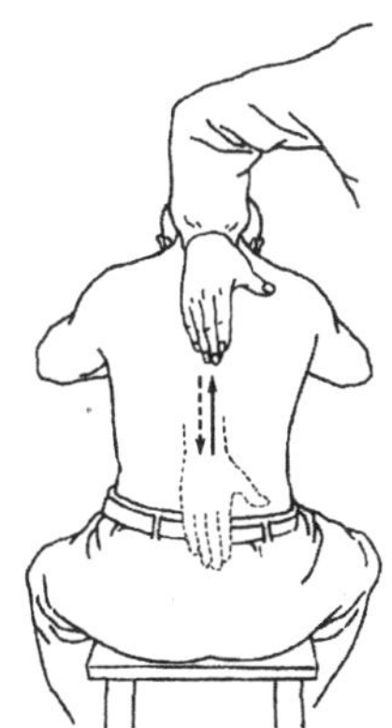

Figure 3-27 Hypothenar-chafing method
图 3-27 小鱼际擦法

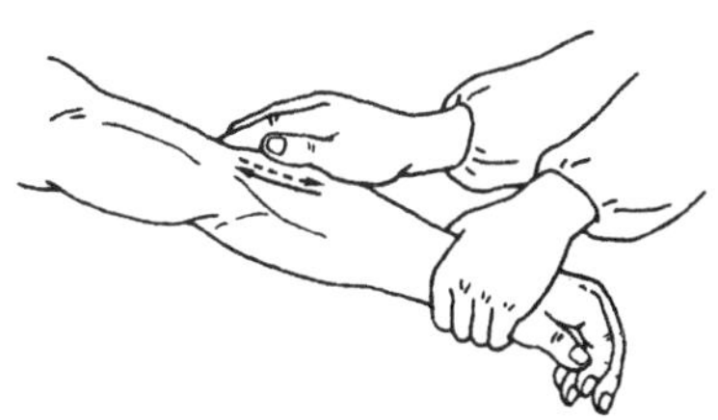

Figure 3-28 Thenar-chafing method
图 3-28 鱼际擦法

Explanation

(1) The frequency is usually 80～120 times per minute. The palm-chafing method is slower and the finger-chafing method is faster.

(2) It is needed to have a chafing action on a straight line, not tortuous and crooked.

(3) It is needed to chafe forcefully both back and forth.

(4) It is needed to lengthen the distance of back-forth operation as much as possible, in order to enhance the velocity within the unit time and increase the heat production.

(5) It is needed to adjust the hand form according to the fluctuation of the body surface, and to have the finger and palm tightly adhered to the body surface, without jumps, and maintain the even pressure in the whole operation.

(6) The amount of force is decided upon the penetration of heat into the skin, without causing skin creases.

(7) It is necessary for the practitioner to breathe naturally and avoid holding up breathing.

(8) The chafing method can be applied on a single layer of clothes or towel. If applied directly on the skin, it is necessary to apply a little sesame oil or evergreen cream on the massage area, in order to help heat penetration and avoid skin lesion.

(9) For the skin already applied with the chafing method, usually it is not advisable to use any other manual techniques, in order to avoid damaging the skin.

(10) It is needed to keep warm in the treatment room, in order to avoid catching cold.

说明

(1) 频率一般为每分钟80～120次。掌擦法较慢，指擦法略快。

(2) 擦法为直线运动，不可扭曲歪斜。

(3) 来回都要用力。

(4) 将往返操作的距离尽可能拉长，可提高单位时间内的运动速度，增加产热量。

(5) 应根据受术体表的起伏形状调整手形，指掌贴实体表，不得跳跃，保持操作全程压力均匀。

(6) 用力大小以热量能渗透而皮肤不起皱褶为度。

(7) 术者自然呼吸，切忌屏气。

(8) 擦法可隔着一层单衣或治疗巾操作，如直接接触皮肤，应先在受术部位涂上少许麻油、冬青膏等润滑介质，既有助于热量深透，也可防止破皮。

(9) 经擦法操作过的皮肤，一般不能在该处再使用其他手法，以免皮肤损伤。

(10) 操作环境应保持温暖，避免着凉。

Application

The chafing method is appropriate for various parts of the whole body. The hypothenar-chafing method is mostly used on the two sides of the spine, upper part of the scapula, and hypochondriac region. The thenar-chafing method is mostly used on the upper limb. The palm-chafing method is appropriate for shoulder and back (Figure 3-29), hypochondriac region (Figure 3-30), chest and abdomen with comparatively larger area and flat part. The finger-chafing method is appropriate for small joints of the four limbs, sterna part and infraclavicular fossa. It is commonly used to chafe the nape, chest, abdomen, back, the bilateral bladder meridian on the back, and hypochondriac region, and chafe Shenshu (BL 23), Mingmen (GV 4), the Governor Vessel, Shangliao (BL 31), Ciliao (BL32), Zhongliao (BL 33), Xialiao (BL 34), Yongquan (KI 1), and for self massage on the lumbosacral region (Figure 3-31) and Yongquan (KI 1) by the palm.

应用

擦法适用于全身各部位。其中小鱼际擦法多用于脊柱两侧、肩胛上部、肋间；鱼际擦法多用于上肢部；掌擦法适用于肩背部（图 3-29）、胁肋部（图 3-30）、胸腹部等面积较大而又较平坦的部位；指擦法适用于四肢小关节及胸骨部、锁骨下窝等处。常用操作法有：擦项部，擦胸部，擦腹部，擦背部，擦背部两侧膀胱经，擦胁肋部，擦肾俞、命门、督脉、八髎、涌泉，以及自我掌擦腰骶部（图 3-31）、涌泉等。

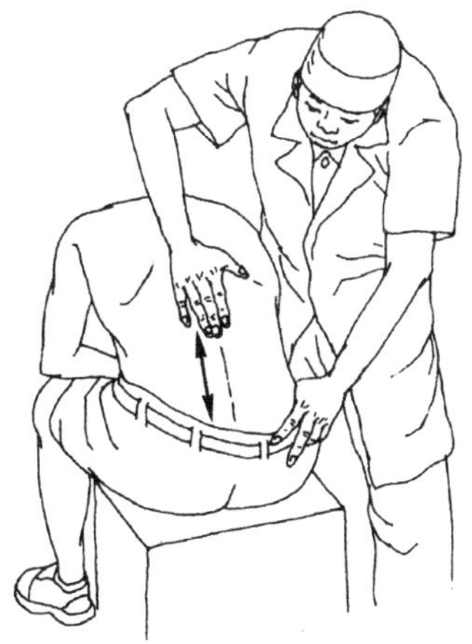

Figure 3-29 Chafe the back by the palm

图 3-29 掌擦背部

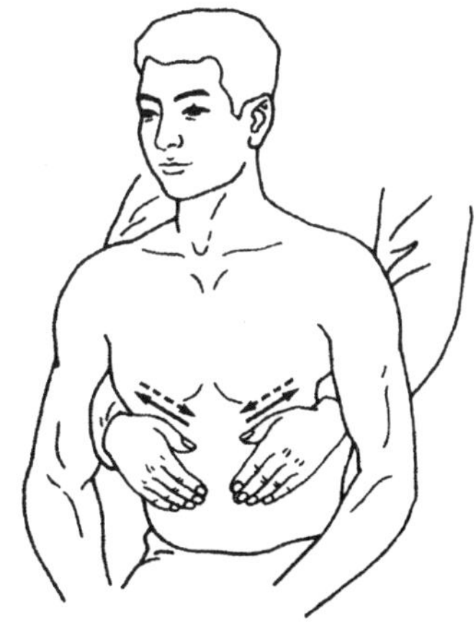

Figure 3-30 Chafe the hypochondriac region by the palm

图 3-30 掌擦胁肋部

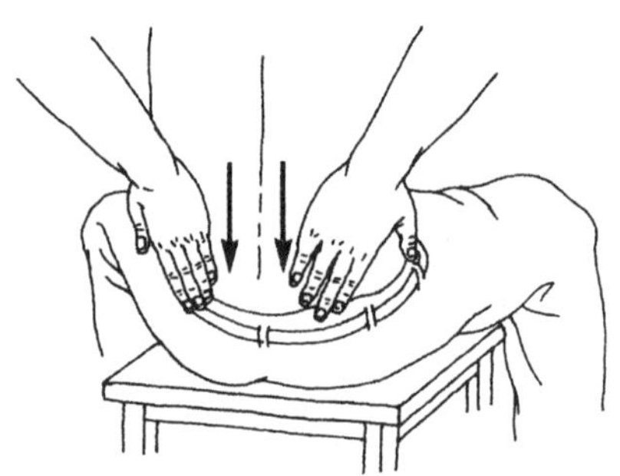

Figure 3-31　Self palm-chafing method on the lumbosacral region

图3-31　自我掌擦腰骶部

12　Wiping method

It refers to the manual technique to push and wipe with the cushion of the thumb or thenar on a straight line or curved line. There are the finger-wiping method and palm-wiping method.

Form

The practitioner adheres to the body surface with the cushion of the thumb or palm, to push and wipe upward and downward, or leftward and rightward in a single direction or back and forth. This method can be operated by the single hand or two hands, and can be moved on a straight line or in a curved migration on the body surface.

Explanation

(1) The wiping method is free in the motion route and can be nimbly applied in accordance with the body surface.

(2) It is needed to be stable and moderate in the wiping method, light without floating tendency and heavy without stagnant tendency.

(3) It is advisable to apply the lubricating medium on the massage area.

Application

The wiping method is gentle and comfortable,

12　抹法

以拇指指纹面或鱼际作直线或弧线推抹，称为抹法。有指抹法和掌抹法两种。

术式

术者用拇指末节指纹面或掌面贴于体表，作上下、左右的单向或往返推抹。可单手操作，也可双手同时操作；可直线移动，也可顺体表形状作弧线移动。

说明

（1）抹法的运动路线比较自由，可根据体表的特点灵活运用。

（2）抹法要求平稳缓和，轻而不浮，重而不滞。

（3）可在操作部位涂以润滑介质。

应用

抹法轻柔舒适，多应用

mostly used on the head, face, chest, abdomen and palm. It is commonly used to wipe the forehead divergently with the thumb (Figure 3-32), the orbit divergently with the thumb, the forehead divergently with the thenar, the intercostal space with the thumb, the palm divergently with the thumb, and wipe the back of the hand divergently with the thenar, etc.

于头面部、胸腹部、手掌部。常用的操作法有:拇指分抹前额(图 3-32),拇指分抹眼眶,鱼际分抹前额,拇指抹肋间,拇指分抹掌心,鱼际分抹手背等。

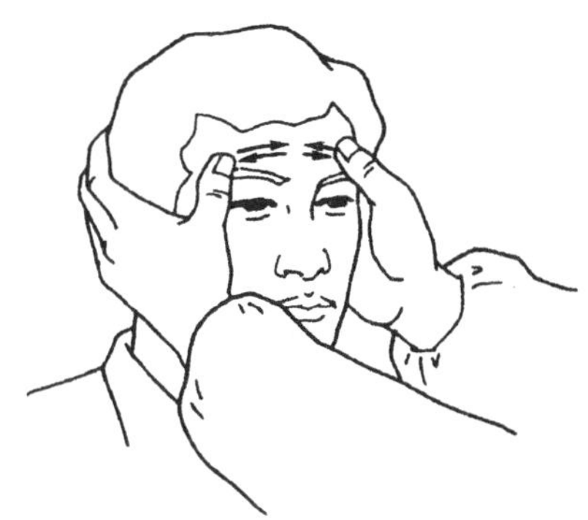

Figure 3-32 Wipe the forehead
图 3-32 抹前额

13 Circular rubbing method

It refers to the manual technique to rub the body surface circularly with the palm or finger. There are the finger-circular rubbing method and palm-circular rubbing method.

13 摩法

用手掌或手指在体表作环形摩擦的手法,称为摩法。有指摩法和掌摩法两种。

Form

The practitioner puts the finger cushion or palm lightly on the massage area or acupoint of the body surface to make a circular and rhythmical rubbing action.

术式

术者用手指指面或手掌面,轻放于体表受术部位或腧穴上,作环形有节律的摩动。

13.1 Finger-circular rubbing method

The practitioner extends and closes the fingers naturally, relaxes and flexes the wrist joint, and touches the body surface with the cushion of the

13.1 指摩法

术者手指自然伸直、并拢,腕关节放松微屈,以中指,或示中二指,或示、中、环

middle finger, or the cushions of the index and middle finger, or the cushions of the index, middle finger and ring finger, to make a circular rubbing action on the body surface by sinking the shoulder, dropping the elbow, with the elbow as a fulcrum, and flexing and extending the forearm slightly, respectively termed the circular rubbing method by the middle finger, the circular rubbing method by the two fingers, and the circular rubbing method by the three fingers (Figure 3-33).

三指末节的指纹面接触体表，沉肩、垂肘，以肘关节为支点，作前臂轻度屈伸，带动手指在体表作环形摩擦，分别称为中指摩法、二指摩法、三指摩法(图 3-33)。

13.2 Palm-circular rubbing method

The practitioner relaxes and extends the wrist joint slightly, with the palm straightened naturally and put on the body surface, to make a circular rubbing action with the palm by the movement of the shoulder and elbow (Figure 3-34)

13.2 掌摩法

术者腕关节放松略背伸，手掌自然伸直，掌心置于体表，以肩肘的运动带动手掌作环旋摩擦(图 3-34)。

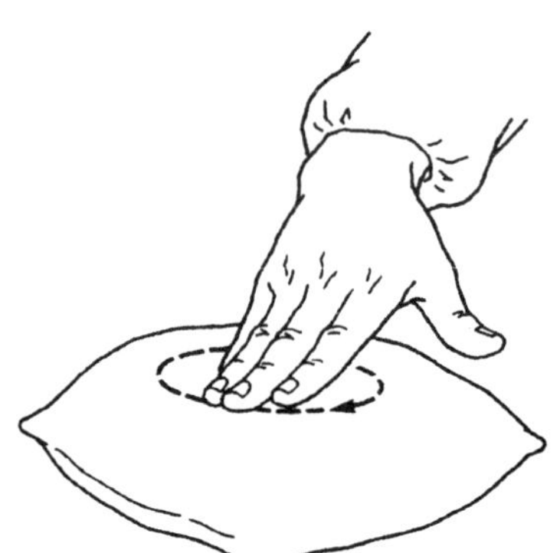

Figure 3-33　Finger-circular rubbing method
图 3-33　指摩法

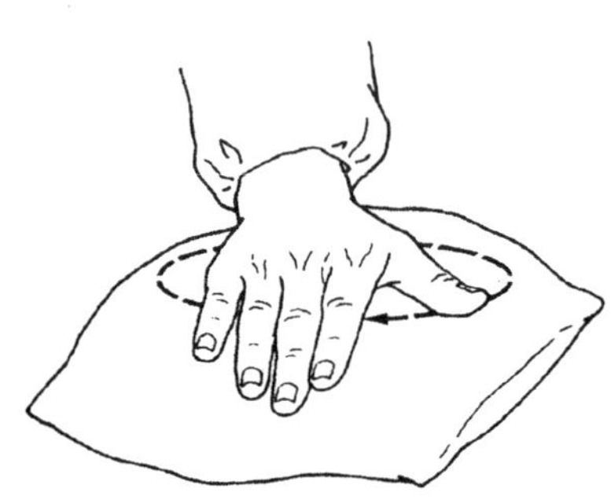

Figure 3-34　Palm-circular rubbing method
图 3-34　掌摩法

Explanation

(1) The frequency is 100～120 times per minute. The palm-circular rubbing method is comparatively slower. The finger-circular rubbing method is slightly faster.

说明

(1) 频率每分钟 100～120 次。掌摩法较慢，指摩法略快。

(2) In doing the circular rubbing method, it is needed to flex and extend the elbow joint in 120°～150°.

(2) 摩法操作时，肘关节的屈伸在120°～150°之间。

(3) If the circular rubbing method is used directly on the skin, it is advisable to apply some lubricating medium on the body surface.

(3) 摩法如直接接触皮肤，可在体表涂以润滑介质。

Application

应用

The circular rubbing method is gentle and comfortable in stimulation, appropriate for various parts of the whole body, mostly used on the abdomen and face. It is often used to circularly rub the abdomen by the palm or three fingers, circularly rub the face by the middle finger or two fingers, circularly rub the chest, hypochondriac region, low back and four limbs by the palm, and circularly rub Yongquan (KI 1) and lower abdomen by the three fingers, or circularly rub Yongquan (KI 1) and Shenshu (BL 23) with the palm by self massage.

摩法刺激柔和舒适，适用于全身各部位，多用于腹部和面部。常用的操作法有：掌摩或三指摩腹，中指摩或二指摩面部，掌摩胸胁、腰背、四肢，三指摩涌泉、丹田，以及自我掌摩涌泉、肾俞等。

If the rubbing method is used together with the herbal paste, it is termed paste rubbing method, the indications of which are related to the pharmaceutical properties of the herbal products.

摩法若与外用中药软膏制剂结合，则称为膏摩法，其主治与摩膏的方药功效有关。

14 Patting method

14 拍法

It refers to the manual technique to pat the body surface with the palm or finger.

用手掌或手指拍打体表的手法，称为拍法。

Form

术式

14.1 Palm-patting method

14.1 掌拍法

The practitioner closes the five fingers, and slightly flexes the metacarpophalangeal joints, with the palm curved into a loose palm and the wrist joint relaxed, to pat the massage area with the palm stably by the flexion and extension of the elbow joint (Figure 3-35)

术者五指并拢，掌指关节微屈，掌心微凹成虚掌，腕关节放松，以肘关节的屈伸发力，使手掌平稳地拍打受术部位(图3-35)。

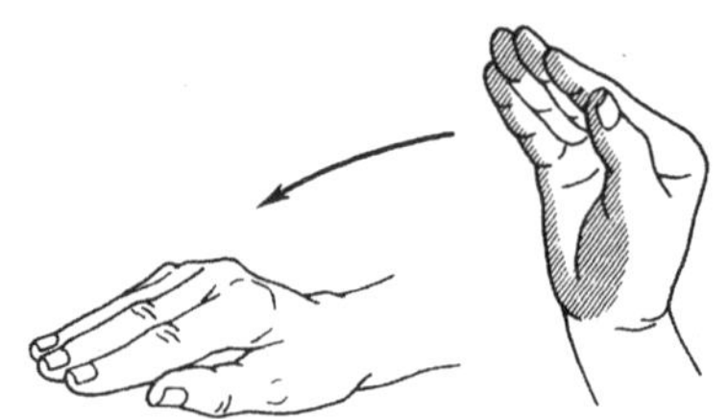

Figure 3-35 Palm-patting method

图 3-35 掌拍法

14.2 Finger-patting method

The practitioner straightens and closes the five fingers to pat the massage area with the finger cushions of middle three fingers lightly and rhythmically by the strength of the forearm.

Explanation

(1) It is needed to pat stably and touch the massage area with finger cushions and palm simultaneously.

(2) It is generally needed to relax the wrist joint and to take the palm with the forearm.

(3) It is needed not to be too large in the movement of the wrist joint, and not to swing the fingers, in order to avoid causing pain in the skin.

(4) It is advisable to pat with the single hand or pat with the two hands in alternation.

(5) The patting method is usually used as the finishing technique for certain body part.

(6) In patting the back with the palm for helping expectoration from the lung, it is necessary to pat upwards and concentrically.

Application

The patting method is appropriate for the shoulder, back, lumbosacral region and lower limbs and is frequently used to pat the upper back with the palm, pat the lumbar region with the two palms, pat the face and sternum with the three fingers.

14.2 指拍法

术者手指伸直并拢，运用前臂力量，以中间三个手指的指腹轻巧有节奏地拍打受术部位。

说明

（1）拍法要求动作平稳，指面和手掌同时接触受术部位。

（2）腕关节一般要求放松，以前臂带动手掌。

（3）腕关节动作不可过大，手指不可甩动，以免受术者表皮疼痛。

（4）可单手操作，也可双手交替拍击。

（5）拍法一般作为某一部位的结束手法。

（6）掌拍背部用于肺部排痰时，要由下而上、由外到内地操作。

应用

拍法适用于肩背部、腰骶部以及下肢等。常用的操作法有掌拍上背部，双手掌拍腰背部，三指拍面部、胸骨部等。

15 Striking method

It refers to the manual technique to strike the body surface with the fist, palm, finger or stick. There are the fist-striking method, the palm-striking method, the finger-striking method, and stick-striking method, etc.

Form

15.1 Fist-striking method

It is advisable to hold a loose fist, with the thumb on the palm heart, and strike the massage area with the lower eye of the fist (hypothenar and ulnar part of the flexed small finger), or heart of the fist (hyperthenar, hypothenar, back of the four fingers) by the active force of the forearm, respectively termed the fist eye-striking method (Figure 3-36) and the fist heart-striking method (Figure 3-37, 3-38). There is another fist back-striking method by the back of the clenched fist (Figure 3-39). In knooking, the wrist joint should be straight, without flexion and extension.

15 击法

用拳、掌、指以及棒状工具叩击体表的手法，称为击法。有拳击法、掌击法、指击法、棒击法等。

术式

15.1 拳击法

手握空拳，拇指置于掌心，腕关节放松，以前臂主动用力，用下拳眼（小鱼际及屈曲的小指尺侧部）或拳心（大鱼际、小鱼际、四指指背）捶打受术部位，分别称为拳眼击法（图 3-36）和拳心击法（图 3-37，3-38）。还有一种以握拳的拳背击打的拳背击法（图 3-39），叩击时腕关节要挺直，不能有屈伸动作。

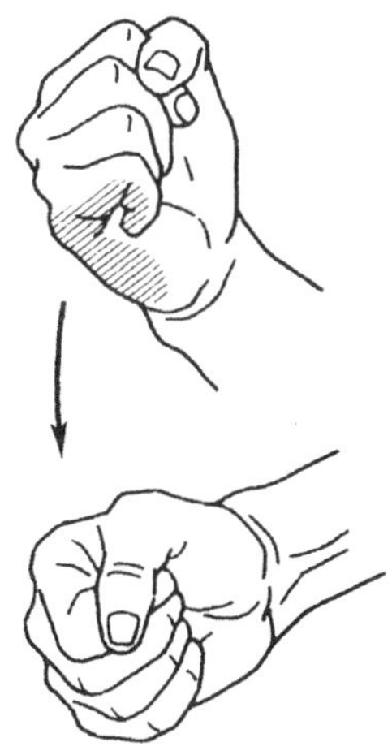

Figure 3-36 The fist eye-striking method
图 3-36 拳眼击法

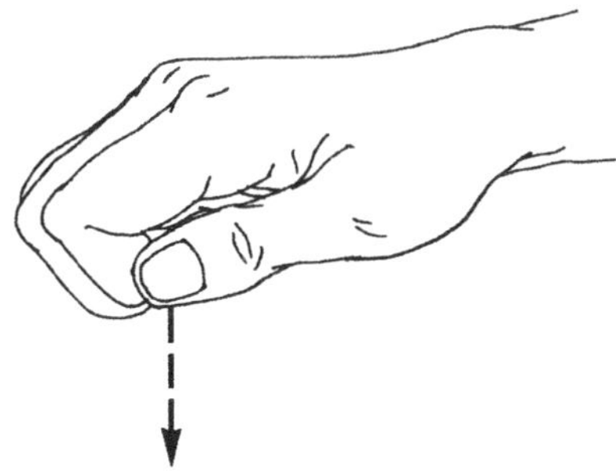

Figure 3-37 The fist heart-striking method
图 3-37 拳心击法

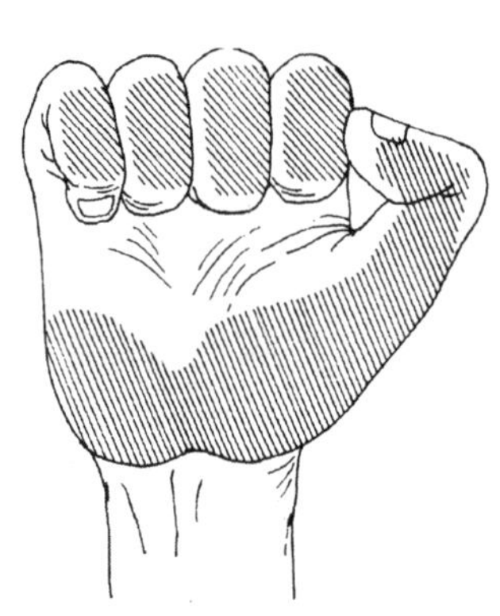

Figure 3-38　The contact part of the fist heart-striking method
图 3-38　拳心击法的接触部位

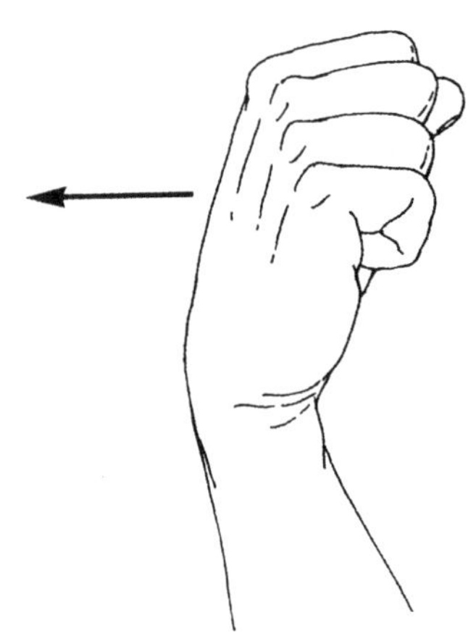

Figure 3-39　The fist back-striking method
图 3-39　拳背击法

15.2　Palm-striking method

The practitioner strikes the massage area with the ulnar side of the palm, palm root or palm center by the strength from the flexion and extension of the elbow joint, respectively termed the palm side-striking method (Figure 3-40), the palm root-striking method (Figure 3-41), and palm center-striking method.

15.2　掌击法

术者运用肘关节屈伸的力量,以手掌尺侧部、掌根或掌心着力,击打受术部位,分别称为掌侧击法(图 3-40)、掌根击法(图 3-41)和掌心击法。

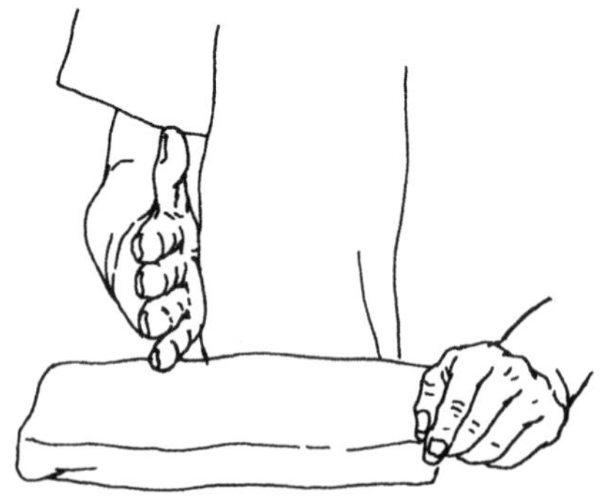

Figure 3-40　The palm side-striking method
图 3-40　掌侧击法

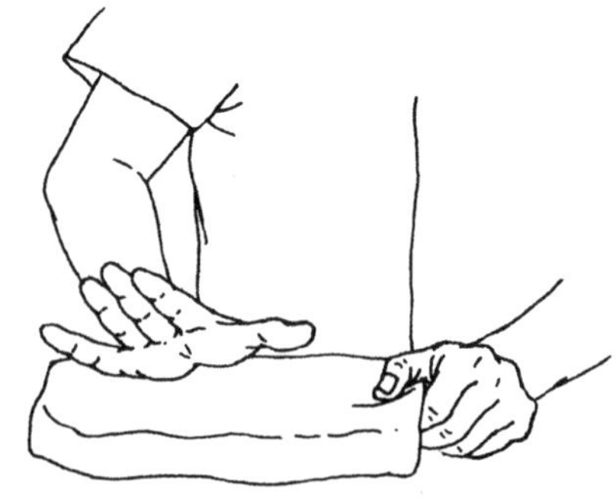

Figure 3-41　The palm root-striking method
图 3-41　掌根击法

It is also advisable to join the two palms to strike with the palm side by the strength from the rotating motion of the forearm, termed the striking method by the joined palms (Figure 3-42).

也可两掌相合，以前臂的旋转运动发力，作掌侧击法，称为合掌击法(图 3-42)。

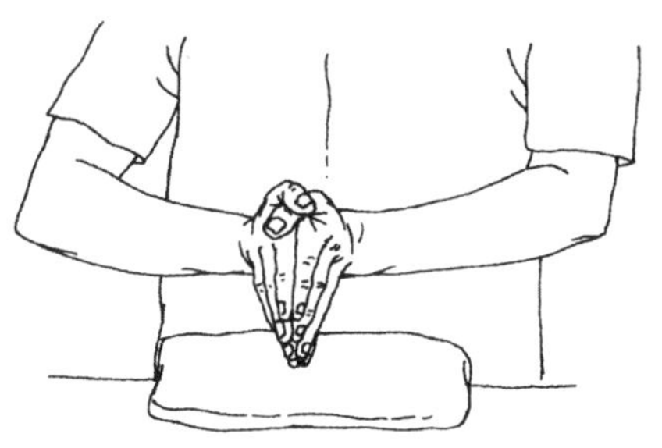

Figure 3-42 The striking method by the joined palms
图 3-42 合掌击法

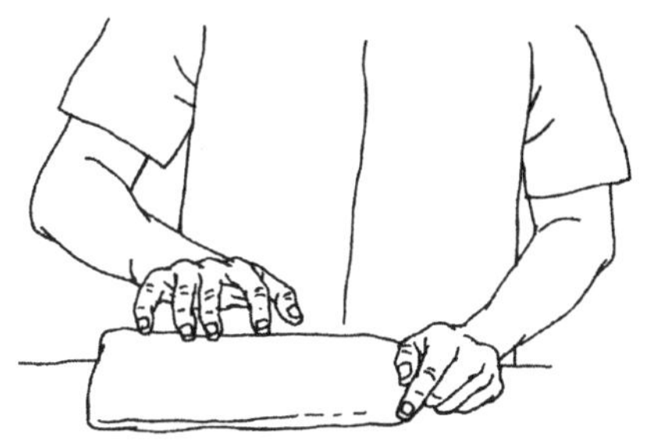

Figure 3-43 The striking method by the fiver finger tips
图 3-43 五指指端击法

15.3 Finger-striking method

The practitioner flexes the finger slightly and spreads the five fingers in a claw form, to strike the massage area with the tips of the five fingers simultaneously by the strength from the flexion and extension of the wrist joint (Figure 3-43).

There is another manual technique with joined palms to strike the massage area with the index and middle finger by the strength from the rotation of the forearm, termed the striking method by the side of two fingers (Figure 3-44).

15.3 指击法

术者手指略弯曲，五指分开成爪形，以腕关节的屈伸发力，五指指端同时叩击受术部位(图 3-43)。

还有一种两掌相合，以前臂的旋转发力，以示中二指叩击受术部位的手法，称为二指侧击法(图 3-44)。

15.4 Stick-striking method

The practitioner holds one end of a specially-made mulberry twig stick to strike the massage area stably with the stick (Figure 3-45).

Explanation

(1) It is needed to avoid the protruded part of the joint in the striking area.

(2) It is needed to be stable in the operation.

15.4 棒击法

术者手握特制的桑枝棒的一端，用棒体平稳击打受术部位(图 3-45)。

说明

(1) 击打部位应避开骨骼关节突起处。

(2) 操作时要平稳。

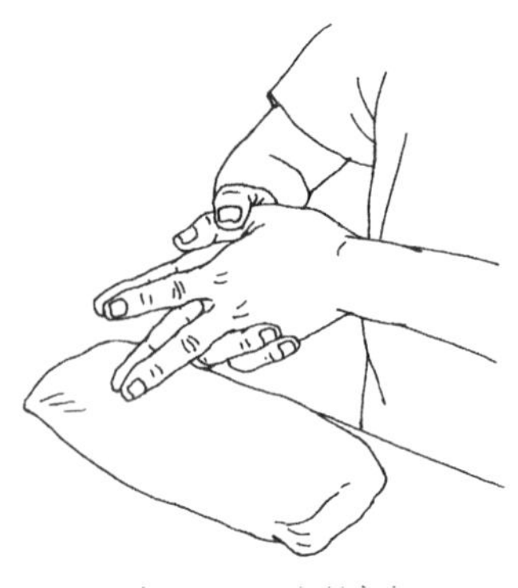

Figure 3-44　The striking method by the side of two fingers
图 3-44　二指侧击法

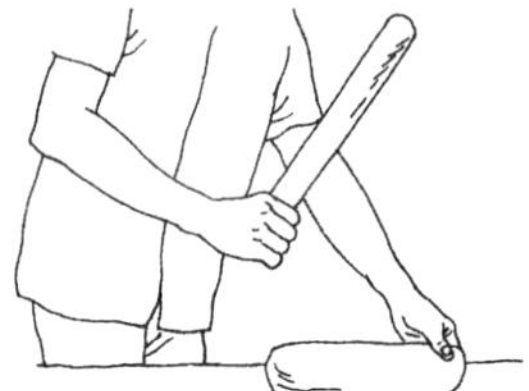
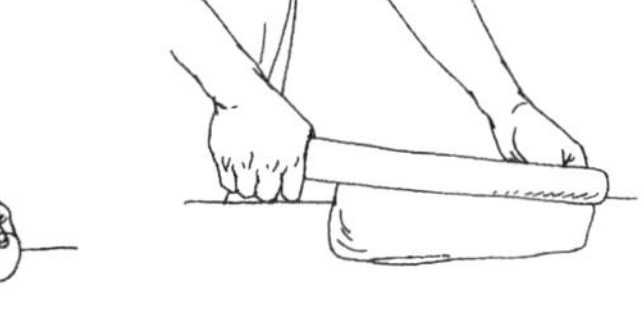

Figure 3-45　The stick-striking method
图 3-45　棒击法

(3) It is advisable to strike with the fist or palm of the single hand or by two hands coordinately.

(3) 拳击和掌击可单手操作,也可双手协同操作。

(4) Before the striking method by the finger tip, it is necessary to cut off the nails, in order to avoid piercing the skin.

(4) 指端击法操作前,指甲应修短,以免刺伤皮肤。

(5) It is needed to have the patient ready, and not to strike suddenly with the fist or stick.

(5) 令受术者作好准备,不施冷拳或冷棒。

(6) In striking with the stick, it is necessary to keep the stick parallel to the limb or muscular direction (except lumbosacral region). It is prohibited to strike the occipital and renal region with the stick. Usually, every part is beat for 3～5 times.

(6) 作棒击时,棒体一般与肢体或肌纤维方向平行(腰骶部除外)。枕部、肾区部位,禁止棒击。一般每个部位击打 3～5 次。

(7) Mulberry twig stick can be made by the following steps: In the hottest days in summer, peel and dry in shadow 12 pieces of mulberry twigs 36～40 cm long and 0.5 cm thick. Firstly, wrap up each mulberry twig with mulberry paper, and then encircle it with cotton thread tightly and densely, and then tighten 12 pieces of the mulberry twigs together and wrap them up with the mulberry paper and tighten it tightly with cotton thread, and finally su-

(7) 桑枝棒可自行制作。方法:在三伏天取长 36～40 厘米,粗 0.5 厘米的嫩桑枝 12 根,去皮阴干。先用桑皮纸(引线纸)包裹每根桑枝,然后用棉线密密环绕一层;将 12 根桑枝合并成一把,再用桑皮纸包裹并用棉线扎紧;最后在外面缝上全棉的

ture it with a cotton cloth externally.

Application

The striking method is mostly used on the shoulder, back and four limbs. It is often used to strike the upper part of the scapula, low back and four limbs by the fist, to strike Dazhui (GV 14) by the back of the fist, to strike the scapular region by the palm root, and to strike Shangliao (BL 31), Ciliao (BL 32), Zhongliao (BL 33) and Xialiao (BL 34) with the back of the fist transversely, and to hit the nape, upper part of the scapular region and vertex with the joined palms, strike the vertex with the five fingers and to strike the forehead with the side of the two fingers, and strike the lower limb with the stick, etc.

布套即可。

应用

击法多应用于肩背、四肢。常用的操作法有：拳击肩胛上部、腰背部、四肢部，拳背击大椎，掌根击肩胛间区，拳背横击八髎，合掌击项部、肩胛上部，五指击头顶，二指侧击前额，棒击下肢等。

16 Vibrating method

It refers to the manual technique to vibrate the massage area quickly with the palm or finger. There are the palm-vibrating method and finger-vibrating method.

Form

16.1 Palm-vibrating method

After the patient takes a sitting or supine position, the practitioner puts the palm naturally and lightly on the massage area and concentrates the mind on the palm, to vibrate quickly and strongly with the arm by the strong and static muscular contraction of the forearm, so as to have the vibration wave function vertically on the massage area via the palm (Figure 3-46).

16.2 Finger-vibrating method

After the patient takes a sitting or supine position, the practitioner puts the tip of the middle fin-

16 振法

以手掌或手指在受术部位作快速振颤的手法，称为振法。有掌振法与指振法两种。

术式

16.1 掌振法

受术者取坐位或卧位，术者将手掌面自然轻放于受术部位，意念集中于掌心，主要靠前臂肌肉作强烈的静止性收缩，使手臂发出快速而强烈的振颤，振动波通过手掌垂直作用于受术部位（图3-46）。

16.2 指振法

受术者取坐位或卧位，术者以中指端轻放于受术部

ger on the massage area lightly, with the flexed index and ring finger holding the middle finger and the mind focused on the tip of the finger, to have a quick and strong vibration in the arm by the strong and static muscular contraction of the forearm and hand, so as to have the vibration wave to transmit to the massage area via the tip of the finger (Figure 3-47). The vibrating method can also be done by piling the index finger on the middle finger.

位,示指和无名指屈曲并夹住中指,意念集中于指端,前臂和手部的肌肉作强烈的静止性收缩,使手臂发出快速而强烈的振颤,使振动波通过指端传递到受术部位(图 3-47)。也可示指叠于中指上作振法。

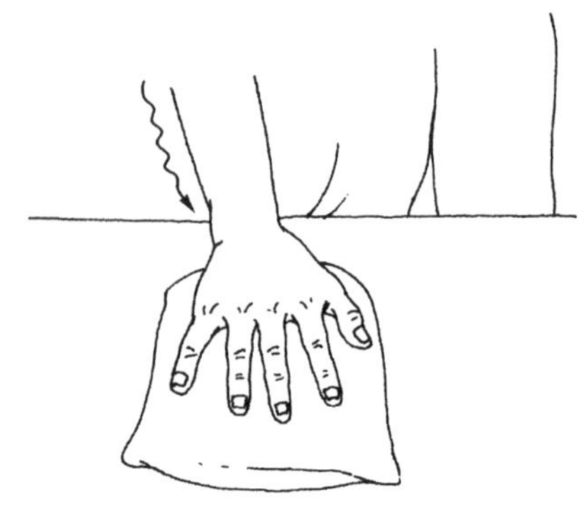

Figure 3-46　The palm-vibrating method
图 3-46　掌振法

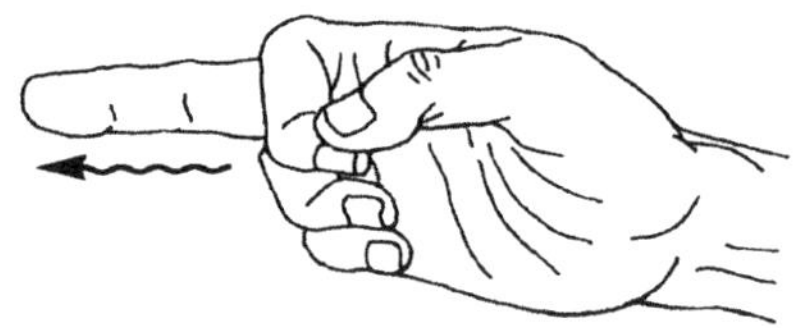

Figure 3-47　The finger-vibrating method
图 3-47　指振法

Explanation

(1) The frequency of the vibration can be as high as 700 times per minute, but is requested to be above 300 times per minute.

(2) It is needed to put the finger or palm on the body surface, and not to press forcefully.

(3) It is needed to focus the concentration on the finger tip or palm center, to breathe naturally and not to hold up breathing.

(4) It is needed to use the force statically in the palm, finger and forearm, i.e. have the muscles of the hand and forearm tensed, without any external active movement in large amplitude.

说明

(1) 振法的频率可高达每分钟 700 次左右,最低要求每分钟 300 次以上。

(2) 指掌部轻置于受术体表,不可用力按压。

(3) 意念集中在指端或掌心,呼吸要自然放松,不可屏气。

(4) 掌、指与前臂须静止性用力,即手部和前臂肌肉绷紧,外观无大幅度的主动运动。

(5) It is needed for the practitioner to keep the flexor muscles and extensor muscles of the upper limb tensed and relaxed in alternation by the repeated flexion and extension of the elbow joint, so as to maintain smooth blood circulation and alleviate fatigue. But, it is necessary to maintain even pressure as much as possible.

(5) 术者可通过肘关节的小幅度反复屈伸,使上肢的屈肌群与伸肌群交替紧张与放松,从而保持血流通畅,以缓解疲劳,但施术压力要尽可能均匀不变。

(6) It is needed to vibrate continuously for over three minutes at least.

(6) 振动应连绵不断,并能持续 3 分钟以上。

Application

应用

The palm-vibrating method is mostly used on the abdomen, back and lumbosacral region. The finger-vibrating method is appropriate for the acupoints of the whole body. It is often used to vibrate the abdomen by the palm, vibrate Shangliao (BL 31), Ciliao (BL 32), Zhongliao (BL 33) and Xialiao (BL 34) and scapular region by the palm, and to vibrate Yintang (Extra) and Yifeng (TE 17) by the finger.

掌振法多用于腹部、背部和腰骶部,指振法适用于全身腧穴。常用的操作法有掌振腹部,掌振八髎和掌振肩胛间区,指振印堂、翳风等。

17 Shaking method

17 抖法

It refers to the manual technique to hold the four limbs of the patient to shake vertically in the small amplitude.

握住受术者的四肢作小幅度的径向抖动,称为抖法。

Form

术式

17.1 Shake the upper limb

17.1 抖上肢

After the patient takes a sitting or supine position, the practitioner holds the wrist or palm of the patient with the two hands or one hand, raise his upper limb slowly forward and laterally about 60°, and shake it slight forcefully and continuously in the small amplitude and high frequency, upward and downward, to transmit the shaking wave upward to the shoulder (Figure 3-48). It can also be shaken by

受术者坐位或仰卧。术者用双手或单手握住受术者的手腕部或手掌部,将其上肢慢慢地向前外侧抬起约 60°,然后稍用力作连续的、小幅度的、频率较高的上下抖动,将抖动波逐渐上传到肩部(图 3-48)。也可单手握手

the single hand transversely. But, it is necessary to transmit the shaking wave gradually to the triceps muscle of the arm (Figure 3-49)

作横向抖动，要求将抖动波逐渐传送到肱三头肌（图 3-49）。

17.2 Shake the lower limb

After the patient takes a supine position, with the lower limb relaxed and straightened, the practitioner stands in front of his feet, holds the ankle of the patient with the two hands, and uplift it and then shake it continuously in the small amplitude upward and downward, to transmit the shaking wave to the quadriceps muscle of the thigh and hip part.

17.2 抖下肢

受术者仰卧位，下肢放松伸直。术者站于其脚后方，用双手握住受术者的踝部，并提起离开床面，然后作连续的、小幅度的上下抖动，使抖动波传送到股四头肌和髋部。

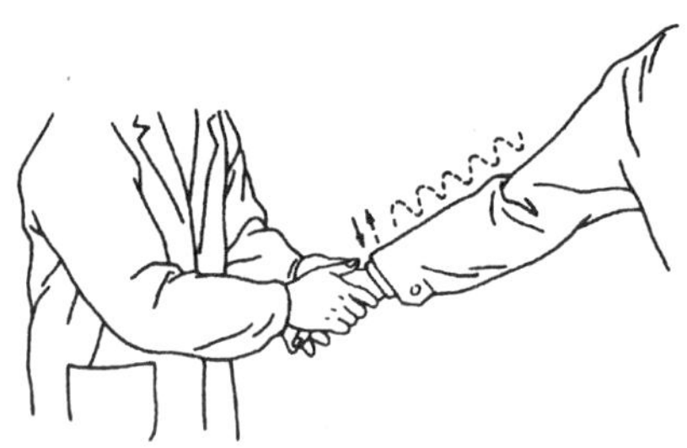

Figure 3-48　Shake the upper limb
图 3-48　抖上肢

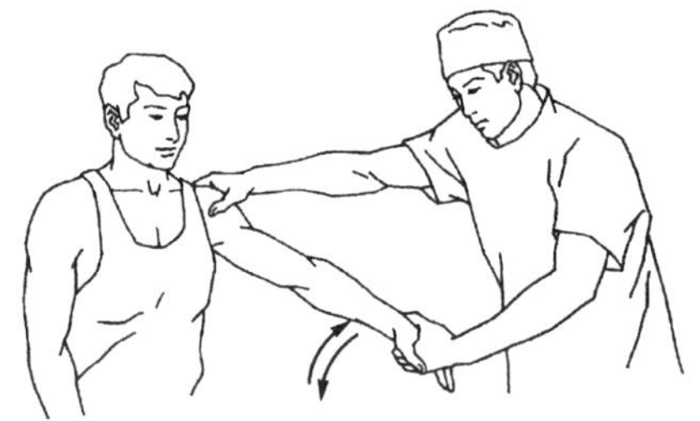

Figure 3-49　Shake the upper limb transversely
图 3-49　横抖上肢

Explanation

(1) The frequency is 200～250 times per minute in shaking the upper limb, and about 100 times per minute in shaking the lower limb.

(2) The patient's limb should be straightened and relaxed naturally.

(3) The amplitude in shaking the upper limb should be controlled in 2～3 cm, and a little bit bigger in shaking the lower limb.

(4) The frequency should be increased.

(5) In the operation, the movement should be continuous.

说明

（1）抖上肢的频率为每分钟 200～250 次，抖下肢的频率为每分钟 100 次左右。

（2）受术者的肢体要自然伸直和放松。

（3）抖上肢的幅度应控制在 2～3 厘米，抖下肢则幅度稍大。

（4）频率要由慢到快。

（5）操作时动作要连续。

(6) It is necessary for the practitioner to breathe naturally and not to hold up breathing.

(7) The four limbs should be shaken after the pulling-stretching method or rubbing method.

(8) The shaking method for the upper limb should be used carefully in the patient with habitual dislocation of the shoulder joint.

Application

The shaking method is mainly appropriate for the four limbs, more frequently for the upper limb. It is usually used as a finishing technique for one body part. It is often used to shake the upper limb, shake the upper limb transversely, and shake the lower limb.

(6) 术者操作时呼吸自然，不可屏气。

(7) 四肢的抖法通常在拔伸法或搓法操作后进行。

(8) 有习惯性肩关节脱位者慎用上肢抖法。

应用

抖法主要适用于四肢，以上肢更为常用。通常作为一个部位的结束手法。常用操作法有抖上肢，横抖上肢，抖下肢等。

18 Pulling-stretching method

It refers to the manual technique to fix one end of the joint or limb and pull and stretch another end along the vertical axis, including the pulling-stretching method for the spine, and joints of the four limbs.

Form

18 拔伸法

拔伸即牵引、拉伸之意。固定关节或肢体的一端而沿纵轴方向牵拉另一端的手法，称为拔伸法。包括脊柱和四肢关节的拔伸方法。

术式

18.1 Pulling-stretching method for the cervical vertebras

(1) The pulling-stretching method by upholding the chin with the hand After the patient takes a sitting position, the practitioner stands behind him, puts the anterior 1/3 of the forearm on the shoulder of the patient, and upholds the two sides of the patient's chin by spreading the hands and holding Fengchi (GB 20) at the occipital bone with the thumbs and other four fingers of the two hands, and then, by his shoulder as a fulcrum, presses downward with the elbow and upholds with the two

18.1 颈椎拔伸法

(1) 虎口托颌拔伸法

受术者坐位。术者站于其后，前臂前 1/3 处搁于受术者肩部，虎口张开，双手拇指抵于枕骨的风池处，其余手指托受术者下颌骨两侧，然后以其肩部为支点，操作者肘部下压，双手上托，将颈部向上牵拉 1～2 分钟（图 3-50）。

hands to pull the neck upwards for 1～2 minutes (Figure 3-50).

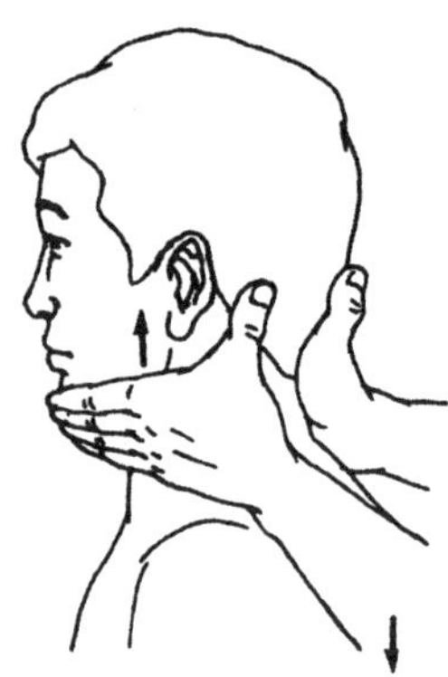

Figure 3-50　The pulling-stretching method for the cervical vertebras (1)
图 3-50　颈椎拔伸法(1)

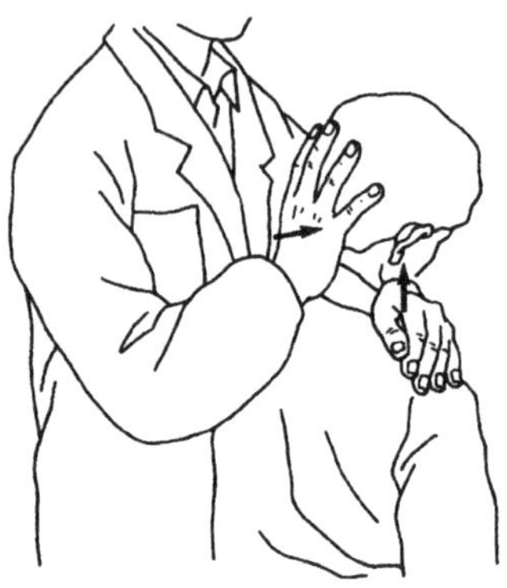

Figure 3-51　The pulling-stretching method for the cervical vertebras (2)
图 3-51　颈椎拔伸法(2)

(2) The pulling-stretching method by the elbow upholding　After the patient takes a sitting position, with the head in the middle position or bending slightly forward, the practitioner stands behind or at the side of the patient, upholds the patient's chin with the elbow after putting one hand on his opposite shoulder in front of his neck, and pushes the patient's occipital part forward with the palm root of another hand, to pulls upward with the two hands in coordination and extend the cervical vertebras for 1～2 minutes (Figure 3-51).

(2) 肘托拔伸法　受术者坐位,头呈中立位或稍前倾位。术者站于受术者后方或侧方,一手从颈前部穿过并搭在对侧肩上,用肘窝部托住受术者的下颏部,另一手掌根将受术者枕部向前推,双手协同向上牵拉,拔伸颈椎 1～2 分钟(图 3-51)。

(3) The pulling-stretching method by the palm upholding　After the patient takes a sitting position, with the head in the middle position or bending slightly forward, the practitioner stands at the side of the patient, upholds the patient's chin with one palm, and holds the patient's occipital part with another palm, to gradually pull and extend the cervical vertebras upward for 1～2 minutes (Figure 3-52).

(3) 掌托拔伸法　受术者坐位,头部呈中立位或稍前倾位。术者站于受术者侧面,一手掌心向上托住受术者下颏部,一手用手掌或张开的虎口住托枕部,然后逐渐运劲向上拔伸颈椎 1～2 分钟(图 3-52)。

(4) The pulling-stretching method in the supine position After the patient takes a supine position, the practitioner stands behind his head, upholds his occipital part with one hand and holds his chin with another hand, and then leans backward with the upper body, and pulls the cervical vertebras continuously with the slow strength of the two hands simultaneously for 1～2 minutes (Figure 3-53).

（4）仰卧拔伸法 受术者取仰卧位。术者位于其头后方，一手托其枕部，另一手钩住其下颏部，然后上身后倾，两手同时缓缓运劲，持续牵拉颈椎 1～2 分钟（图 3-53）。

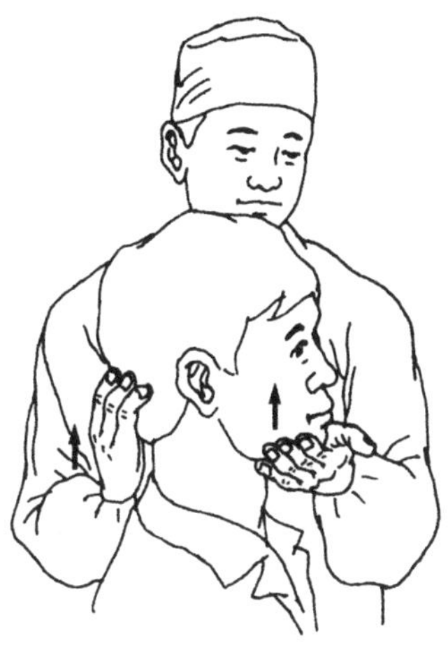

Figure 3-52 The pulling-stretching method for the cervical vertebras (1)
图 3-52 颈椎拔伸法(1)

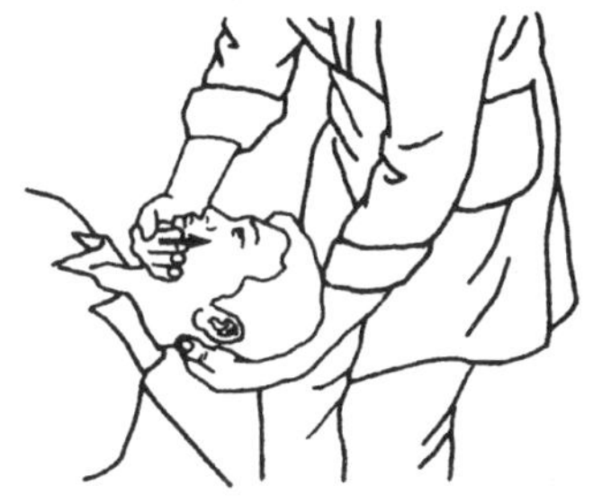

Figure 3-53 The pulling-stretching method for the cervical vertebras (2)
图 3-53 颈椎拔伸法(2)

18.2 Pulling-stretching method for the lumbar vertebras

After the patient takes a prone position, grabbing the bed sides next to the head with the two hands (or the assistant seizes the two armpits of the patient to pull in opposite direction), the practitioner stands in front of his feet, straightens the two arms, and holds and raises his two ankles respectively with the two hands, with an angle of 20° between the leg and bed and the knees slightly away from the bed, and then pulls the lower limbs of the

18.2 腰椎拔伸法

受术者俯卧位，双手抓住头端床沿（或助手抓住受术者两腋部对抗牵拉）。术者站于其足后，两臂伸直，双手分别握住两踝部抬起，使小腿与床面约成 20°，膝部微微抬离床面，然后身体后倾，利用足蹬（或膝顶）和躯干腰背肌力量，将受术者下肢向

patient backward with the strength by leaning backward, stamping the ground (or poking with the knee) and from the muscles of the body trunk and low back, continuously for 1～2 minutes (Figure 3-54). In order to decrease the intensity of the operation, it is advisable to wrap up the patient's ankles with the towel and to grab the towel and pull and extend. The practitioner can also hold the patient's two ankles with the two armpits to pull and extend.

远端牵拉，持续 1～2 分钟(图 3-54)。为减轻操作强度，也可用毛巾或治疗巾缚住受术者双踝，术者抓住毛巾拔伸。术者也可以两腋夹住受术者两足踝部拔伸。

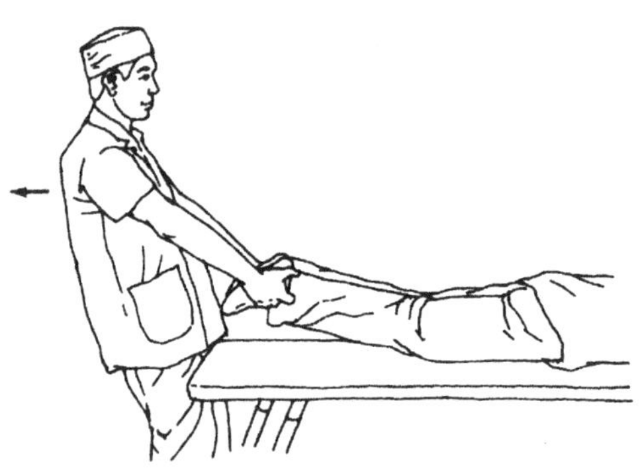

Figure 3-54 The pulling-stretching method for the lumbar vertebras
图 3-54 腰椎拔伸法

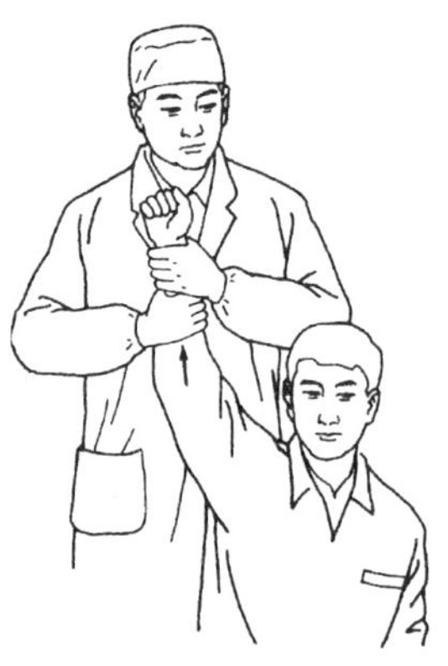

Figure 3-55 The pulling-stretching method for the shoulder (1)
图 3-55 肩部拔伸法(1)

18.3 Pulling-stretching method for the shoulder

(1) The pulling-stretching method by upholding the shoulder After the patient takes a sitting position in a low stool, the practitioner stands behind and lateral to the patient, holds his wrist with the two hands and upholds it slowly upward to its utmost, to maintain the shoulder in an upward continuous traction for a while (Figure 3-55). If the stool is comparatively high, the practitioner can hold the lower part of the patient's upper arm with the two hands to pull and extend (Figure 3-56).

18.3 肩部拔伸法

(1) 肩上举拔伸法 受术者坐于低凳上。术者站于其侧后方，双手握住其腕部，慢慢向上作上举运动至最大限度停止，使肩部保持向上持续性牵拉，停留片刻(图 3-55)。如凳子较高，术者可双手握住上臂下段近肘部拔伸(图 3-56)。

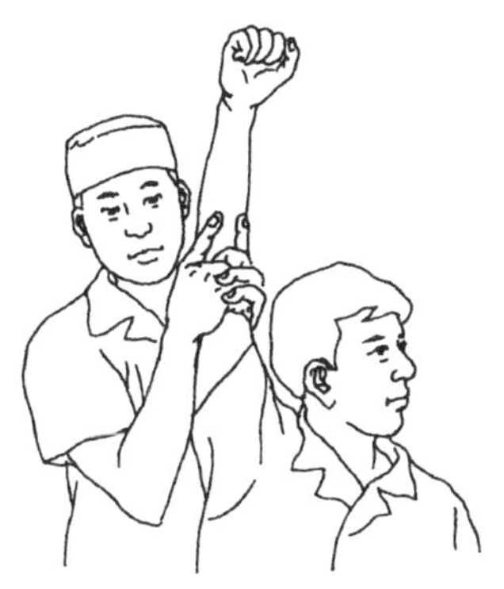

Figure 3-56 The pulling-stretching method for the shoulder (2)
图 3-56 肩部拔伸法(2)

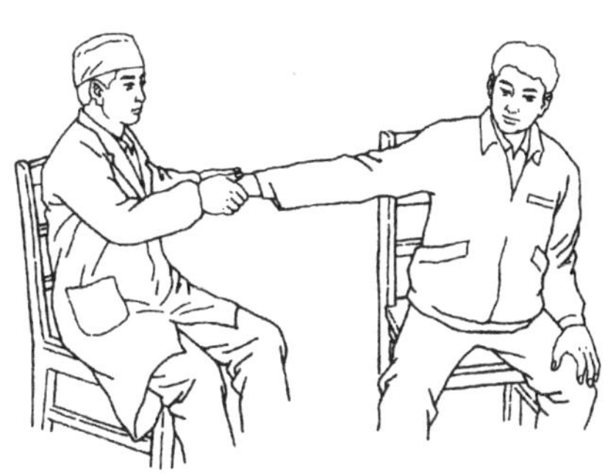

Figure 3-57 The pulling-stretching method for the shoulder (3)
图 3-57 肩部拔伸法(3)

(2) The pulling-stretching method by abducing the shoulder After the patients takes a sitting position, the practitioner holds the patient's wrist or upper part of the his forearm with the two hands respectively, to stretch his shoulder outward for 60° and pull gradually and forcefully, and at the same time tells the patient to lean to the opposite side (or the assistant helps to fix his body), for resisting the pulling-stretching power, continuously for 1～2 minutes (Figure 3-57).

(2) 肩外展对抗拔伸法

受术者坐位。术者双手分别握住其腕部或前臂上段，肩关节外展 60°，逐渐用力牵拉，同时嘱其身体向对侧倾斜(或由助手协助固定其身体)，以与拔伸之力相对抗，持续拔伸 1～2 分钟(图 3-57)。

18.4 Pulling-stretching method for the wrist joint

The practitioner stands face to face with the patient, holds the middle section of his forearm with one hand, and holds his palm with another hand, to pull and stretch his wrist in the opposition direction by the two hands simultaneously, gradually and forcefully (Figure 3-58).

18.4 腕关节拔伸法

术者与受术者相对。以一手握住其前臂中段，另一手握其手掌部，两手同时逐渐用力向相反方向拔伸腕部(图 3-58)。

18.5 Pulling-stretching method for the fingers

The practitioner holds the patient's wrist or palm with one hand, and holds his fingers with another hand, to pull and stretch the metacarpopha-

18.5 手指拔伸法

术者一手握住受术者腕部或手掌，另一手捏住受术者手指，两手同时向相反方

langeal joints in the opposite direction by the two hands simultaneously (Figure 3-59), or grab the proximal phalanges with one hand and grab the distal phalanges with another hand, to pull and stretch the interphalangeal joints in the opposite direction by the two hands simultaneously.

向用力，拔伸掌指关节（图3-59），或者一手捏住手指近端指骨，另一手捏住同一手指的远端指骨，两手同时向相反方向用力，拔伸指骨间关节。

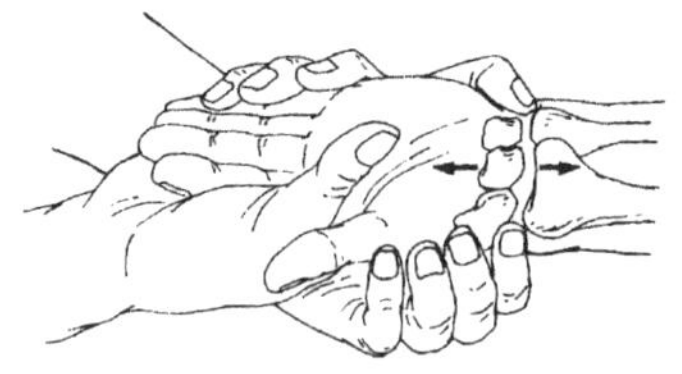

Figure 3-58　The pulling-stretching method for the wrist joint

图 3-58　腕关节拔伸法

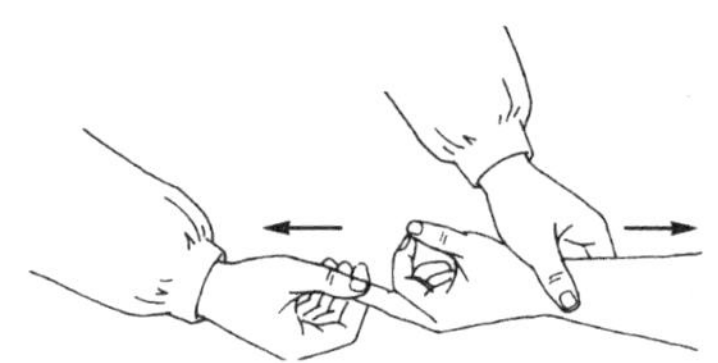

Figure 3-59　The pulling-stretching method for the fingers

图 3-59　手指拔伸法

18.6　Pulling-stretching method for the hip joint

After the patient takes a supine position, with a soft pillow at this perineum, the practitioner holds his ankle of one leg with the two hands, steps on the soft pillow at the patient's perineum with another foot, and then leans backward in the upper body and pulls the lower limb forcefully with the two hands for 1～2 minutes (Figure 3-60). The pulling and stretching power of this method can function on the hip joint and also on the sacroiliac joint.

18.6　髋关节拔伸法

受术者仰卧位，会阴部垫一软枕。术者双手握住其一腿的踝部，一足底置于受术者会阴部的软枕上，然后上身后仰，双手用力将下肢向远端牵引1～2分钟(图3-60)。此法的拔伸力主要作用于髋关节，也作用到骶髂关节。

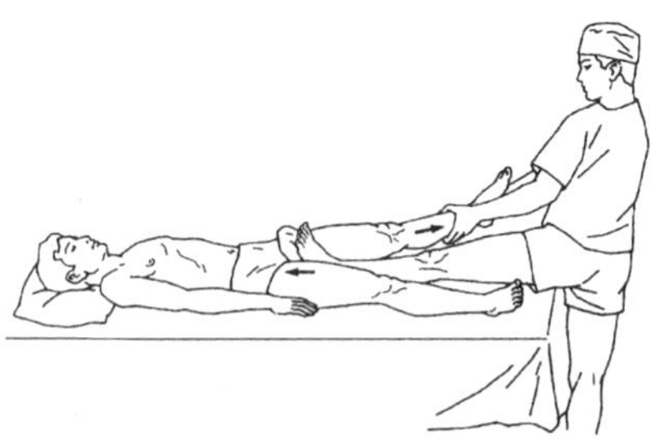

Figure 3-60　The pulling-stretching method for the hip joint

图 3-60　髋关节拔伸法

18.7 Pulling-stretching method for the knee joint

After the patient takes a prone position, with the knees flexed in 90°, the practitioner stands at one side, and presses his posterior aspect of the thigh near the popliteal fossa with the knee (or asks the assistant to press), and holds his ankle with the two hands, to pull and stretch his knee joint upward.

Another method: After the patient takes a supine position, with the lower limb naturally straightened, the practitioner holds his ankle joint of one leg, to pull and stretch continuously along the direction of the vertical axis (Figure 3-61). In the operation, it is also advisable to resist the patient's the sole of another lower limb with the knee. This method can be used to pull and stretch the hip joint and knee joint at the same time.

18.8 Pulling-stretching method for the ankle joint

After the patient takes a supine position, the practitioner holds his heel with one hand, and holds the foot side or toes with anther hand, to pull forcefully and gradually with the two hands simultaneously (Figure 3-62)

18.7 膝关节拔伸法

受术者俯卧位，屈膝90°。术者站于一侧，用膝部压住其股后部近腘窝部（或请助手按压），双手握住其踝部，向上拔伸膝关节。

一法：受术者仰卧位，下肢自然伸直。术者双手握住一侧下肢的踝关节部，沿下肢的纵轴方向持续拔伸（图3-61）。也可在操作时用膝部顶住受术者另一侧下肢的足底。此法可同时拔伸髋关节、膝关节。

18.8 踝关节拔伸法

受术者仰卧，术者用一手托住其足跟，另一手握住脚掌侧面或脚趾，两手同时用力，逐渐牵拉（图3-62）。

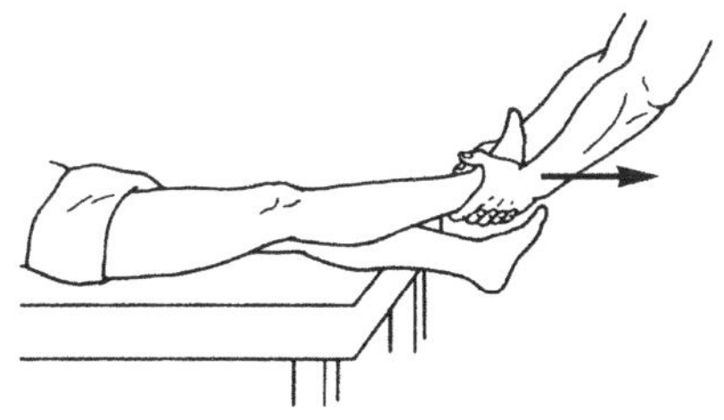

Figure 3-61 The pulling-stretching method for the knee joint
图3-61 膝关节拔伸法

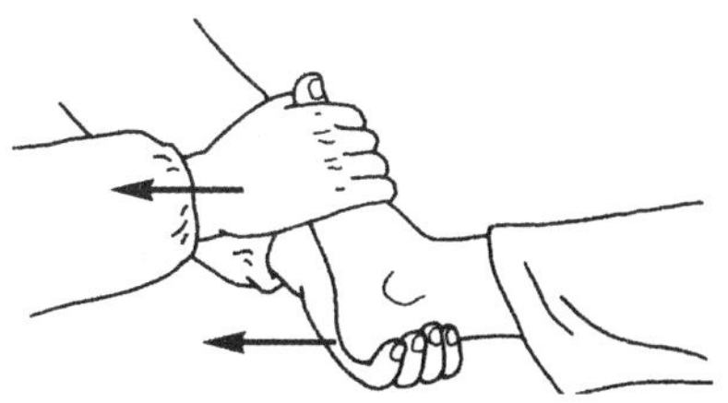

Figure 3-62 The pulling-stretching method for the ankle joint
图3-62 踝关节拔伸法

Explanation

(1) It is needed to control the pulling power and direction in accordance with the different positions and symptoms. For instance, in pulling and stretching the cervical vertebras, the head should be maintained in the middle position or leaning forward a little bit, not backward.

(2) In accordance with the different positions and therapeutic purposes, it is needed to maintain enough pulling and stretching time, usually 1～2 minutes.

(3) It is needed to use the strength continuously and stably. No satisfactory therapeutic effect can be achieved by intermittent pulling power.

(4) It is needed not to use awkward force, and not to pull with sudden force.

(5) It is needed to breathe naturally, and not to hold up breathing.

(6) It is needed to use the strength from the big group of muscles, in order to reduce fatigue and avoid strain. For instance, in pulling and stretching the low back, it is needed to straighten the elbow joint, by leaning backward in the upper body and stamping with the lower limb, not just to pull and stretch only by flexing the biceps muscle of the arm.

(7) Before pulling and stretching the cervical and lumbar vertebras, it is needed to relax the local soft tissues by massage first.

Application

The pulling-stretching method is appropriate for the cervical vertebras, lumbar vertebras and joints of the four limbs. It is frequently used to pull and stretch the cervical vertebras and lumbar vertebras, pull and stretch the shoulder joint, fingers,

说明

（1）要根据不同的部位和症状，控制拔伸力量和方向。如拔伸颈椎时，头部要保持中立位或略前倾位，不要后仰。

（2）根据不同的部位和治疗要求，维持足够的拔伸时间，通常需要1～2分钟。

（3）持续平稳用力。时断时续的拔伸力难以取得满意的疗效。

（4）不可使用蛮力，一般不要瞬间发力牵拉。

（5）自然呼吸，不可屏气。

（6）尽量运用大肌肉群用力，以减轻疲劳，避免劳损。如拔伸腰部时术者的肘关节应尽量伸直，靠上身后倾和下肢的蹬力操作，不可以肱二头肌屈曲用力为主拔伸。

（7）颈椎、腰椎等部位拔伸前，应该先推拿放松局部软组织。

应用

拔伸法适用于颈椎、腰椎，以及四肢关节。常用操作法有拔伸颈椎，拔伸腰椎，拔伸肩关节，拔伸手指，拔伸髋关节，拔伸踝关节等。

hip joint and ankle joint, etc.

19 Rotating method

It refers to the manual technique to make a rotating motion of the joint along the direction of the motor axis.

Form

19.1 Rotating method for the cervical vertebras

One method: After the patient takes a sitting position, with the neck relaxed and flexed forward a little bit, the practitioner holds his occipital part with one hand, and holds his chin with another hand, to shake his head circularly to rotate his cervical vertebras (Figure 3-63).

Another method: The practitioner upholds the patient's occipital part with the hand holding his occipital part, and holds his chin with another hand (please refer to the pulling-stretching method for the cervical vertebras), to rotate the cervical vertebras by maintaining an upward pulling state (Figure 3-64).

19 摇法

将关节沿其运动轴的方向作环转运动的手法，称为摇法。

术式

19.1 颈椎摇法

一法：受术者坐位，颈项放松，略前屈。操作者用一手扶住其顶枕部，另一手托住下颏，双手协同，环转摇动受术者头部，带动颈椎摇转（图 3-63）。

一法：扶住其顶枕部的手可以托住受术者的枕项部，另一手托住其下颏部（参见颈椎掌托拔伸法），在保持一定向上牵引力的状态下作颈椎摇法（图 3-64）。

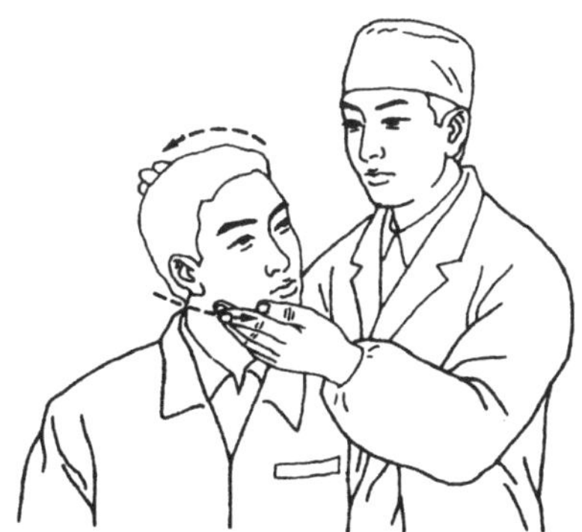

Figure 3-63 The rotating method for the cervical vertebras (1)

图 3-63 颈椎摇法(1)

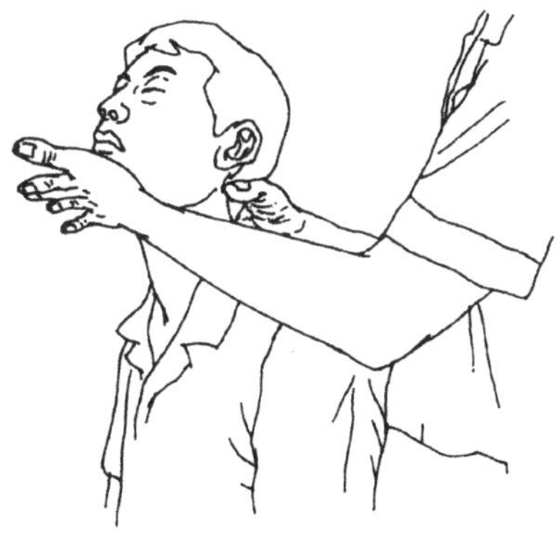

Figure 3-64 The rotating method for the cervical vertebras (2)

图 3-64 颈椎摇法(2)

19.2 Rotating method for the lumbar vertebras

(1) The rotating method for the lumbar vertebras in the sitting position After the patient takes a sitting position, with the ten fingers of the two hands crossed and holding the occipital part, the practitioner sits or stands behind and lateral to the patient, presses his lumbar region with one hand, and holds his nape with another hand underneath his armpit, to slowly rotate his low back by the two hands in coordination (Figure 3-65).

(2) The rotating method for the lumbar vertebras in the supine position After the patient takes a supine position, with the knee and hip flexed and two knees closed, the practitioner presses his two knees with one hand, and holds the lower part of his two legs with the other hand, to make a rotating motion in the two lower limbs to take the patient's pelvic and lumbar vertebras for a rotating motion (Figure 3-66).

19.2 腰椎摇法

(1) 坐位腰椎摇法 受术者坐位，双手十指交叉相扣勾住枕项部。术者坐或站于其侧后方，一手按住其腰部，另一手从受术者腋下穿过扣住其项部，两手协同用力，缓缓摇转其腰部(图 3-65)。

(2) 仰卧位腰椎摇法 受术者仰卧，屈膝屈髋，双膝并拢。操作者一手按其两膝部，另一手托两小腿下端，作两下肢环转摇动，带动受术者骨盆与腰椎产生环转运动(图 3-66)。

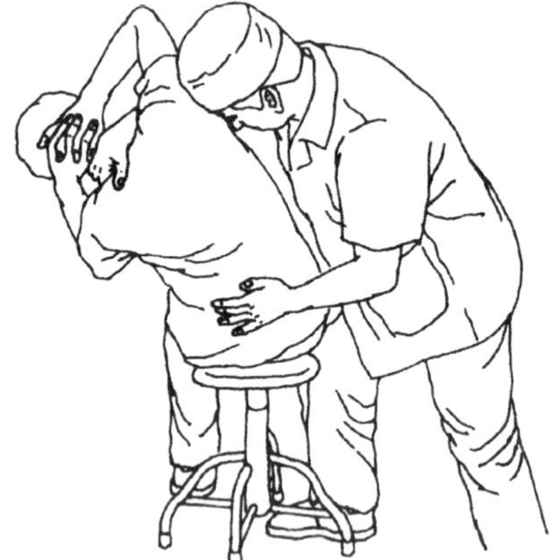

Figure 3-65 The rotating method for the lumbar vertebras (1)
图 3-65 腰椎摇法(1)

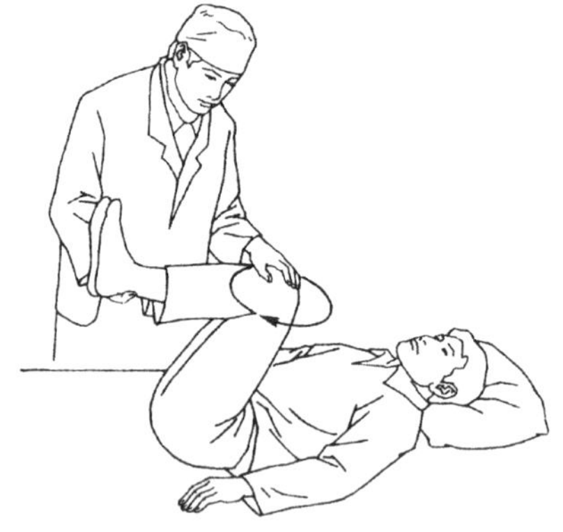

Figure 3-66 The rotating method for the lumbar vertebras (2)
图 3-66 腰椎摇法(2)

(3) The rotating method for the lumbar vertebras in the prone position After the patient takes a prone position, the practitioner presses his low back with one palm, and raise his lower limb with the other hand under his two knees, and then slowly rotate his low back in the backward leaning state by the two hands in coordination (Figure 3-67).

(3) 俯卧位腰椎摇法 受术者俯卧。术者一手掌按其腰部,一手从其双膝下穿过并将下肢抬起,然后两手协同用力,在腰部后伸状态下缓缓摇转其腰部(图 3-67)。

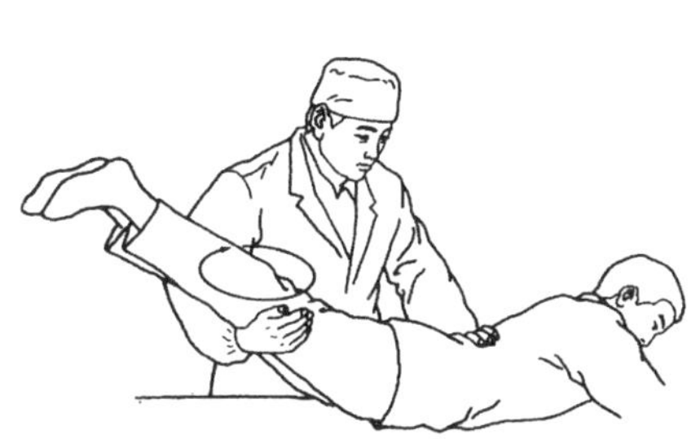

Figure 3-67 The rotating method for the lumbar vertebras (3)
图 3-67 腰椎摇法(3)

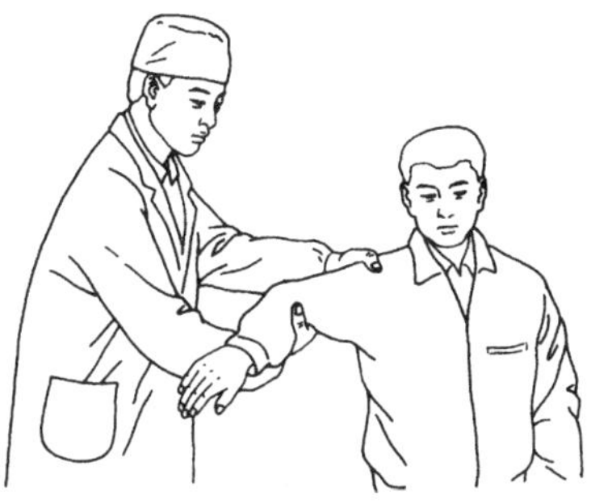

Figure 3-68 The rotating method for the shoulder (1)
图 3-68 肩部摇法(1)

19.3 Rotating method for the shoulder

(1) The rotating method for the shoulder by upholding the elbow After the patient takes a sitting position or supine position, the practitioner stands at his side, and holds the upper part of his shoulder joint with one hand, and upholds the patient's flexed elbow with another hand (with his forearm relaxed and put on the forearm of the practitioner), to rotate the shoulder joint slowly clockwise or counterclockwise (Figure 3-68). It is also advisable to rotate the shoulder joint by upholding the elbow and forearm respectively with the two hands.

(2) The rotating method for the shoulder by holding the elbow After the patient takes a sitting

19.3 肩部摇法

(1) 托肘摇肩法 受术者取坐位或仰卧位。术者站于其侧,一手扶住其肩关节上部,另一手托起受术者屈曲的肘部(使其前臂放松搭于术者的前臂),然后作缓慢的顺时针或逆时针方向的肩关节环转摇动(图 3-68)。也可双手分别托住肘部和前臂摇动。

(2) 扶肘摇肩法 受术者坐位,肩关节放松,上肢自

position, with the shoulder joint relaxed and the upper limb naturally flexed, the practitioner stands behind and lateral to the patient, presses the upper part of the proximal shoulder lightly and holds the patient's elbow with another hand, to make a rotating motion of the shoulder joint (Figure 3-69).

然屈肘。术者站于受术者侧后方,一手轻按近侧肩上部,另一手扶住受术者肘部,作肩关节的环转运动(图3-69)。

(3) The rotating method for the shoulder by holding the hand　After the patient takes a sitting position or supine position, with the upper limb naturally relaxed and dropped, the practitioner stands at the lateral side of the patient, holds his shoulder with one hand and holds his hand with another hand, to pull the upper limb a little bit and then make a rotating motion of the shoulder joint in a small amplitude (Figure 3-70).

(3) 握手摇肩法　受术者取坐位或仰卧位,上肢自然放松、下垂。术者站于受术者侧方,一手扶住其肩部,另一手握住其手,将其上肢稍加牵拉,然后作肩关节的小幅度环转摇动(图3-70)。

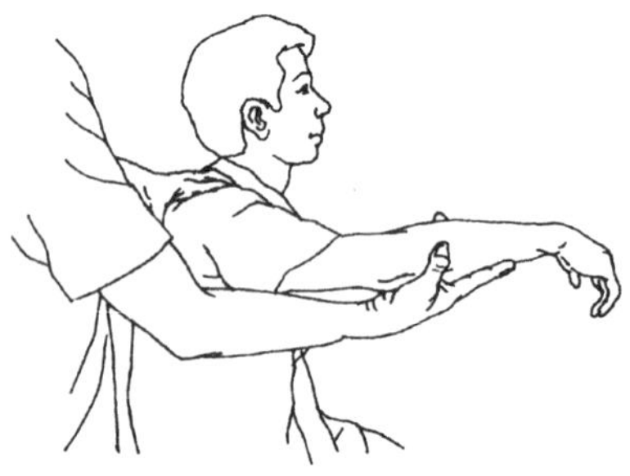

Figure 3-69　The rotating method for the shoulder (2)
图3-69　肩部摇法(2)

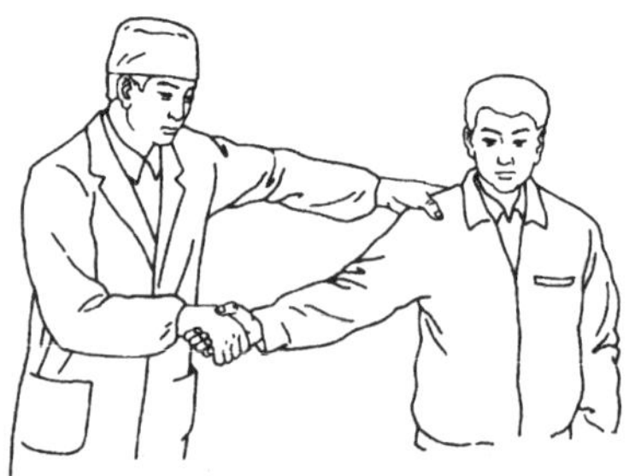

Figure 3-70　The rotating method for the shoulder (3)
图3-70　肩部摇法(3)

(4) The rotating method for the shoulder in large amplitude　After the patient takes a sitting position, with the upper limb relaxed and dropped, the practitioner stands at the side of the patient with a T-step, holds the patient's wrist with the two hands (Figure 3-71a), then upholds his upper limb upward and forward slowly, and turns the palm gradually with the hand below (Figure 3-71b),

(4) 大幅度摇肩法　受术者取坐位,上肢放松下垂。术者以丁字步站于受术者体侧,两手夹住受术者的腕部(图3-71a);然后慢慢地将其上肢向上向前托起,位于下方的手逐渐翻掌(图3-71b),当前上举至最高点时(图3-71c),一手

while raising to the utmost, holds his wrist downward with one hand and wipe lightly with the part between the thumb and index finger from the wrist, along the upper arm to the shoulder, then turns the part between the thumb and index finger in 180°, and guides the patient's arm to rotate downward continuously, and at the same time continuously wipe light upward from the upper limb to the wrist with the part between the thumb and index finger. This procedure can be repeated.

虎口向下握住其腕部,另一手以虎口部从腕部沿上肢轻抹至肩部,随即虎口转 180°;一手继续引导受术者手臂环转向下,同时一手虎口继续轻抹上肢至腕部。如此周而复始。

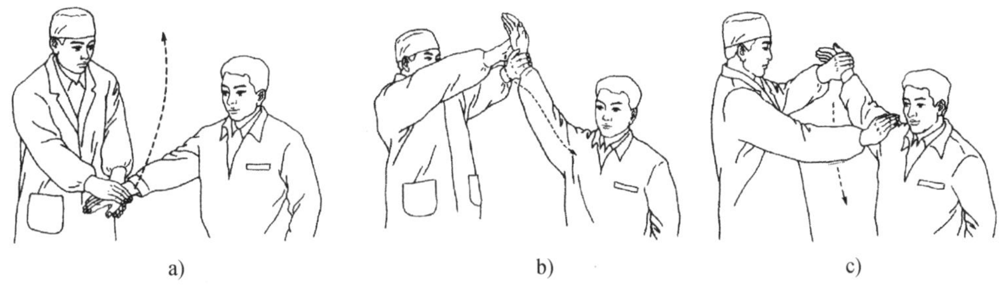

a) b) c)

Figure 3-71 The rotating method for the shoulder (4)

图 3-71 肩部摇法(4)

19.4 Rotating method for the elbow joint

After the patient takes a sitting position or supine position, the practitioner upholds his elbow with one hand and grabs his wrist with the other hand, to make a rotating motion of the elbow joint (Figure 3-72).

19.4 肘关节摇法

受术者取坐位或仰卧位。术者一手托住其肘部,另一手握住腕部,作肘关节的环转运动(图 3-72)。

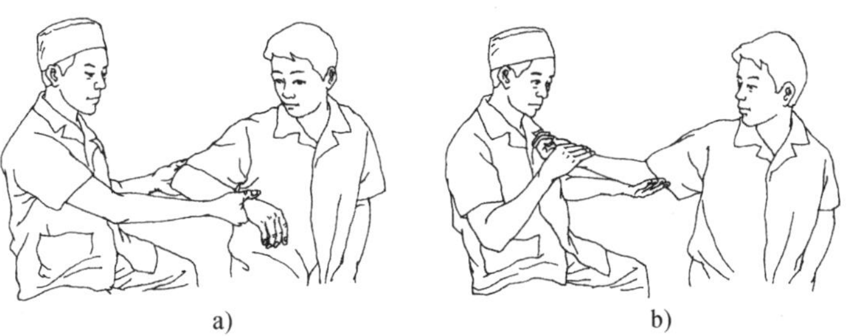

a) b)

Figure 3-72 The rotating method for the elbow joint

图 3-72 肘关节摇法

19.5 Rotating method for the wrist joint

After the patient takes a supine position or sitting position, the practitioner holds the upper part of the patient's wrist joint with one hand, and grabs his palm or finger with the other hand, to pull the wrist joint slightly first and then make a bidirectional rotating motion of the wrist joint, or the practitioner holds the patient's forearm with one hand and clasps the patient's five fingers with the five fingers of the other hand, to make a bidirectional rotating motion of the wrist joint (Figure 3-73).

19.5 腕关节摇法

受术者仰卧或坐位。术者一手握住受术者腕关节的上端，另一手握住其手掌或手指，先略作腕关节的拔伸，而后将腕关节作双向环转摇动。或术者一手握住受术者的前臂，另一手五指分开与受术者的五指相扣，将其腕关节作双向环转摇动（图3-73）。

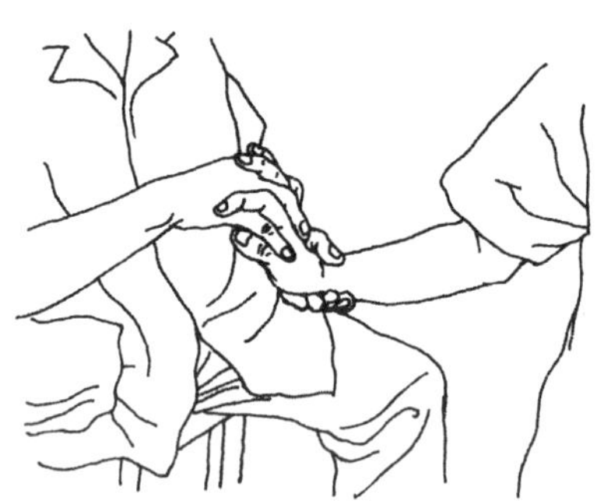

Figure 3-73 The rotating method for the wrist joint

图3-73 腕关节摇法

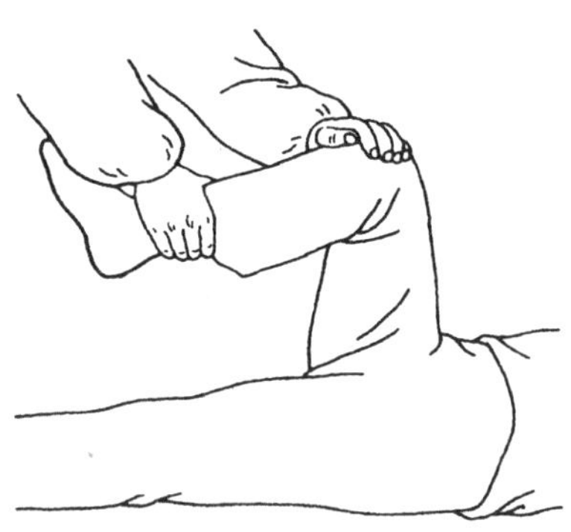

Figure 3-74 The rotating method for the hip joint (1)

图3-74 髋关节摇法(1)

19.6 Rotating method for the hip joint

After the patient takes a supine position, the practitioner stands at his body side, with the hip and knee flexed in one leg, holds his knee with one hand, and grabs his heel with the other hand, to flex his hip joint about 90°, and then make a bidirectional rotating motion (Figure 3-74), or thrust one hand underneath the patient's popliteal fossa to hold the patient's knee to make a rotating motion with the two hands (Figure 3-75).

19.6 髋关节摇法

受术者取仰卧位。术者站于其体侧，先将其一腿屈髋屈膝，一手扶住其膝部，另一手握住其足跟部，在将其髋关节屈曲至90°左右后，作双向环转摇动(图3-74)。或一手从受术者腘窝下穿过，双手抱住受术者膝部作环转摇动(图3-75)。

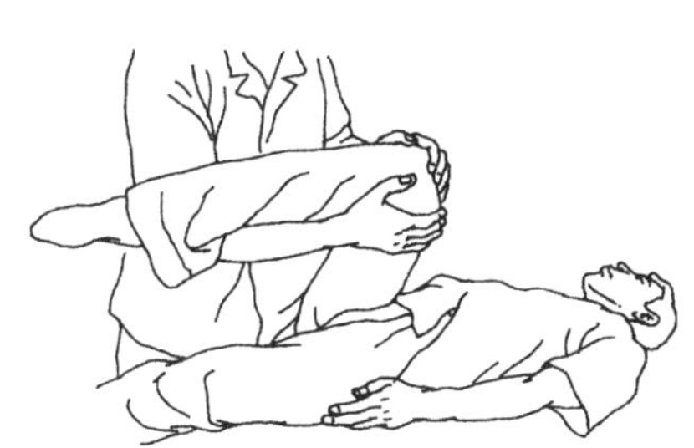

Figure 3-75 The rotating method for the hip joint (2)
图 3-75 髋关节摇法(2)

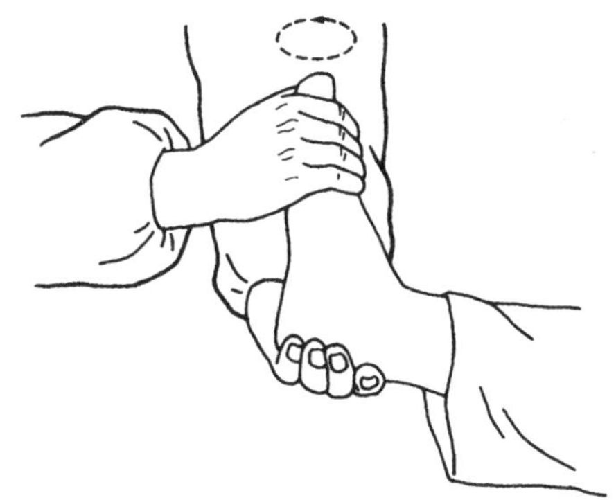

Figure 3-76 The rotating method for the ankle joint
图 3-76 踝关节摇法

19.7 Rotating method for the ankle joint

After the patient takes a supine position or sitting position, with the lower limb straightened, the practitioner stands in front of his foot, upholds patient's heel with one hand, and holds the dorsum of the foot with another hand, to pull the ankle joint a little bit and make a rotating motion of the ankle joint at the same time (Figure 3-76), or stands at his side, holds the upper part of the ankle joint with one hand, and holds and rotates the foot with another hand.

Explanation

(1) The rotating motion should be increased from small amplitude to large amplitude, and should be restricted within the normal physiological scope as much as possible, or within the tolerance of the patient.

(2) In accordance with the pathological situation, the rotating amplitude should be properly adjusted and must be applied exactly upon the actual circumstances.

19.7 踝关节摇法

受术者取仰卧位，或取坐位，下肢伸直。术者站于其足后，一手托住受术者足跟，另一手握住其足背，在略作踝关节拔伸的同时，作踝关节的环转摇动(图 3-76)。或站立其侧，一手握住踝关节上部，另一手握住脚掌摇动。

说明

(1) 摇转的幅度应由小到大，且尽量限制在正常关节生理活动范围之内，或在受术者能忍受的范围内进行。

(2) 根据病情恰如其分地掌握摇转幅度的大小，做到因势利导，适可而止。

(3) The rotating motion must be stable and coordinative and the rotating speed must be slow.

(4) This rotating method must be prohibited for habitual dislocation of the joint, cervical spondylosis in vertebral artery type, and fracture of the cervical vertebras.

Application

The rotating method is appropriate for the cervical vertebras, lumbar vertebras, and shoulder joint, elbow joint, wrist joint, hip joint, ankle joint and joints of the four limbs. The commonly used methods are the rotating method for the cervical vertebras, rotating method for the lumbar vertebras, rotating method for the shoulder joint, rotating method for the wrist joint, rotating method for the hip joint and rotating method for the ankle joint.

(3) 摇转动作要平稳协调，摇动速度宜缓慢。

(4) 对习惯性关节脱位、椎动脉型颈椎病及颈椎骨折等病症禁止使用该部的关节摇法。

应用

摇法适用于颈椎、腰椎，以及肩关节、肘关节、腕关节、髋关节、踝关节等四肢关节。常用的操作法有颈椎摇法，腰椎摇法，肩关节摇法，腕关节摇法，髋关节摇法，踝关节摇法等。

20　Pulling method

It refers to the manual technique to produce the passive rotating, flexing, extending, abducting and adducting motion of the joint by "inch-strength" functioning on the joints to have a sudden compression.

20　扳法

以"寸劲"作用于关节，使其瞬间突然受力，而产生被动的旋转、屈伸、展收等关节运动的手法，称为扳法。

20.1　Pulling method for the spine

Form

(1) The oblique pulling method for the cervical vertebras　After the patient takes a sitting position, with the neck slightly bent, the practitioner stands behind the patient, upholds the patient's chin with one palm, puts the other palm on the patient's occipital part, by coordination of the two hands, to rotate the patient's head to the limited direction to the elastic limited position, and then make a sudden and controlled pull by "inch-strength" for enlarging the rotation in $3^\circ \sim 5^\circ$ amplitude (Figure 3-77).

20.1　脊柱扳法

术式

(1) 颈椎斜扳法　受术者坐位，颈部微屈，操作者站立于受术者身后，一手掌托受术者下颏，另一手掌面置于受术者枕部，两手协同，先使受术者头颈向旋转受限侧旋转至弹性限制位，然后用"寸劲"作一突发有控制的扳动，扩大旋转幅度 $3^\circ \sim 5^\circ$(图3-77)。

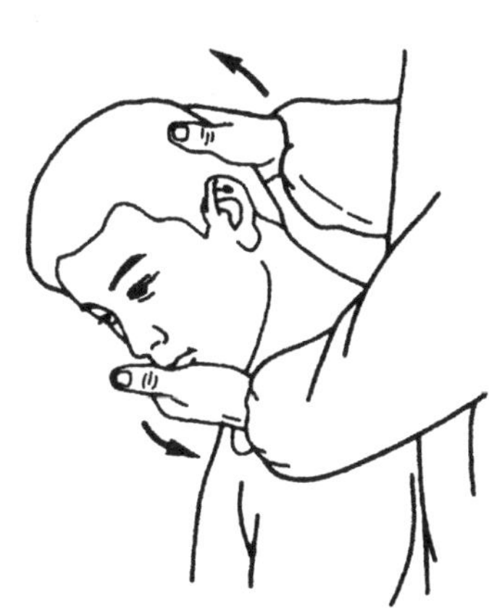

Figure 3-77 The oblique pulling method for the cervical vertebras
图 3-77 颈椎斜扳法

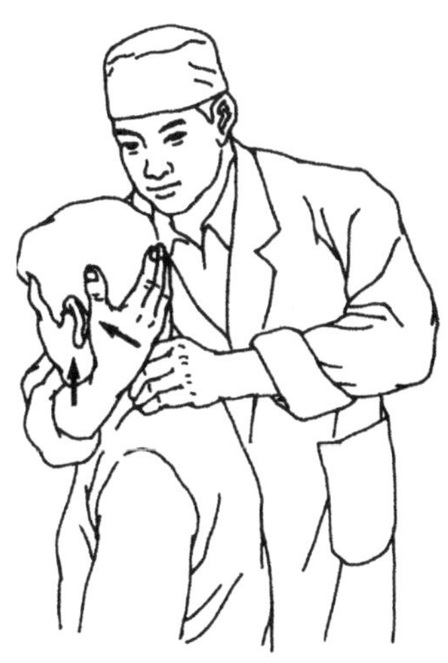

Figure 3-78 The pulling method by positioning and rotation for the cervical vertebras
图 3-78 颈椎定位旋转扳法

(2) The pulling method by positioning and rotation for the cervical vertebras After the patient takes a sitting position, the practitioner stands laterally and posterior to the patient, with the elbow joint flexed, upholds the patient's chin with the palm side of the elbow joint, and encircles the opposite occipital part with the palm, and pokes the protruded side of the spinous process of the cervical vertebra with the thumb of the other hand, guided by the upper limb holding the head, to gradually flex the patient's neck passively to the superior space of the protruded spinous process, and maintain the flexion of the neck, and rotate the neck passively toward the protruded spinous process to the elastic limited position, and hold it for a while, and then make a sudden and controlled pull of the enlarged rotation (2°～3°), and at the same time push and poke the spinous process toward the opposite side of the protrusion with the thumb of another hand (Figure 3-78).

（2）颈椎定位旋转扳法 受术者坐位。操作者站立于受术者侧后方，同侧肘关节屈曲，肘关节掌侧托住受术者下颌，手掌环抱对侧枕部，另一手拇指顶推颈椎棘突偏凸侧；在抱头之上肢引导下，逐渐被动屈曲受术者颈部至偏凸棘突上位间隙分离，维持颈部屈曲幅度，向棘突偏凸侧被动旋转颈部至弹性限制位，略作停顿，作一突发有控制的扩大旋转幅度的扳动（2°～3°），同时另一手拇指向偏凸对侧协调推顶棘突（图 3-78）。

(3) The resisting and repositioning method for the thoracic vertebras After the patient takes a sitting position, with the two hands crossed behind the nape, the practitioner stands behind the patient, extends the two hands respectively underneath the armpits of the patient, in front of his upper arms, and grabs the lower portion of his forearms. Then, the practitioner stands on one foot, and props up the lower border of the spinous process of the thoracic vertebras with the lifted knee, by the force from the coordination of the two hands, to extend the body trunk of the patient backward passively to the elastic limited position, and make a sudden and short pull backward and upward by the two hands while the patient almost finishes his exhalation (Figure 3-79)

(3) 胸椎对抗复位法 受术者坐位，两手指交叉扣于项后。操作者站于受术者身后，双手分别从受术者腋下伸出，经其上臂之前，从后方握住其前臂下段，然后操作者单足站立，用上提的膝部顶住偏凸的胸椎棘突下缘，双手协调用力，使受术者躯干被动后伸至弹性限制位，在受术者呼气末双手向后上方作突发短促的扳动(图 3-79)。

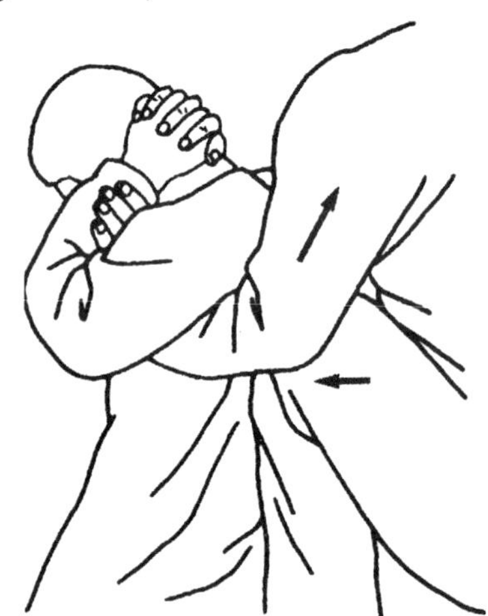

Figure 3-79 The resisting and repositioning method for the thoracic vertebras

图 3-79 胸椎对抗复位法

(4) The pulling method by positioning and rotation for the thoracic vertebras After the patient sits on a stool, and the assistant stands in front of the patient, holding the patient's thigh at the healthy side with the two legs and putting the two

(4) 胸椎定位旋转扳法 受术者坐于凳上，助手站于受术者面前，双腿夹住受术者健侧大腿固定骨盆，两手分置受术者两肩前后方。操

hands respectively on the anterior and posterior part of the patient's shoulder, the practitioner stands (or sits) behind and lateral to him, pokes the spinous process of the dislocated vertebra toward the protruded side with the thumb of one hand, hold the patient's nape and shoulder with another hand in front of the chest below the proximal armpit, and fell the patient to bend the body forward fill the intervertebоal space of the sick segment opens and then rotates the spine with the hand to the elastic limited position, to make a sudden and controlled pull for enlarging the rotation in 3°～5°, at the same time poke the spinous process forcefully obliquely upward for adjusting the dislocated spinal joint (Figure 3-80).

作者站(或坐)于其侧后方,一手拇指自偏凸侧推顶错缝椎体棘突,另一手经近侧腋下胸前,抓握受术者项肩部,嘱受术者躯干主动前屈至病变节段棘间隙张开,然后以手带动脊柱旋转至弹性限制位,作一突发有控制的扳动,扩大扭转幅度 3°～5°,同时拇指用力向斜上方顶推棘突,调整错缝的脊椎关节(图 3-80)。

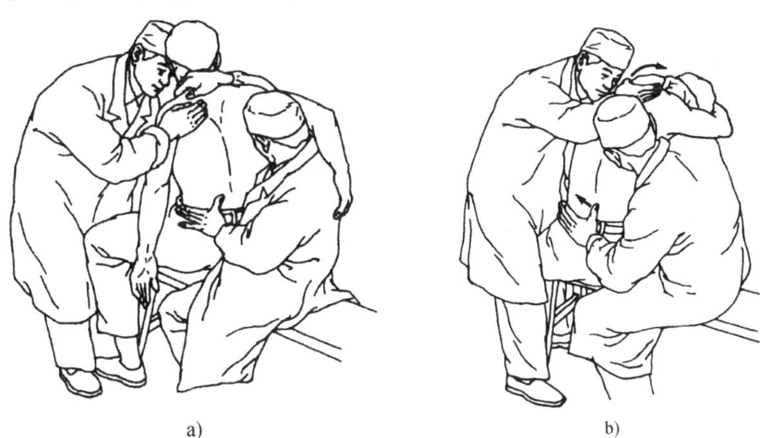

Figure 3-80 The pulling method by positioning and rotation for the thoracic vertebras

图 3-80 胸椎定位旋转扳法

(5) The oblique pulling method for the lumbar vertebras After the patient takes a lateral recumbent position on the healthy side, with the hip joint of the healthy side flexed, the lower limb straightened and knee and hip joint of the sick side flexed and the medial malleolus under the popliteal fossa of the healthy lower limb, the practitioner stands be-

(5) 腰椎斜扳法 受术者健侧卧位,健侧髋关节微屈,下肢伸直,患侧膝髋关节屈曲,内踝置于健侧下肢腘窝处。操作者站于其面前,通过调整健侧下肢角度来调整腰椎位置,操作者斜向上

side him and adjusts the position of the lumbar vertebras by adjusting the angle of the healthy lower limb. The practitioner pulls the healthy lower limb of the patient obliquely and upward, to have the rotating center of the spine exactly on the segment of the pathological lumbar vertebras to lock the segment to be adjusted, and then push the patient's shoulder backward with the other hand, with the elbow of another limb half flexed, by poking the buttocks with the upper portion of the forearm to pull forward, and after rotating the spine to the elastic limited position, to make a sudden and controlled pull for enlarging the rotation in 3°～5° (Figure 3-81).

牵拉受术者健侧上肢，使脊柱的扭转中心正好落于病变腰椎节段，锁定调整节段；然后以一手按受术者肩前部向后推，另一上肢肘部半屈，以前臂上段抵住臀部向前扳，将脊柱扭转至弹性限制位后，作一突发有控制的扳动，扩大扭转幅度 3°～5°（图3-81）。

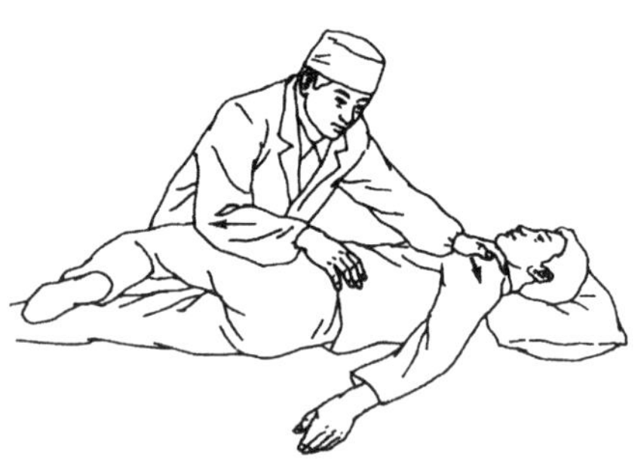

Figure 3-81　The oblique pulling method for the lumbar vertebras

图 3-81　腰椎斜扳法

(6) The pulling method by positioning and rotation for the lumbar vertebras　After the patient takes a lateral recumbent position on the healthy side (hereafter, take the right recumbent position as an example), the practitioner stands face to face with the patient, puts the thumb of the right hand between the two spinous processes of the dislocated segment, removes (bends) the patient's upper body forward with the left hand till the thumb feels the upper and lower vertebras loosened and the space enlarged. Then, the practitioner puts the thumb of

（6）腰椎定位斜扳法　受术者健侧卧位（以下以右侧卧位为例）。术者面对受术者而站，右手拇指置于错位节段的两个腰椎棘突之间，左手将受术者上半身向前搬动（弯腰），直至右手拇指感觉到上下棘突松动、间隙扩大，即停止前屈；将左手拇指置于原来右手拇指触摸的棘突间隙中；以右手将受

the left hand on the space of the spinous processes the thumb of the right hand touches before, straightens and removes (flexes the hip) the patient's right lower limb forward till the thumb of the left hand feels the space between the upper and lower spinous processes is further enlarged. Then, the practitioner flexes the knee and hip joint of the patient's left lower limb as much as possible, and puts the thumb of the right hand back to the original space of the spinous processes, and at the same time presses the patient's hip with the right forearm to fix his pelvis, and then asks the patient to hold his own right shoulder with the left hand and hold his own left shoulder with the right hand. After squatting down a little bit, the practitioner upholds the patient's right elbow with the left palm and rotates the patient's body leftward to the elastic limited position, to make a controlled and sudden pull for slightly enlarging the amplitude. In this moment, the practitioner can feel a bouncing sensation in the space of the spinous processes the thumb of the right hand touches, and hear a "clicking" sound. The manual technique is finished (Figure 3-82).

术者的右下肢伸直后向前搬动(屈髋),至左手拇指感觉上下棘突间隙进一步张开为止;将受术者的左下肢尽量屈膝屈髋;将右手拇指放回原来的棘突间隙中,同时右手前臂压住受术者臀部以固定其骨盆;然后令受术者先左手抱住右肩,再右手抱住左肩;术者略下蹲,用左掌托住受术者右肘,使受术者上身向左旋转,至弹性限制位时,作一有控制的、稍增大幅度的突发性扳动。此时术者可感觉右手拇指所在的棘突间隙有弹动感,并可听到"喀"一声响,手法结束(图 3-82)。

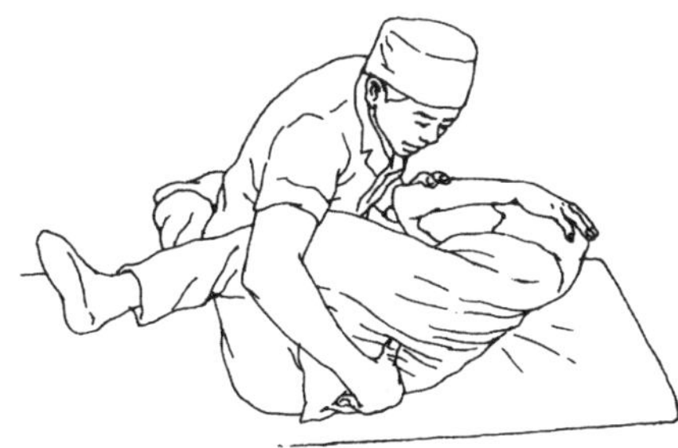

Figure 3-82 The pulling method by positioning and rotation for the lumbar vertebras

图 3-82 腰椎定位斜扳法

(7) The pulling method by positioning and rotation for the lumbar vertebras in the sitting position After the patient sits on the treatment table with a horse-riding posture, with the two legs on the two sides of the table to fix the pelvis (If sitting on a stool, the assistant should press his leg to fix the pelvis), the practitioner sits lateral to and behind the patient, pokes the protruded spinous process with the thumb of one hand, and extends another hand underneath the proximal armpit to hold his nape, so as to bend the patient's lumbar vertebras forward till the intervertebral space opens superior to the vertebra to be adjusted (Figure 3-83a), then rotate toward the side of the protruded spinous process to the elastic limited position, forcefully by the two hands in coordination, to make a sudden and controlled pull for enlarging the amplitude in 3°～5°, and at the same time poke the protruded spinous process with the thumb to the opposite direction (Figure 3-83b).

(7) 坐位腰椎定位旋转扳法　受术者以骑马式坐于治疗床上，两腿跨于床的两侧以固定骨盆（如坐在方凳上，应由助手按住其一侧大腿以固定骨盆），操作者坐于受术者侧后方，一手拇指抵住偏凸之棘突，另一手从近侧腋下穿过，扣握其项部，使受术者腰椎前屈至需调整椎体上位椎间隙张开（图3-83a），然后向棘突偏突侧旋转至弹性限制位，双手协调用力，作一突发有控制的扳动，扩大扭转幅度3°～5°，同时拇指向偏凸对侧推顶棘突（图3-83b）。

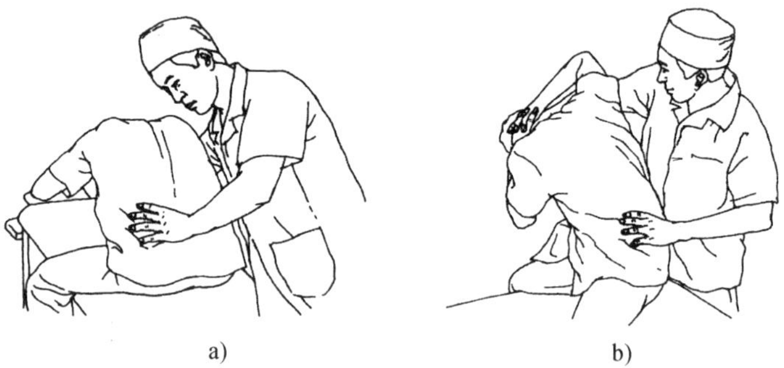

a)　　b)

Figure 3-83　The pulling method by positioning and rotation for the lumbar vertebras in the sitting position

图3-83　坐位腰椎定位旋转扳法

(8) The pulling method by backward extension for the lumbar vertebras After the patient takes a

(8) 腰椎后伸扳法　受术者俯卧。操作者站于腰椎

prone position, the practitioner stands at the side with the protrusion of the lumbar vertebras, presses the protruded spinous process with the pisiform bone of the palm root of one hand, holds the remote end of the opposite thigh with the other hand to pull upward to the elastic limited position, to make in a proper moment a sudden and controlled pull and enlarge the amplitude of backward extension in 3°～5°, and at the same time presses the spinous process with the pisiform bone of the palm root (Figure 3-84). The practitioner can also press the lumbosacral region with one hand, and uphold the two legs with the forearm of the other hand under the thighs, to shake and extend backward to the limited position, and then make a sudden and controlled pull.

棘突偏凸侧，一手掌根豌豆骨部按抵偏凸之棘突，另一手托住对侧大腿远端向上扳到弹性限制位，然后适时作一突发有控制的扳动，扩大脊柱后伸幅度3°～5°，掌根豌豆骨同时推压棘突（图3-84）。也可用一手按住腰骶部，另一手前臂从大腿下方托起两腿，边作摇动边后伸至限制位，再向上作一突发有控制的扳动。

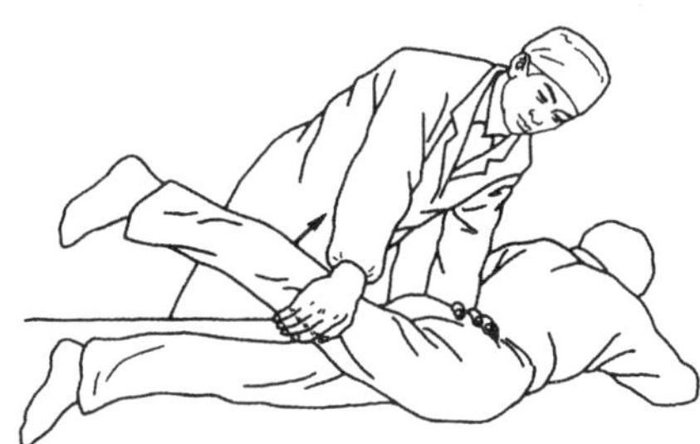

Figure 3-84 The pulling method by backward extension for the lumbar vertebras

图3-84 腰椎后伸扳法

Explanation

(1) Before the operation of the pulling method for the spine, it is necessary to have the good knowledge about the spine anatomy and understand clearly the structure features and physiological activities of the spinal joints.

(2) "Inch-strength" in the pulling method refers to a short and forceful strength, a controlled

说明

（1）脊柱扳法操作前，必须要有很好的脊柱解剖学知识基础，并且要对脊柱关节的结构特征、生理活动范围有清晰的了解。

（2）扳法的"寸劲"，是指短促有力的发力，是目的明

strength with clear purpose. It is needed to release and withdraw this strength at any time, and stop as soon as the effect appears. This kind of work can only be obtained after repeated training and clinical practice. Before the assurance, it is prohibited to try on the human body.

确的、有控制的发力，要求随发随收，点到即止、中病即止。这种功夫，要靠反复训练和临床实践才能获得。在没有把握之前，切忌在人体上试验。

(3) In the operation, it is needed not to go beyond the physiological scope of the articular activities. The pulling method for the cervical and thoracic vertebras must be operated very carefully. Otherwise, it might damage the spinal cord, cauda equine, and nerve root tissues.

(3) 操作时不可逾越关节运动的生理活动范围。否则可能伤及脊髓、马尾及神经根组织，颈、胸部扳法操作时尤当谨慎。

(4) It is prohibited to use the violent force and brute force.

(4) 不可使用暴力和蛮力。

(5) It is not forced to hear the clicking sound in the joint.

(5) 不可强求关节弹响。

(6) The pulling method is prohibited for the traumatic injury of the spine and spinal symptoms, if the diagnosis is not confirmed.

(6) 诊断不明确的脊柱外伤及有脊髓症状、体征者禁用扳法。

(7) The pulling method must be used carefully or prohibited for the elderly with serious hyperosteogeny, and osteoporosis. The pulling method is prohibited for bone tuberculosis and bone tumors.

(7) 老年人有较严重的骨质增生、骨质疏松者慎用或禁用扳法。对于骨关节结核、骨肿瘤者禁用扳法。

(8) In the operation of the oblique pulling method for the cervical vertebras, it must not be operated by the brute force, if the arm of force is longer and positioning is poor, in order to avoid causing damage.

(8) 颈椎斜扳法操作时力臂较长，定位性较差，不可强力操作，避免造成损伤。

(9) The pulling method by rotation and position for the cervical vertebras is better than the oblique pulling method in the segmental positioning. The key in the operation of the manual technique is to regulate the cervical vertebras to the elastic limited position and use the force by the two hands in co-

(9) 颈椎旋转定位扳法的节段定位性较斜扳法好，调整颈椎至弹性限制位和双手协调用力是手法操作的要点。

ordination.

(10) The sudden backward pull by the two hands must not be too powerful in the resisting and repositioning method for the thoracic vertebras, in order to avoid causing damage to the prethoracic soft tissues of the patient. At the same time, in order to avoid the uncomfortable sensation in the patient's spine, it is necessary to put a thin cushion between the practitioner's knee and patient's spine.

(10) 胸椎对抗复位法双手向后的突发扳动不可力量过大,以免造成受术者胸前软组织的损伤。同时,为避免受术者脊柱的不适感,可在术者膝部与受术者脊柱之间加一薄垫。

(11) The pulling method by rotation and positioning for the thoracic vertebras is comparatively complicated. The anteflexion of the patient's body trunk is active, but the rotation is passive. The assistant must cooperate with the practitioner. If this method is operated by single person, it is advisable to tell the patient to ride on the treatment table to fix the pelvis.

(11) 胸椎旋转定位扳法的操作较复杂,受术者躯干前屈为主动运动,旋转则是被动运动。助手与术者动作应协调。本法如单人操作,可令受术者骑跨于治疗床上以固定骨盆。

(12) In the operation of the pulling method by positioning and rotation for the lumbar vertebras in the sitting position, the key to lock the target segment is to tell the patient to bend forward first and rotate afterward.

(12) 坐位腰椎定位旋转扳法操作时,令受术者腰椎先前屈后旋转,是锁定目标节段的要点。

(13) The mechanism of the oblique pulling method by positioning for the lumbar vertebras is to bend the patient's spine to an angle before the operation, in order to focus the rotating stress of the upper and lower segments of the spine on the target segment. Therefore, in pushing the patient's upper body for the pulling method, his upper body can only be rotated and cannot be straightened. Otherwise, all the efforts in the previous preparatory phase would be wasted. In the lateral recumbent position, the patient must lie down backward as much as possible, in order to avoid influencing the prepar-

(13) 腰椎定位斜扳法的定位机制,是在扳动前将受术者的脊柱屈折成角,使脊柱上下两段的旋转应力能集中于目标节段。因此最后推动受术者上身作扳法时,只能使其上身旋转而不可使其脊柱伸直,否则前期准备阶段的所有努力将前功尽弃。受术者侧卧时应尽量靠后睡,以免影响以后的弯腰屈髋准备动作。托住肘部旋转

atory movements in bending the body and flexing the hip. The method to uphold the elbow for rotating the upper body can be replaced by the method to push and press the shoulder directly.

上身的方法也可改为直接推按肩部。

(14) In the operation of the pulling method by backward extension for the lumbar vertebras, this method is inappropriate, if the patient's symptom of nerve irritation is aggravated due to the reduction of the intraspinal volume.

(14) 腰椎后伸扳法操作时，椎管内容积缩小，如引起受术者神经刺激症状加重，则不宜使用该法。

Application

应用

The pulling method for various spinal segments is appropriate for the corresponding spinal segments. The commonly used ones are the oblique pulling method for the cervical vertebras, the pulling method by positioning and rotation for the cervical vertebras, the resisting and positioning method for the thoracic vertebras, the pulling method by positioning and rotation for the thoracic vertebras, the oblique pulling method for the lumbar vertebras, the pulling method by positioning and rotation for the lumbar vertebras in the sitting position, the oblique pulling method by positioning for the lumbar vertebras, and the oblique pulling method by backward extension for the lumbar vertebras, etc.

脊柱各节段的扳法适用于相应脊柱的节段。常用操作法有颈椎斜扳法，颈椎定位旋转扳法，胸椎对抗复位法，胸椎定位旋转扳法，腰椎斜扳法，坐位腰椎定位旋转扳法，腰椎定位斜扳法，腰椎后伸扳法等。

20.2 Pulling method for the four limbs

20.2 四肢扳法

Form

术式

(1) The pulling method for the shoulder joint the pulling method by anterior upholding action, the pulling method by abduction and upholding action, the pulling method by abduction, the pulling method by adduction, and the pulling method by anterior rotation and adduction, etc.

(1) 肩关节扳法：有前上举扳法、外展上举扳法、外展扳法、内收扳法、旋前内收扳法等。

1) The pulling method by abduction for the shoulder joint　After the patient takes a sitting po-

1) 肩关节外展扳法　受术者取坐位，肩关节放松。

sition, with the shoulder relaxed, the practitioner stands in front of or behind the patient's shoulder, presses his shoulder as a fulcrum with one palm, and holds his elbow (or upholds his elbow with the forearm) with the other hand, to make a abduction of the shoulder joint to 90°, and then do the pulling method by abduction for the shoulder joint, by pressing and lifting action with the coordinative strength of the two hands (Figure 3-85).

术者站于受术者肩前面或者后侧，一手掌按住其肩部为支点，另一手握住其肘部(或者用前臂托住其肘部)，作肩外展运动，至 90°时，两手协同用力，一按一提，作肩关节外展扳法(图 3-85)。

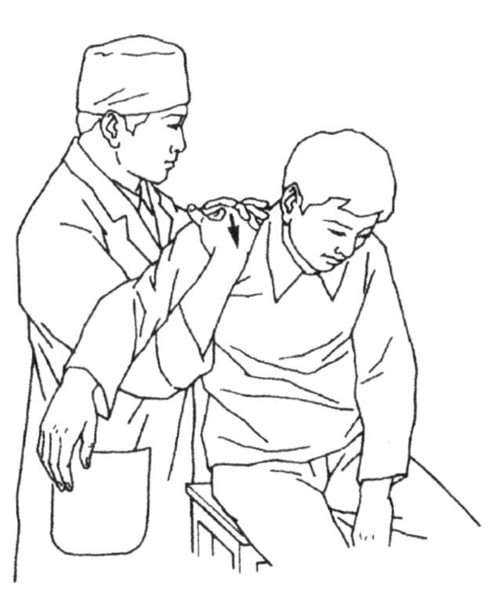

Figure 3-85 The pulling method by abduction for the shoulder joint
图 3-85 肩关节外展扳法

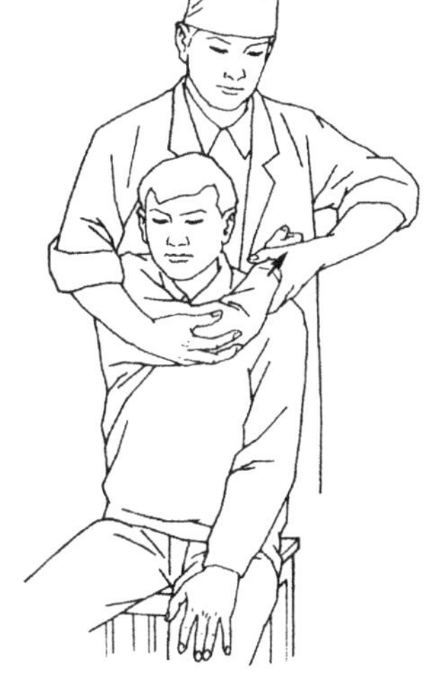

Figure 3-86 The pulling method by adduction for the shoulder joint
图 3-86 肩关节内收扳法

2) The pulling method by adduction for the shoulder joint After the patient takes a sitting position, with the elbow joint flexed, and sick limb in front of the chest, the practitioner stands behind him, close to his back, to stabilize his body, and holds the sick shoulder with the hand at the same side of the sick shoulder, and upholds the elbow of the sick limb with another hand to adduct the shoulder joint to its utmost, and then do the pulling method by

2) 肩关节内收扳法 受术者取坐位，屈肘关节，将患肢放于胸前。术者站于其后侧，紧靠其背部，稳住其身体，用自己与患肩同侧的手扶住患肩；另一手托住患肢的肘部作肩关节内收至有阻力时，两手同时用力作肩关节内收扳动(图 3-86)。

adduction for the shoulder joint forcefully with the two hands at the same time (Figure 3-86).

3) The pulling method by abduction and upholding action for the shoulder joint　After the patient takes a sitting position, the practitioner stands lateral-anterior or lateral-posterior to the patient, upholds the patient's upper limb with the upper arm, and presses the patient's shoulder with the palm at the same time, and presses the dorsum of the palm with the other palm, to have a abduction in the shoulder joint. When the shoulder joint is abducted and upheld to its certain limit, press downward with the palm, abduct the forearm, and at the same time pull the shoulder upward with "inch-strength" (Figure 3-87).

3) 肩关节外展上举扳法　受术者取坐位，术者站于受术者侧前方或侧后方。用上臂托起受术者上肢，同时用手掌按住受术者肩部，另一手掌按于手掌背上，作肩关节外展，待肩关节外展上举到一定限度时，手掌下按，前臂外展，同时用“寸劲”向上扳动肩部(图 3-87)。

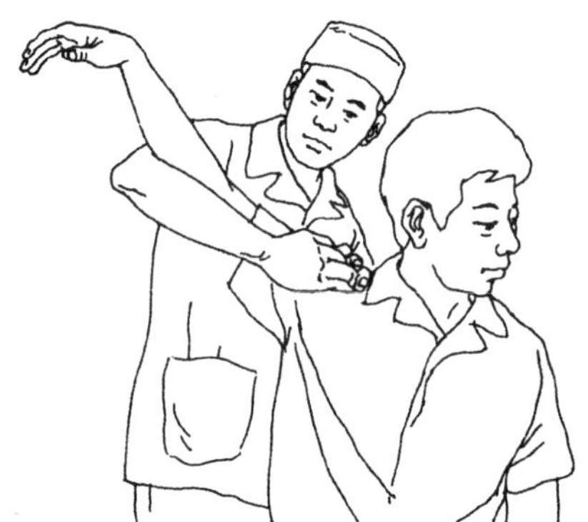

Figure 3-87　The pulling method by the abduction and upholding action for the shoulder joint (1)

图 3-87　肩关节外展上举扳法(1)

4) The pulling method by anterior upholding action for the shoulder joint　After the patient takes a sitting position, the practitioner gets down anteriorly and laterally to the patient, straightens the patient's upper limb, and puts the forearm on the practitioner's shoulder. The practitioner presses the sick shoulder with the two hands, with the sick

4) 肩关节前上举扳法　受术者取坐位，术者以半蹲位站于受术者前侧方，受术者上肢伸直，前臂放于术者肩上。术者用双手按住其患肩，以患肩为支点，慢慢地用肩将患肢抬起，作前屈上举

shoulder as a fulcrum, slowly raises the sick limb with the shoulder and makes a passive anterior flexing and upholding movement. To the utmost, the practitioner makes a pulling method by anteflexion and upholding action forcefully with the two hands in coordination (in this method, the practitioner stands laterally to thc patient, doing the pulling method by abduction and upholding action, Figure 3-88). Or the practitioner presses the sick shoulder with one hand, and holds the elbow of the sick shoulder with the other hand, to raise it slowly (flex forward and raise) to its utmost, and then pulls the shoulder with the two hands in coordination (Figure 3-89). This method can also be done in the supine position.

被动运动,至有阻力时,双手协同用力,作肩关节前屈上举扳法(此法术者站于侧方,也可作外展上举扳法,见图3-88);或术者一手按住患肩,另一手握住患肢的肘部,缓缓上提(作前屈上举)至最大限度时,两手协同用力扳动肩部(图3-89)。此法还可以仰卧位操作。

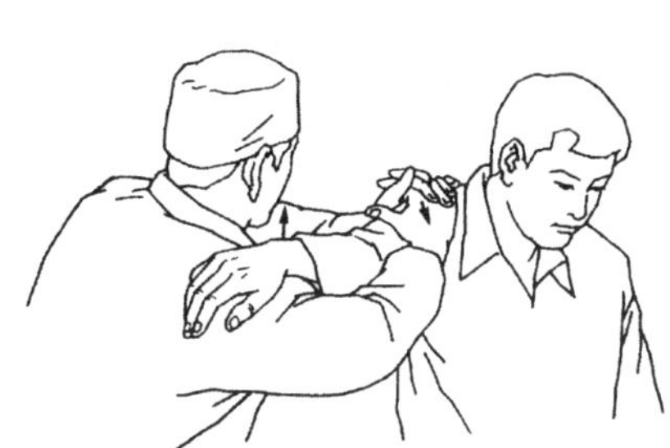

Figure 3-88 The pulling method by the abduction and upholding action for the shoulder joint (2)
图 3-88 肩关节外展上举扳法(2)

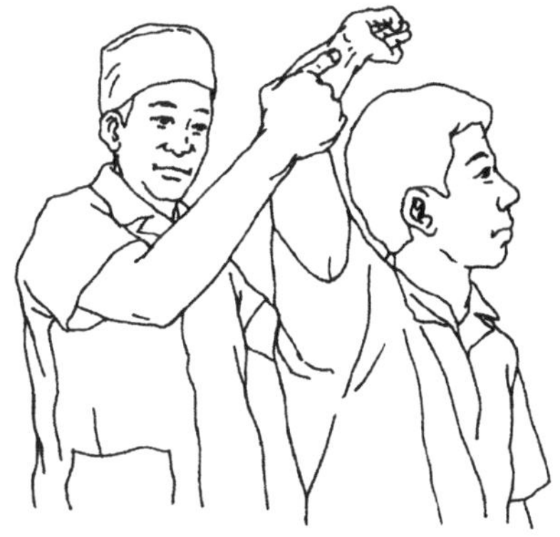

Figure 3-89 The pulling method by the abduction and upholding action for the shoulder joint
图 3-89 肩关节前上举扳法

5) The pulling method by the anterior rotation and adduction for the shoulder joint After the patient takes a sitting position, with the hand and forearm of the upper limb at the one side, flexed at the lumbosacral region, the practitioner stands lat-

5) 肩关节旋前内收扳法 受术者坐位,一侧上肢的手与前臂屈肘置于腰骶部。术者立于其侧方。以一手扶按该上肢肩部以固定,另一手

erally to the patient, presses and fixes the shoulder of this upper limb with one hand, and holds wrist with the other hand to raise it slowly along the back for gradually abducting the shoulder. To its utmost, the practitioner makes a quick and controlled movement by the "inch-strength" to raise his forearm, so as to adduct his shoulder in a position of anterior rotation for moving the back of the hand upward along the lumbar vertebras for 1 cm and then let it go immediately. This movement can be repeated for 3～5 times (Figure 3-90).

握住腕部将其前臂沿腰背部缓缓上抬，以使其肩关节逐渐内收，至有阻力时，以"寸劲"作一快速的、有控制的上抬其前臂动作，以使其肩关节产生旋前位的内收的扳动，使其手背沿着腰椎上移1厘米左右，迅即放松。重复3～5次(图3-90)。

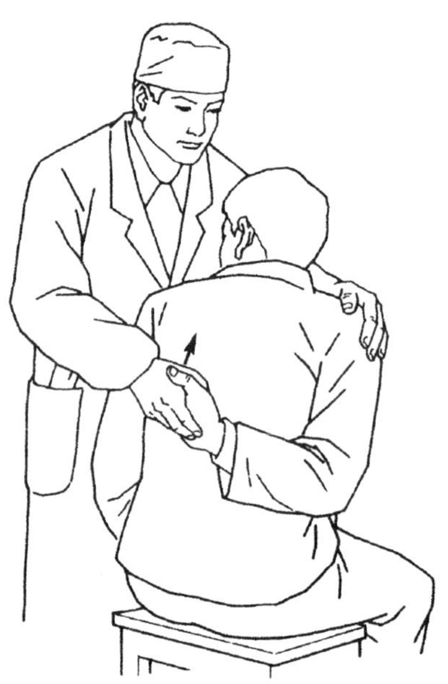

Figure 3-90 The pulling method by the anterior rotation and adduction for the shoulder joint
图3-90 肩关节旋前内收扳法

(2) The pulling method for the wrist joint: There are three types of the pulling method by flexing the wrist, the pulling method by extending the wrist, and the pulling method by lateral flexion for the wrist.

(2) 腕关节扳法：有屈腕扳法、伸腕扳法和腕侧屈扳法三种。

1) The pulling method by flexing the wrist The practitioner sits face to face with the patient, holds and fixes the lower portion of the forearm with one hand, and holds the fingers and palm with another hand, to make the flexion and extension of the wrist joint repeatedly, and puts and presses the wrist joint on the flexed position to its utmost, and then makes a sudden flexion of the wrist joint by "inch-strength", repeatedly for several times.

1) 屈腕扳法 术者与受术者相对而坐。以一手握住前臂下端以固定,另一手握住指掌部,先反复做腕关节的屈伸活动,然后将腕关节置于屈曲位加压,至有阻力时以"寸劲"作一突发的、稍增大幅度的屈腕动作。反复数次。

2) The pulling method by extending the wrist The practitioner sits face to face with the patient, with the fingers crossed with the five fingers of the patient, puts the wrist joint in the position of back extension, and presses it continuously, to its utmost and makes a pushing action by "inch-strength" in a comparatively large amplitude, repeatedly for several times.

2) 伸腕扳法 术者与受术者相对而坐。术者与受术者五指外相叉,先其腕关节置于背伸位,不断加压,至有阻力时,以"寸劲"作一稍增大幅度的推动,反复数次。

3) The pulling method by lateral flexion for the wrist The practitioner sits face to face with the patient, holds the lower end of the patient's forearm with one hand, and holds his hand with the other hand to pull and extend the wrist joint, and then pulls and flexes the wrist joint leftward and rightward by "inch-strength" (Figure 3-91).

3) 腕侧屈扳法 术者与受术者相对而坐。一手握住受术者前臂的下端,另一手握住其手掌部,先将腕关节拔伸,然后以"寸劲"在拔伸的基础上作腕关节的左右侧屈扳动(图 3-91)。

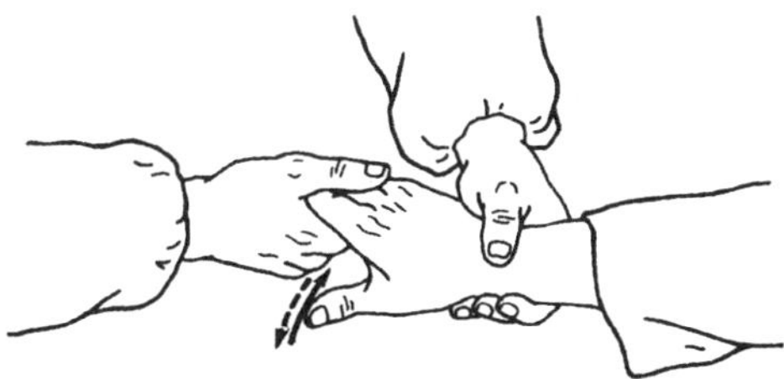

Figure 3-91 The pulling method by lateral flexion for the wrist

图 3-91 腕侧屈扳法

(3) The pulling method for the ankle joint:

(3) 踝关节扳法:主要有

There are mainly the pulling method by plantar flexion, and the pulling method by back extension.

1) The pulling method by plantar flexion for the ankle joint　After the patient takes a supine position, with the two lower limbs straightened, the practitioner sits facing to his sole, upholds his heel with one hand and holds the dorsum of the foot with the other hand, to have a plantar flexion of the ankle joint forcefully by the two hands in coordination, to its utmost, and to pull for a plantar flexion in a comparatively large amplitude by " inch-strength" (Figure 3-92a).

2) The pulling method by back extension for the ankle joint　After the patient takes a supine position, with the two lower limbs straightened, the practitioner sits facing to his sole, upholds his heel with one hand and holds the dorsum of the foot with the other hand, to extend the ankle joint backward, to its utmost, and to make a backward extension in a comparatively large amplitude by "inch-strength" (Figure 3-92b).

The pulling method for the ankle joint can be done by holding the heel with one hand and holding the back of the foot with the other hand, to pull outward and inward (Figure 3-92c, Figure 3-92d).

跖屈扳法和背伸扳法。

1）踝关节跖屈扳法　受术者仰卧，两下肢伸直，术者面向其足底而坐。以一手托住其足跟部，另一手握住脚掌部，两手协调用力，在踝关节跖屈至有明显阻力时，以"寸劲"作一增大幅度的跖屈扳动（图 3-92a）。

2）踝关节背伸扳法　受术者仰卧，两下肢伸直，术者面向其足底而坐。以一手托住其足跟部，另一手握住脚掌部，两手协调用力，在踝关节背伸至有明显阻力时，以"寸劲"作一增大幅度的背伸扳动（图 3-92b）。

踝关节扳法还可一手握足跟，另一手握足跗部，进行外翻或内翻扳动（图 3-92c，3-92d）。

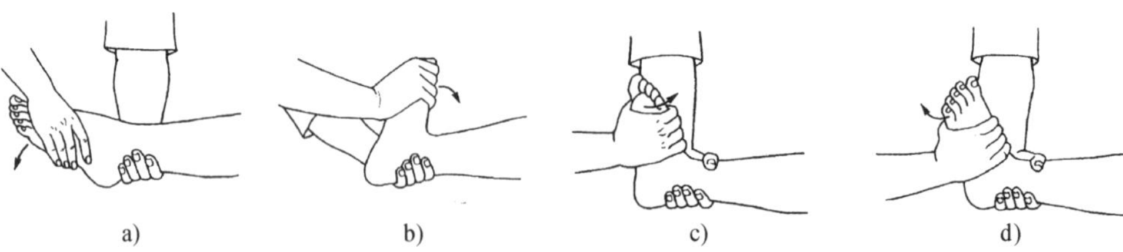

Figure 3-92　The pulling method for the ankle joint

图 3-92　踝关节扳法

Explanation

(1) The pulling method for the four limbs should be decided for the concrete method in accordance with the direction and degree of the limited articular functions.

(2) There is usually no clicking sound in the pulling method for the four limbs.

(3) It is necessary not to use the violent force, in order to avoid accidents of soft tissue injury of the muscles and ligaments and bone fracture.

(4) The pulling method must be used carefully or prohibited for the elderly with serious hyperosteogeny, and osteoporosis. The pulling method is prohibited for bone tuberculosis and bone tumors.

(5) In the application of the pulling method for scapulohumeral periarthritis with long-term duration and serious adhesion, it is not appropriate to resolve adhesion for just once, in order to avoid tearing the articular capsule and aggravating the pathological situation.

Application

The pulling method for the four limbs is mainly used for the shoulder joint, wrist joint and ankle joint. The commonly used ones are the pulling method for the shoulder joint, and the pulling method for the ankle joint, etc.

说明

（1）四肢的扳法应该根据关节功能受限的方向和程度决定具体的扳法。

（2）四肢的扳法通常没有关节弹响声。

（3）切忌暴力，以免发生肌肉、韧带等软组织损伤和骨折等意外事故。

（4）老年人有较严重的骨质增生、骨质疏松者慎用或禁用扳法。对于骨关节结核、骨肿瘤者禁用扳法。

（5）病程日久、粘连严重的肩关节周围炎在实施扳法时不宜一次性分解粘连，以免关节囊撕裂而加重病情。

应用

四肢扳法主要用于肩关节、腕关节和踝关节。常用操作法有肩关节扳法，踝关节扳法等。

Section 4 Specific techniques

第4节 特殊手法

1 Sweeping method

It refers to the manual technique to wipe and rub quickly back and forth with the radial side of

1 扫散法

用拇指桡侧部和其余四指指端自头颞部向耳后快速

the thumb and the tips of other four fingers from the temple to the back of the ear.

地来回推擦，称扫散法。

Form

The practitioner stands face to face with the patient, holds the patient's opposite head with one hand, and stretches the other hand, with the thumb straightened, other fingers closed and the interphalangeal joints flexed, and puts the radial side of the thumb and the tips of the rest four fingers on the temple to wipe and rub back and forth by the active flexion of the elbow joint taking the four fingers, and at the same time, push upward, backward and downward along the pathway of the gallbladder meridian at the side of the head in one direction (Figure 3-93).

术式

术者面向受术者站立，以一手扶住受术者对侧头部，另一手虎口张开，拇指伸直，其余四指并拢、指骨间关节屈曲，将拇指桡侧缘及其余四指指端置于头颞部，肘关节作主动屈伸带动五指在颞部来回推擦，同时沿头侧的胆经循行部位从前上向后下方单向推动(图 3-93)。

Explanation

(1) The frequency of the sweeping method is about 200 times per minute.

(2) In the operation, it is necessary to hold the patient's head with one hand, in order to avoid over shaking of the patient's head.

(3) It is needed to push in predominance, and to be light when the hand comes back.

(4) It is needed to move backward and downward, along the meridian in single direction.

(5) The route in each sweeping action is about 3～4 cm, not too long, and it is needed to sweep backward and downward.

(6) The practitioner should be relaxed in the wrist joint, persistent in the movement, proper in the speed, and appropriate in pressure, and complete once.

(7) If the patient's hair is too long, it is needed to thrust the five fingers into the hair to sweep, in

说明

(1) 扫散法的频率约每分钟 200 次。

(2) 操作时应注意一手固定受术者头部，勿使受术者头部过度摇晃。

(3) 来回推擦以向前推动为主，回来时用力较轻。

(4) 移动的路线为前上到后下，顺经单向操作。

(5) 每次推擦的路线一般为 3～4 厘米，不宜过长，边扫散边向后下方移动。

(6) 术者腕关节放松，动作连贯，快慢适度，轻重有致，一气呵成。

(7) 受术者头发较长时，可将五指伸入发间操作，避

order to avoid pulling the hair and causing pain.

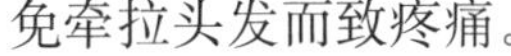

免牵拉头发而致疼痛。

(8) To stretch the hand is a specific requirement in the internal-works tuina school, and it can also be simplified to operate with the tips of the five fingers, and even with the radial side of the thumb.

（8）上述虎口张开的操作方法是内功推拿流派的特殊要求，亦可简化为五指指端着力，甚至仅以拇指桡侧缘着力操作。

Application

This method is effective to expel wind, disperse cold, balance the liver, suppress the yang, wake up the brain, promote the spirit, dredge the collaterals and stop pain, and is often used for headache, migraine, heavy sensation in the head, vertigo, blurred vision, hypertension, insomnia, low spirit and tiredness, etc.

应用

本法具有祛风散寒、平肝潜阳、醒脑提神、通络止痛之功用，常用于治疗头痛，偏头痛、头重如裹、眩晕、视物模糊、高血压、失眠、神疲倦怠等病症。

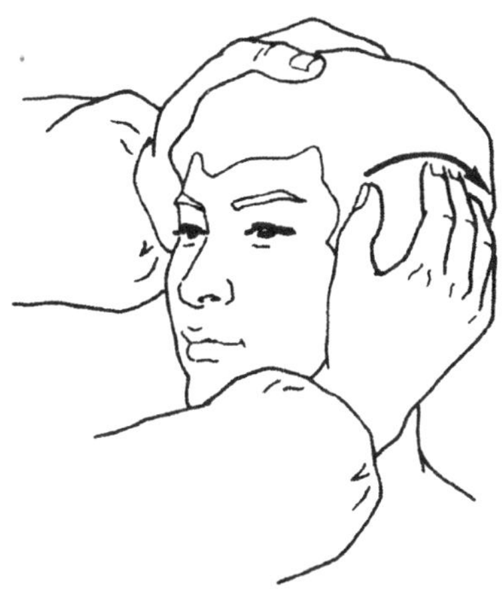

Figure 3-93 The Sweeping Method
图 3-93 扫散法

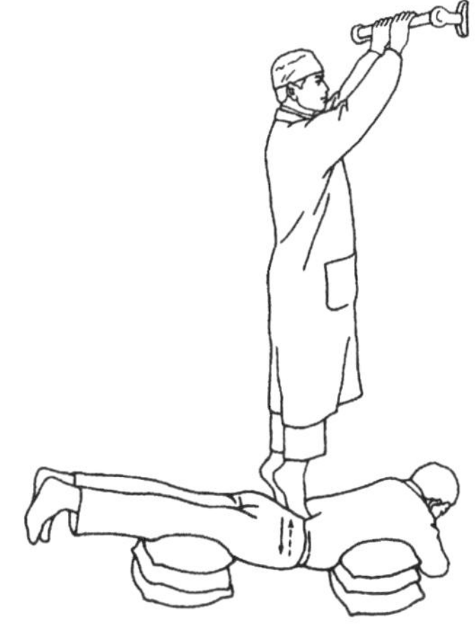

Figure 3-94 The Treading Method
图 3-94 踩蹻法

2 Treading method

It refers to a method to step and tread the patient's body. Hereafter, a treading method for the lumbar region is introduced.

2 踩蹻法

术者用足部踩踏受术者身体一定部位的方法，称踩蹻法。这里仅介绍一种腰部踩蹻法。

Form

After the patient takes a prone position, with the pillow under the chest and thighs respectively, to suspend the abdomen (usually about 10 cm away from the table), the practitioner holds the hand rail (hanging rod, crossbar on the wall, or floor plank), to control the self bodyweight and regulate the treading power, and at the same time step the patient's lumbar region with the two feet, and make certain springing movement. In the operation, it is necessary to lift the heel, step on the lumbar region with the anterior part of the foot, so as to pounce with the body up and down and produce a pouncing and pressing rhythmical stimulation on the lumbar region, by the flexion and extension of the knee joint and hip joint in small amplitude (Figure 3-94). Usually, it is needed to pounce with the body continuously for 10～20 times.

术式

受术者俯卧，在胸部和股前部垫枕，使腹部腾空（一般离床 10 厘米左右）。术者双手抓住扶手（悬吊的拉杆，墙上的横木，或落地式支架），以控制自身体重和调节踩踏的力量，同时用双足踩踏受术者腰部，并作适当的弹压动作。踩踏时，足跟提起，以足前部着力于腰部，运用膝关节和髋关节的小幅度屈伸运动，使身体一起一落，对腰部作一弹一压的节律性刺激（图 3-94）。一般可连续弹压 10～20 次。

Explanation

(1) It is needed to adjust the treading power, and pouncing amplitude and times in accordance with the body condition or pathological situation of the patient.

(2) In pouncing up, the foot tip must not leave the low back and jump up completely.

(3) The strength and velocity of the treading technique must be even and rhythmical.

(4) The treatment table should be proper in hardness.

(5) The patient should be told not to hold up breathing, and told to breathe naturally with the pouncing movement, and told to inhale in pouncing up and to exhale in treading down.

(6) The patient should be told not to take any

说明

（1）根据受术者的体质或病情，调整踩踏力量和弹压幅度和操作次数。

（2）弹起时足尖不可离开腰部而完全腾空。

（3）踩踏的力量和速度，要均匀而有节奏。

（4）推拿床要软硬适中。

（5）嘱受术者不要屏气，应随着弹压动作自然呼吸，弹起时吸气，踩踏时呼气。

（6）嘱受术者施术前一

food and not to drink too much water within one hour prior to the treatment.

小时内不要进食和过多饮水。

(7) During the treatment, because the lumbar spinal canal becomes small due the enlarged backward extension of the low back, nerve irritation might be aggravated in some patients. If the patient is unable to tolerate pain, it is necessary to stop this technique immediately.

(7) 在施术过程中,因腰部后伸度加大而腰椎管容积变小,可能导致部分病人神经刺激症状加重,若受术者疼痛难忍,应立即停止操作。

(8) Because this technique is strong in stimulation, it must be used carefully. This technique cannot be used for those patients with high age, weak constitution, serious cardiovascular diseases, intervertebral problems, osteoporosis, or pathological change in the spinal column.

(8) 本法刺激量大,应用时必须谨慎,对年老体弱、有较严重的心血管疾病、椎管内疾病、骨质疏松或脊椎骨质有病变者均不可使用本法。

Application

应用

This technique has the effects to soothe the meridians, dredge the collaterals, regulate the tendons, promote restoration, circulate qi and stop pain, characterized by strong pressure, good permeation and strength-saving feature, appropriate for shoulder, back, lumbar region and buttocks, and often used for chronic intractable lumbar soft tissue pain, lumbar muscular spasm and stiffness, posterior articular disturbance of the lumbar vertebras, and chronic lumbar strain.

本法具有舒筋通络、理筋整复、行气止痛的作用,并具有压力大、渗透性好和省力的优点。适用于肩背、腰臀等部位,常用于治疗慢性顽固性腰部软组织疼痛、腰部肌肉痉挛僵硬、腰椎后关节紊乱、慢性腰肌劳损等病症。

The treading technique can also be used for healthcare massage and unformed diseases. In treading the lumbar region, this technique can be combined with the pressing-kneading technique, sliding-pushing technique, divergent pushing technique, and striking technique for heel, and kneeling-kneading technique for the knee, and can also be applied on the back and posterior aspect of the lower limbs.

踩蹻也可用于保健按摩和治未病。踩踏腰部时可配合按揉、滑推、分推、足跟叩击、膝部跪揉等足部技法,并可扩大应用于背部、下肢后部等部位。

Chapter 4 Practice on the human body

第 4 章 推拿人体操作

Section 1 Brief introduction to practice on the human body

第 1 节 推拿人体操作概述

1 Tuina operating method and tuina practice on the human body

The tuina basic techniques applied on the human body are termed tuina practicing methods. Tuina practicing methods are composed of the two components, i. e. tuina techniques and tuina areas (including meridians and acupoints).

The tuina practice on the human body refers to the training course to further practice the training skills on the human body, after the basic skills of the tuina techniques are learnt.

The main training contents of the tuina practice on the human body include:

(1) Training of various tuina basic techniques on different body parts.

(2) Training of routine sets of the commonly used tuina techniques on every body part.

1 推拿操作法与推拿人体操作

推拿基本手法在人体上的运用称为推拿操作法。推拿操作法由两个要素组成，即推拿手法和受术部位（包括经络、腧穴）。

推拿人体操作，是在学习了推拿手法的基本技巧后，进一步在人体上进行的推拿操作练习的技能训练课程。

推拿人体操作的主要训练内容包括：

（1）各种推拿基本手法在人体不同部位的操作技巧训练。

（2）每个部位常用的手法操作常规套路训练。

2 Targets of tuina practice on the human body

The basic target of tuina practice on the human body is supposed to build up a bridge between the basic tuina manual techniques and its clinical application, preliminarily competent for the simulated practice of tuina clinical prescription. By the training of the manual skills on various body parts, it can help to realize the goals to

(1) Master the skill for practice of tuina manual techniques on various body parts.

(2) Obtain the two practical experiences to offer and receive the commonly used manual techniques.

(3) Be familiar with routine practicing procedure on various body parts.

(4) Select proper tuina practicing methods in accordance with the morphostructure of various body parts.

(5) Store up the spare practicing methods of various body parts.

(6) Understand the commonly used practicing methods and styles of some tuina schools.

2 推拿人体操作课程的目标

推拿人体操作课程的基本目标是搭建从基本推拿手法到推拿临床应用的桥梁，能初步胜任推拿临床处方的模拟操作。通过在人体不同部位的技能操作训练，能够：

（1）掌握在人体不同部位实施推拿手法的技巧。

（2）获得常用操作法的施术和受术两种实际体验。

（3）熟悉各个部位的常规操作套路。

（4）根据不同部位的形态结构特点选择恰当的推拿操作法。

（5）储备每个部位多种备用操作法。

（6）了解部分推拿流派的常用推拿操作法及其风格特点。

3 The learning methods of tuina practice on the human body

(1) Review the basic manual techniques.

(2) Review the knowledge on human anatomy and meridians and acupoints.

(3) Train the location of the basic manual techniques on the human body, the practice on the fixed areas and train practice along the meridians.

(4) Train on various body parts.

3 推拿人体操作的学习方法

（1）复习推拿基本手法。

（2）复习人体解剖学知识和经络腧穴学知识。

（3）基本手法的人体定点、定位练习和循经操作训练。

（4）各个部位的推拿人

体操作训练。

(5) Train the routine procedure of the practice on the whole body.

（5）全身性推拿常规套路训练。

(6) Train the simulated clinical probation and tuina prescriptions

（6）推拿科临床见习和推拿处方模拟训练。

4 Basic requirements of tuina practice on the human body

4 推拿人体操作的基本要求

(1) It is needed to take off watch and ring before practice, in order to avoid damaging the patient.

（1）操作训练前必须解除手表、戒指，以免伤及受术者。

(2) It is needed to wash the hands before class, and maintain personal sanitation and hygiene.

（2）上课前必须洗手，保持个人清洁卫生。

(3) In accordance with the clinical requirements, it is needed to spread the sheet and towel, and tidy up the treatment table and stool.

（3）按照临床的要求，垫铺床单和治疗巾，以及整理推拿床和凳子。

(4) It is needed to take off shoes before stepping on the table, and take off the belt for practice on the lumbar region, back and abdomen.

（4）上床必须脱鞋，腰背部、腹部操作必须去掉皮带。

(5) It is needed to tide up the sheet and towel upon the requirements after practice is finished.

（5）操作完成后必须按规定整理床单、治疗巾。

(6) It is necessary for every student to posses the spirit to serve the classmates and help each other, and to practice on other students and also to be the receiver of the practice from other students.

（6）每个学生都应该有为同学服务的精神和互助精神，在为别人施术的同时还应主动当好受术者。

(7) In the training, it is needed to keep quiet in the classroom.

（7）操作训练时保持教室安静。

(8) In the training, it is needed to concentrate the mind, and prohibit laughing and playing and carelessness.

（8）操作时必须集中精力，不可嬉笑和漫不经心。

(9) It is needed to adjust the intensity of the stimulation from the manual techniques in accordance with the subject's reaction (facial expression, change in the muscular tension, etc).

（9）学会根据受术者的反应（面部反应、肌张力变化等）调整手法的刺激量。

(10) It is needed to be able to practice with two hands, i.e. practice with the two hands in alternation or practice with the two hands in coordination.

(10) 尽量做到每个操作法双手都能操作，即能左右手交替操作或双手协同操作。

(11) It is needed to complete the classroom training items based upon the teaching process with the guidance of the teachers, and not to try rashly or train in advance those techniques have not been demonstrated, in order to avoid accidents.

(11) 在教师的指导下，按照教学进度完成课堂训练项目，不要轻易尝试或提前操作没有示范过的操作法，以免发生意外。

(12) It is needed to review and train subjectively the contents of each lecture.

(12) 每次上课的内容课后都应自觉复习、训练。

(13) It is needed to review the knowledge in relation to the relevant courses on human anatomy, and meridians and acupoints.

(13) 及时补习与课程相关的人体解剖学和经络腧穴学知识。

Section 2 Massage practice on various body parts

第2节 人体不同部位的推拿操作

1 Practice on the head and face (supine position)

After the patient takes a supine position, mainly: ① open the heavenly gate, ② push the forehead divergently, ③ knead the forehead and cheek with the thenar, ④ push the orbit with the side of the thumb, ⑤ hook and knead Zanzhu (BL 2) with the two fingers, ⑥ knead Yingxiang (LI 20), Xiaguan (ST 7), Tinggong (SI 19), and Yifeng (TE 17) with the middle finger, ⑦ knead Taiyang (Extra) with the thumb, ⑧ press the orbit with the thumb, ⑨ press Yintang (Extra) to Baihui (GV 20) with the finger, ⑩ knead the bilateral temple regions with the four fingers, ⑪ uphold and knead the nape

1 头面部操作(仰卧位)

患者取仰卧位，主要操作：①开天门；②分推前额部；③鱼际揉前额与面颊部；④一指禅偏锋推眼眶；⑤二指勾揉攒竹穴；⑥中指揉迎香、下关、听宫、翳风；⑦拇指揉太阳穴；⑧拇指按眼眶；⑨指按印堂穴—百会穴；⑩四指揉两侧头颞部；⑪四指托揉项部；⑫仰卧拔伸颈椎；⑬指击前额部。

with the four fingers, ⑫ pull and stretch the cervical vertebras in the spine position, ⑬ pat the forehead with the finger.

2　Practice on the head and face (sitting position)

After the patient takes a sitting position, mainly: ① open the heavenly gate, ② wipe the forehead and orbit (with the two hands), ③ knead the forehead with the thenar, ④ sweep the temple, and ⑤ grasp the five meridians.

2　头面部操作(坐位)

患者取坐位,主要操作:①开天门;②抹前额、眼眶(双手);③鱼际揉前额;④扫散颞部;⑤抓五经。

3　Practice on the nape (prone position)

After the patient takes a prone position, mainly: ① push the nape with the thumb, ② grasp the nape, ③ hook and knead bilateral Fengchi (GB 20) with the middle fingers of the two hands, ④ knead the superaspinous fossa with the palm, ⑤ roll the nape and shoulder, ⑥ pluck the superior scapular angle and medial border of the scapula, ⑦ press the first and second lateral lines of the bladder meridian with the finger, ⑧ press the superaspinous fossa, ⑨ push the nape divergently with the thumb, ⑩ grasp Jianjing (GB 21), and ⑪ pat the nape and shoulder.

3　颈项部操作(俯卧位)

患者取俯卧位,主要操作:①一指禅推项部;②拿项部;③双手中指勾揉两侧风池穴;④掌揉冈上窝;⑤㨰项肩部;⑥弹拨肩胛上角和肩胛骨内侧缘;⑦指按膀胱经第一、二侧线;⑧指按冈上窝;⑨拇指分推项肩部;⑩拿肩井;⑪叩击项肩部。

4　Practice on the nape (sitting position)

After the patient takes a sitting position, mainly: ① push the nape with the thumb, ② roll the shoulder and back, ③ combine the rolling method with the passive movement of the nape (forward flexion, backward extension, leftward flexion, rightward flexion, and horizontal rotation), ④ press and knead the nape with the thumb, ⑤ knead the shoulder and back with the palm, ⑥ pull and stretch the cervical vertebras (the pulling method by palm up-

4　颈项部操作(坐位)

患者取坐位,主要操作:①一指禅推项部;②㨰肩背部;③㨰法配合颈部被动运动(前屈后伸、左右侧屈、水平旋转);④拇指按揉项部;⑤掌揉肩背部;⑥拔伸颈椎(掌托拔伸法,肘托拔伸法);⑦拿风池;⑧拿项部;⑨拿肩井,按天宗;⑩拳背击大椎、

holding action, the pulling method by elbow upholding action), ⑦ grasp Fengchi (GB 20), ⑧ grasp the nape, ⑨ grasp Jianjing (GB 21) and press Tianzong (SI 11), ⑩ strike Dazhui (GV 14) with the back of the fist, and pat the shoulder and back, and ⑪ rub and knead the back.

叩击肩背部;⑪搓揉肩背部。

5 Practice on the shoulder and upper limb (prone position)

After the patient takes a sitting position, mainly: ① push the shoulder with the thumb, ② roll the shoulder, ③ combine the rolling method with the passive movement of the shoulder joint (abduction, abduction and upholding, anterior flexion and upholding, adduction, backward bending), ④ grasp the deltoid muscles with the two hands, ⑤ grasp the triceps muscle of the arm, ⑥ pull and stretch the shoulder joint, ⑦ rotate the shoulder joints (the shoulder-rotating method by upholding the elbow, the shoulder-rotating method by holding the elbow, and the shoulder-rotating method in a large amplitude), ⑧ rotate the elbow joint, ⑨ hold and rotate the shoulder and rub the upper limb, and ⑩ rotate the upper limb.

5 肩与上肢部操作(坐位)

患者取坐位,主要操作:①一指禅推肩部;②㨰肩部;③㨰法配合肩关节被动运动(外展、外展上举、前屈上举、内收、后弯);④双手拿三角肌;⑤拿肱三头肌;⑥拔伸肩关节;⑦摇肩关节(托肘摇肩法、扶肘摇肩法、大幅度摇肩法);⑧摇肘关节;⑨抱揉肩部和搓上肢;⑩抖上肢。

6 Practice on the lumbar region (prone position)

After the patient takes a prone position, mainly: ① knead the lumbar region by piled palms, ② roll the lower back, ③ pluck the two sides of the lower back by the piled thumbs, ④ press the first and second lateral pathways of the bladder meridian at the back, ⑤ press the spine with the piled palms (lower portion of the thoracic vertebras, lumbar vertebras and sacral vertebras), ⑥ push the Governor Vessel with the palm, ⑦ push the bladder meridian at the back with the elbow, ⑧ pull and

6 腰背部操作(俯卧位)

患者取俯卧位,主要操作:①叠掌揉腰背部;②㨰腰背部;③叠拇指弹拨腰背部两侧;④指压腰背部膀胱经第一、二侧线;⑤叠掌按脊柱(下段胸椎、腰椎与骶骨);⑥掌推督脉;⑦肘推背部膀胱经;⑧拔伸腰椎;⑨斜扳腰椎(侧卧位);⑩横擦腰部;⑪叩击腰背部。

stretch the lumbar vertebras, ⑨ pull the lumbar vertebras obliquely (in lateral recumbent position), and ⑩ strike the lower back.

7 Posterior aspect of the lower limb (supine position)

After the patient takes a prone position, mainly: ① knead the buttocks with the palm, ② roll the buttocks from the posterior aspect of the lower limb to the heel, ③ roll the buttock in combination of the passive movement of the hip joint (backward extension, abduction, inward rotation and outward rotation of the hip joint), ④ roll the buttocks and lateral aspect of the lower limb (abduction and outward rotation of the hip joint, and knee flexion), ⑤ grasp the posterior aspect of the lower limb, ⑥ push the posterior aspect of the lower limb with the palm, and press the lower limb, and ⑦ rub and grasp the thigh.

7 下肢后部(俯卧位)

患者取俯卧位,主要操作:①掌揉臀部;②㨰臀部、下肢后面至跟腱部;③㨰臀部并配合髋关节被动运动(髋关节后伸;外展;旋内、旋外)。④㨰臀部以及下肢外侧(髋关节外展、旋外并屈膝位);⑤拿下肢后部;⑥掌推下肢后面并撑压下肢;⑦搓拿大腿。

8 Anterior aspect of the lower limb (supine position)

After the patient takes a supine position, mainly: ① press the anterior aspect of the thigh with the palm, ② grasp the quadriceps muscle of the thigh with the two hands, ③ press and knead Zusanli (ST 36) and Yanglingquan (GB 34) with the thumb, ④ grasp the posterior aspect of the leg to the heel (in position with the knee and hip flexed), ⑤ pull and stretch the lumbar vertebras, ⑥ rotate the hip joint, and ⑦ rub and shake the lower limb.

8 下肢前部(俯卧位)

患者取仰卧位,主要操作:①掌按股前部;②双手拿股四头肌;③拇指按揉足三里、阳陵泉;④拿小腿后部至跟腱(屈膝屈髋位);⑤拔伸腰椎;⑥摇髋关节;⑦搓抖下肢。

9 Practice on the abdomen (supine position)

After the patient takes a supine position, mainly: ① push the infraclavicular fossa divergently with the thumb, ② chafe the upper chest trans-

9 胸腹部操作(俯卧位)

患者取仰卧位,主要操作:①拇指分推锁骨下窝;②横擦上胸部;③一指禅偏

versely, ③ push the anterior midline of the chest and abdomen with the side of the thumb, ④ push the abdomen with the thumb, ⑤ circularly rub the abdomen with the palm, ⑥ knead the abdomen with the palm, ⑦ press Qihai (CV 6), Shenque (CV 8) and Zhongwan (CV 12) with the palm, ⑧ vibrate the lower abdomen with the palm, and ⑨ push the abdomen divergently.

锋推胸腹部前正中线；④一指禅推腹部；⑤掌摩腹部；⑥掌揉腹部；⑦掌按气海、神阙、中脘；⑧掌振小腹部；⑨分推腹部。

Twelve Regular Meridinas 十二正经

1. Lung Meridian of Hand-Taiyin 手太阴肺经
2. Large Intestine Meridian of Hand-Yangming 手阳明大肠经
3. Stomach Meridian of Footv-Yangming 足阳明胃经
4. Spleen Meridian of Foot-Taiyin 足太阴脾经
5. Heart Meridian of Hand-Shaoyin 手少阴心经
6. Small Intestine of Hand-Taiyang 手太阳小肠经
7. Bladder Meridian of Foot-Taiyang 足太阳膀胱经
8. Kidney Meridian of Foot-Shaoyin 足手阴肾经
9. Pericardium Meridian of Hand-Jueyin 手厥阴心包经
10. Triple Energizer Meridian of Hand-Shaoyang 手少阳三焦经
11. Gallbladder Meridian of Foot-Shaoyang 足少阳胆经
12. Liver Meridian of Foot-Jueyin 足厥阴肝经

Eight Extraordinary Meridians 奇经八脉

1. Governor Vessel 督脉
2. Conception Vessel 任脉
3. Thoroughfare Vessel 冲脉
4. Belt Vessel 带脉
5. Yin Heel Vessel 阴跷脉
6. Yang Heel Vessel 阳跷脉
7. Yin Link Vessel 阴维脉
8. Yang Link Vessel 阳维脉

Chapter 5 General theory on tuina therapy

第5章 推拿治疗总论

Section 1 Therapeutic effects of tuina therapy

第1节 推拿的治疗作用

In terms of the local areas of the limbs, the therapeutic effects of tuina therapy are supposed to circulate qi, activate blood, disperse blood stasis, diminish swelling, soothe the tendons and alleviate spasm, treat pain by relaxation, regulate and lubricate the joints, and adjust the spine for reposition, and in terms of the whole body, are supposed to dredge the meridians and collaterals, regulate and harmonize qi and blood, balance yin and yang, regulate Zangfu organs, support the constitution, correct deficiency, protect the body surface and expel the pathogens.

推拿的治疗作用，对于肢体局部而言，有行气活血、化瘀消肿，舒筋缓急、以松治痛，调利关节、整脊复位的作用。对于全身整体而言，有疏通经络、调和气血，平衡阴阳、调理脏腑，扶正补虚、卫外祛邪的作用。

1 Local effects

1 局部作用

1.1 Circulate qi, activate blood, disperse blood stasis and diminish swelling

1.1 行气活血，化瘀消肿

The mechanical stimulation or warm stimulation from the manual techniques function on the specific areas or acupoints of the body surface, to directly excite the meridian qi, improve the microcirculation and regulate the circulation of qi and

推拿手法的机械刺激或温热刺激，作用于体表特定部位或腧穴，可直接激发经气，改善微循环，调整局部的气血运行。推拿治疗软组织

blood in the local areas. tuina therapy has the obvious effects to activate blood, disperse blood stasis, diminish swelling and stop pain in the treatment of soft tissue injury.

损伤有明显的活血化瘀、消肿止痛作用。

The mechanical stimulation from the power of the manual techniques functions on the soft tissues, can promote the reflux of the venous blood and lymphatic fluid, improve the local blood circulation, accelerate the absorption of blood stasis and effusion, and quickly eliminate the local pain and tumefaction.

手法力的机械刺激作用于软组织,可促进静脉血和淋巴液的回流,改善局部的血液循环,加快瘀血和渗出液的吸收,能较快地消除局部的疼痛和肿胀。

The warm stimulation from the manual techniques also has the effects to warm up the meridians, dredge the collaterals, circulate qi and stop pain. There is such a description that "the heat sensation would appear by pressure. As soon as heat sensation arrives, pain would stop" in *Essential Questions* (Su Wen). It is said in *Savior General Compendium* (Sheng Ji Zong Lu) that, "the obstruction can be removed, once blood and qi are warmed up".

推拿手法的温热刺激,也有温经通络、行气止痛的作用。《素问·举痛论》篇有"按之则热气至,热气至则痛止矣"的描述。《圣济总录》云:"血气得温则宣通。"

There are many manual techniques to promote the circulation of qi and blood. In addition to the techniques to press and knead the specific acupoints by the finger, frequently there are the techniques to push the four limbs centripetally, pinch and grasp the four limbs, pat and strike and press the artery, in combination of the heat compress, etc.

促进气血流通的推拿操作法很多,除了指压、按揉特定腧穴外,常用的有向心性推四肢、捏拿四肢、拍打叩击、按压动脉、手法配合热敷等。

1.2 Soothe the tendons and alleviate spasm, treat pain by relaxation

1.2 舒筋缓急,以松治痛

The tendons refer to the muscular tendons in Chinese medicine, mainly the soft tissues of skeletal muscles and fascia. To soothe the tendons means to relax the soft tissues. To alleviate spasm means to e-

筋,是中医的经筋,主要指骨骼肌、筋膜等软组织。舒筋,指放松软组织;缓急,指解除肌肉的痉挛。肌肉痉

liminate the muscular spasm. Muscular spasm is often the self protective reaction of the organism to the harmful stimulation of pain. Spasm and pain interact as both cause and effect, forming the vicious circle.

挛，往往是肌体对疼痛等伤害性刺激的自我保护反应。痉挛与疼痛可以互为因果，并形成恶性循环。

Clinically, there are mainly two types of the manual techniques to block the vicious circle of "spasm-pain". One type of the manual techniques is the stimulating technique of local soft tissue by pain as the acupoint, such as pressing-kneading technique, pressing technique, springing-plucking technique, and stick-striking technique, etc. The muscles are relaxed by the analgesic effect. The muscles can be relaxed without pain. This type of the manual techniques has also the effects to relieve the adhesion of the soft tissues, and eliminate the nervous compress. Another type of the manual techniques, such as the pulling-stretching method, passive movement of the joint, is used to quickly relax the muscle for alleviating the muscular spasm by prolonging the spasmodic muscles, so as to improve the blood supply of the injured soft tissues, eliminate the aseptic inflammation of soft tissue and treat pain by relaxation.

推拿临床阻断"痉挛－疼痛"恶性循环的操作手法，主要有两类。一类是以痛为腧的局部软组织刺激手法，如按揉、点按、弹拨、棒击等，通过镇痛而放松肌肉，不痛则松。这类手法还有松解软组织粘连，解除神经卡压的作用。另一类是拉伸手法，如拔伸法、关节被动运动等，通过拉长痉挛的肌肉能迅速放松该肌肉以缓解其痉挛，进而改善损伤软组织的血液供应，消除软组织无菌性炎症，以松治痛。

1.3 Regulate and lubricate the joints, and adjust the spine for reposition

1.3 调利骨节，整脊复位

Tuina therapy has the effects to correct dislocation and lubricate the joints.

推拿具有整复错缝，滑利关节的作用。

Various acute and chronic injuries can induce in different degrees the laceration, local hemorrhage, organization of hematoma muscles, and hence adhesion in the muscles, tendons, ligaments and articular capsules around the joints of the four limbs, further resulting in the symptoms of acute or chronic

各种急慢性损伤，都可能不同程度地引起四肢关节周围的肌肉、肌腱、韧带、关节囊的撕裂伤，局部出血、血肿机化而产生粘连，并进而产生急慢性疼痛和关节活动

pain and functional disturbance of the articular activities. The reasons of closed-plaster method after fracture and paralysis can also induce the sequela of the functional disturbance of the articular activities. tuina therapy can be used to treat articular dislocation, joint displacement and their functional disturbance, and restore the normal functions of the joints and can be used in different stages of the treatment and rehabilitation.

功能障碍症状。骨折石膏固定、瘫痪卧床不起等原因也可造成关节活动功能障碍的后遗症。推拿能治疗关节脱位、骨错缝及其功能失衡,能使受限的关节恢复正常的活动功能,可应用于治疗和康复的不同阶段。

In addition to the manual techniques to relax the soft tissues around the joints for lubricating the joints by tuina therapy, there are the commonly used methods, such as the flexion-extension method, the pulling-stretching method, the pulling method, the rotating method, the shaking method, and the treading method, or the rolling method in combination of the passive movements of the patient's joint. It is advisable to guide the patient to train Shaolin internal works and the tendon-changing exercises, etc.

推拿滑利关节除了放松关节周围软组织的手法以外,常用的手法还有屈伸法、拔伸法、扳法、旋转法、摇法、抖法、踩蹻法等,或在㨰法等手法操作中配合患者的关节被动运动。还可以指导病人自我锻炼少林内功、易筋经等功法。

The tuina manual techniques can effectively be used to relax the soft tissues around the spine, and correct the minor dislocation of the posterior spinal joints, and treat neck pain and low back pain induced by the disturbance of the posterior spinal joints. There are the specific manual techniques, such as pressing-kneading method along the spine, the pulling-stretching method for the cervical vertebras, the pulling-stretching method for the lumbar vertebras, the oblique pulling method for the lumbar vertebras, the pulling method by rotation for the cervical vertebras, and the spine-setting technique by resistance and traction for the thoracic vertebras, etc.

推拿手法还能有效地放松脊柱周围的软组织,整复脊柱后关节的轻微错缝,治疗脊柱后关节紊乱引起的颈项疼痛和腰背痛。针对性手法有脊柱沿线的按揉法、颈椎拔伸法、腰椎拔伸法,以及腰椎斜扳法、颈椎旋转扳法、胸椎对抗复位法等整脊手法。

2 Holistic functions

2.1 Dredge the meridians and collaterals, regulate and harmonize qi and blood

The meridians are the pathways for the circulation of qi and blood inside the human body, and pertain to Zangfu organs internally and communicate with the joints externally and integrate the organs, tissues and four limbs into an organic entity, for regulating the functions of the various internal organs of the whole body. Once the functions of the meridians are abnormal in the human body, disturbance will surely take place in the circulation of qi and blood, leading to various diseases. Just as it is said in Su Wen: "if qi and blood are not in harmony, hundreds diseases may occur due to their changes."

In addition to "the finger replacing the needle", similar to the acupuncture stimulation on the acupoints and meridians, tuina therapy in dredging the meridians and collaterals can further directly excite qi and blood, function on the meridians, and promote the circulation of qi and blood. The function to dredge the meridians and collaterals by tuina therapy was mentioned earliest in Su Wen: "Frequent fear and fright are usually related to the obstruction of the meridians and collaterals, manifested by numbness, and should be treated with massage and medicated wine." In tuina therapy, pattern identification based upon the theory of the meridians is highly emphasized, and the manual techniques are often given to "push the acupoints and go through the meridians." Its theoretic foundation is exactly what the forefathers mentioned: "where the

2 整体作用

2.1 疏通经络，调和气血

经络是人体运行气血的通道，内属脏腑，外络肢节，将人体的组织器官、四肢百骸联络成一个有机的整体，以调节全身各部脏腑器官的机能。一旦人体经络功能失常，气血运行必然发生障碍，因而发生各种疾病。正如《素问・调经论》所说："气血不和，百病乃变化而生。"

推拿的疏通经络作用，除了"以指代针"，类似于针刺刺激腧穴和经络以外，更能直接激荡气血，作用于经脉，推动气血运行。《素问・血气形志》篇最早提出了按摩的疏通经络作用："形数惊恐，经络不通，病生于不仁，治之于按摩醪药。"中医推拿十分重视经络辨证，手法所施，主张"推穴道，走经络"，其理论依据，就是前人总结出来的"经脉所过，主治所及"。用于疏通经络的推拿操作，主要是循经取穴，指压、按揉、点穴、叩击、向心性推等手法均可运用。

meridians go, where the problems will be." The manual techniques for dredging the meridians are mainly the selection of the acupoints based upon the meridians, finger-pressing, pressing-kneading, acupoint-pressing, striking, and centripetal-pushing method, etc.

Tuina therapy is able to regulate qi and blood, and also able to regulate the functions of the heart and lung and promote the circulation of qi and blood in the whole body by the meridian system.

推拿能调和气血，还在于通过经络系统调整心、肺等脏腑功能，推动全身的气血运行。

2.2 Balance yin and yang, and regulate Zangfu organs

2.2 平衡阴阳，调理脏腑

The theory of yin and yang is an ancient philosophic concept in China and is a high summary of the mutually related objects or phenomena of mutual opposition in the natural world. The theory of yin and yang belongs to one of the core contents in the basic theory of Chinese medicine. Physiologically, yin and yang are used to divide the body parts, term the meridians, and explain the various physiological phenomena of the human body and their relationship with Zangfu organs. Pathologically, occurrence, development and transmission of diseases are all related to yin and yang. In terms of the body parts, the body surface is yang and the interior body is yin. The upper body is yang and the lower body is yin. The back is yang and abdomen is yin. In terms of Zangfu organs, six hollow organs belong to yang and five solid organs belong to yin. In terms of qi and blood in the human body, qi is yang and blood is yin. In terms of the functions and substances, the function is yang and the substance is yin. In terms of the states of the functional activities, the excitement is yang and the inhibition is yin, and the activ-

阴阳是中国古代哲学概念，是对自然界相互关联的事物或现象对立双方属性的高度概括。阴阳学说是中医基本理论的核心内容之一。生理上，阴阳用于人体部位的划分，用于经络的命名，用于阐释人体各种生理现象，及脏腑之间的关系；病理上，疾病的产生、发展与传变无不与阴阳有关。就人体部位而言，体表为阳、体内为阴；上部为阳、下部为阴；背部为阳、腹部为阴。就脏腑而言，六腑为阳、五脏为阴。就人体气血而言，气为阳、血为阴。就功能与物质而言，功能为阳、物质为阴。就功能活动的状态而言，兴奋为阳、抑制为阴；活动为阳、静止为阴；增长为阳、减退为阴。就气机运行而言，上升为阳、下

ity is yang and tranquility is yin, and the increase is yang and the decrease is yin. In terms of qi dynamics, ascension is yang and descending is yin, and the outward is yang and the inward is yin.

降为阴；向外为阳、向内为阴等。

Zangfu organs are the important organs to produce and transform qi and blood, regulate and dredge the meridians and collaterals, and maintain the life activities of the human body. The dysfunction in Zangfu organs will lead to various diseases.

脏腑是生化气血、通调经络、维持人体生命活动的主要器官。脏腑功能失调会发生各种疾病。

Tuina therapy to balance yin and yang and regulate Zangfu organs is realized based upon the premise for dredging the meridians and harmonizing qi and blood by the manual techniques on the meridians, acupoints, dynamic and static status and operating direction. For instance, to stimulate the specific Front-Mu acupoints, Back-Shu acupoints and other adjuvant acupoints by the light and gentle one-thumb pushing method, kneading method and rubbing method can deal with yin deficiency, yang deficiency or deficiency of both yin and yang in the corresponding internal organs. When the rubbing, chafing or pressing manual techniques of the strong power are used, they are able to expel pathogens and reduce the excess. For diseases in pattern of cold and deficiency, it is advisable to operate on the treatment areas by the slow and gentle and rhythmical manual techniques for a comparatively long time, so as to have the patient warming sensation in the deep layer, for realizing the effects to warm up yang and benefit qi. Besides, to chafe the lower back lightly is able to nourish yin and reduce fire, for clearing away deficient heat from blood. To push the Governor Vessel lightly from Dazhui (GV 14) to the sacral vertebras is able to clear away ex-

推拿平衡阴阳、调整脏腑是以疏通经络、调和气血为前提的，主要通过手法、经络、穴道、动静状态、操作方向等实现。如应用轻柔缓和的一指禅推法、揉法与摩法，刺激特定的募穴、俞穴及其他配穴，能补益相应脏腑的阴虚、阳虚或阴阳两虚，而使用力量较强的摩擦或挤压类手法，则能祛邪泻实；对阴寒虚冷的病证，要用较慢而柔和的节律性手法在治疗部位上作较长时间的操作，使患者产生深层的温热感，则有温阳益气的作用。此外，轻擦腰部，能养阴泻火，以清血中虚热；自大椎至尾椎轻推督脉，可清气分实热，在同一路线上重推督脉，则能清热凉血，以泻血分实热。手法操作时，方向向上，顺其阳升之势，能助阳上升；而方向向下，顺其阴降之势，则有降逆安神之功。

cessive heat from Qi-energy phase. To push the Governor Vessel on the same route strongly can help to clear away heat and cool blood, for reducing the excessive heat from Xue-blood phase. In the application of the manual techniques, by upward direction, it is able to follow the rising tendency of yang, for assisting yang to rise. By downward direction, it is able to follow the descending tendency of yin, for correcting the reverse flow and calming the mind.

Tuina therapy has a better bipolar regulation for Zangfu organs. Its principle is the direct effect on one hand, i.e. stimulate the body surface by the manual techniques to directly influence the functions of Zangfu organs, and the indirect effect on the other hand, i.e. to realize the effect by the relationship between the meridians and Zangfu organs.

推拿对脏腑功能具有良好的双向调节作用。其原理一是直接作用,即通过手法刺激体表而直接影响脏腑功能;二是间接作用,即通过经络与脏腑间的联系来实现。

For instance, in replenishing the kidney, tuina is often applied on the low back, especially on the local acupoints of Mingmen (GV 4), Yaoyangguan (GV 3), Shenshu (BL 23), Qihaishu (BL 24), Dachangshu (BL 25), and Guanyuanshu (BL 26). Qihai (CV 6), Guanyuan (CV 4) and Dantian (Extra) are also the important acupoints to replenish the kidney. In the selection of the acupoints along the meridians, Yongquan (KI 1) and Taixi (KI 3) are mainly selected from the kidney meridian, and massaged mostly by the manual techniques of the rubbing method and chafing method. In combination of the manual techniques and medicinal stuffs, paste massage therapy can also be used to replenish the kidney.

如推拿补肾,常在腰部施术,特别是在腰部的命门、腰阳关、肾俞、气海俞、大肠俞、关元俞等腧穴局部取穴,小腹部的气海、关元、丹田也是补肾要穴。循经远道取穴,则以涌泉、太溪等肾经腧穴为主。手法多取摩法、擦法等。还可运用膏摩法,手法结合药物,而发挥补肾作用。

Tuina therapy is specifically advantageous in regulating the spleen and stomach. Its therapeutic

调理脾胃是推拿疗法的特长。其治法一是在腹部局

methods are just supposed to process local massage on the abdomen and to select Back-Shu acupoints or select acupoints along the meridians, practically by the operating methods to rub the abdomen circularly, push the abdomen with one thumb, and press and knead Tianshu (ST 25), Guanyuan (CV 4) and Zhongwan (CV 12), and press Pishu (BL 20), Weishu (BL 21), Dachangshu (BL 25) and Zusanli (ST 36), and vibrate the abdomen with the palm, and chafe the bladder meridian at the back. For constipation caused by reduced peristalsis of the stomach and intestines, it is advisable to rub and knead along the direction of peristalsis for digesting food and removing food retention.

部操作，一是取背俞穴或循经取穴。操作法有摩腹，一指禅推腹部，按揉天枢、关元、中脘，点按脾俞、胃俞、大肠俞、足三里，掌振腹部，擦背部膀胱经等。对于胃肠蠕动功能减弱所致的便秘不通，多顺肠蠕动方向揉摩，以消食导滞。

The specific advantage in the treatment of pulmonary diseases by tuina therapy is to dissolve phlegm and release phlegm. For instance, the vibrating method by the palm and the patting method by the palm on the upper back can help to vibrate and clean away phlegm and fluid from the air passage, accelerate its outward motion, and dissolve release phlegm. This method has the therapeutic or auxiliary effect on many types of pulmonary diseases, such as cough and asthma, and can also stimulate Feishu (BL 13), Dingchuan (Extra), Zhongfu (LU 1), Yunmen (LU 2), and Lieque (LU 7) via the meridian system for playing a role in the pulmonary system.

推拿治疗肺系病证的独特之处，在于化痰排痰。如在上背部施以掌振法、掌拍法，可振荡气道内的痰涎，加速其由内向外运动，而有化痰排痰之功。此法对咳嗽、哮喘等多种肺系病证有治疗或辅助治疗作用。也可刺激肺俞、定喘、中府、云门、列缺等腧穴通过经络系统而对肺系起作用。

Tuina therapy can regulate the cardiac functions. Chest pain (coronary heart disease) induced by obstruction of the heart blood and blockage of heart meridian can be treated by kneading Xinshu (BL 15) and Jueyinshu (BL 14). To stimulate Neiguan (PC 6) by the strong pressing method and

推拿可以调节心脏的功能，按揉心俞、厥阴俞可治疗由于心血淤阻、血脉不通而引起的胸痹（冠心病）等疾病。用较强的按法、拿法刺激内关，可使心率加快，用于

grasping method can speed up the heartbeat, used for treatment of bradycardia. To stimulate Neiguan (PC 6) by the weak pressing method and kneading method can also slow down the heartbeat, used for the treatment of tachycardia.

治疗心动过缓;用较弱的按法、揉法刺激内关,又可使心率减慢,用于治疗心动过速。

The posterior spinal joint disturbance can induce local pain of the spine and can also influence the physiological functions of various systems of the human body. Therefore, it is termed "spinal diseases". The manual techniques for the posterior spinal joints and soft tissues around the spine are also specifically advantageous in balancing yin and yang, and regulating Zangfu organs.

脊柱后关节紊乱除了引起脊柱局部的疼痛外,还可影响人体各系统的脏腑功能,因而被称为"脊柱源性疾病"。针对脊柱后关节及其脊柱周围软组织的手法,也是推拿平衡阴阳、调理脏腑的独特之处。

2.3 Support the constitution and correct deficiency, and defend the body surface and expel pathogens

2.3 扶正补虚,卫外祛邪

To support the constitution means to support and assist the constitutional energy and strengthen the anti-pathogenic ability of the human body. To expel pathogens means to dissipate the pathogenic factors. tuina therapy has better effects to support the constitution and expel pathogens. It is believed in Chinese medicine: as soon as the constitutional energy exists inside, the pathogenic factors cannot do anything. If the pathogenic factor can impact the body, the constitutional energy is surely deficient. To support the constitution and expel pathogens means to correct deficiency and purge excess.

扶正,是扶助人体正气,增强抗病能力;祛邪,指祛除致病因素。推拿有很好的扶正祛邪作用。中医认为:正气存内,邪不可干;邪之所凑,其气必虚。扶正祛邪,就是补虚泻实。

To support the constitution and correct deficiency is just for deficient patterns of the human body. It is said in *Inner Canon* (Nei Jing) that, the reinforcing technique should be used for deficiency, and the benefiting technique should be used for depletion. The reinforcing technique can excite or

扶正补虚,是针对人的虚证。《内经》说"虚则补之""损者益之"。补法能焕发或振奋人体各部器官组织,使其机能旺盛。推拿作为一种外治法,其补虚的机制与中

boost the various organs and tissues of the human body, flourishing the physiological functions. As an external therapy, tuina therapy is different in the mechanism of deficiency correction from the reinforcing technique by oral administration of herbal drugs. First of all, Zangfu organs are regulated holistically for realizing the effect to correct deficiency. By the holistic regulatory effect of the meridians and the specific effects of the acupoints, the kidneys can be benefited and the spleen can be strengthened to excite the functions of Zangfu organs. The typical tuina techniques are supposed to rub the abdomen, rub the lower abdomen, vibrate the lower abdomen by the palm, vibrate Xinshu (BL 15) by the palm, press and knead Shenshu (BL 23), Pishu (BL 20), Xinshu (BL 15), Feishu (BL 13), Shenshu (BL 23), Zhongwan (CV 12), Qihai (CV 6) and Guanyuan (CV 4), etc. Secondly, qi and blood are circulated locally for realizing the effect to correct deficiency. By the effects of tuina manual techniques to circulate qi and activate blood, blood in the whole body can be allocated once again to solve the symptoms of local blood deficiency. It was pointed out by WU Shiji of the Qing Dynasty in *Parallel Prose on Theory* (Li Yue Pian Wen) that "the circulation of qi and blood is exactly a reinforcement, not just by Radix Ginseng (Ren Shen) and Sclerotium Poria (Fu Ling)" in the external therapy. For instance, the one-finger pushing method, grasping method, and pulling-stretching method applied on the nape can improve blood supply to the brain, used for treating dizziness induced by insufficient blood supply in the brain. Thirdly, the topical application of the herbal stuffs can be adopted to re-

药内服之补法有所不同。首先是通过整体调整脏腑而发挥补虚作用。通过经络的整体调整作用和腧穴的特异性作用,可起到益肾、健脾等振奋脏腑机能的作用。典型的推拿操作法有摩腹,摩丹田,掌振丹田,掌振心俞,按揉肾俞、脾俞、心俞、肺俞、肾俞、中脘、气海、关元等。其次是通过局部流通气血而发挥补虚作用。通过推拿手法的行气活血效应,使得全身血液重新分配,解决局部血虚症状。清代吴师机《理瀹骈文》提出了外治法"气血流通即是补,非必以参苓为补也"的观点。如颈项部的一指禅推法、拿法、拔伸法可改善脑部的血液供应,治疗脑部供血不足之眩晕等。第三是借助药物外治而发挥补虚作用。膏摩是推拿疗法的特色之一。借助有补益作用的摩膏,以手法助药力,使药物经皮吸收,亦可起到补益作用。

alize the effect to correct deficiency. Paste massage is one of tuina therapies. By the paste with tonic effect, the manual techniques can be used to assist the herbal potency, so as to have the herbal stuffs absorbed through the skin for playing a tonic role.

Tuina therapy in the effect to support the constitution and correct deficiency is also reflected in the treatment of unformed diseases, and has been extensively used for sub-health group.

推拿的扶正补虚作用，还体现在推拿的治未病方面，而被广泛应用于亚健康人群。

To defend body surface and expel pathogens belongs to the reducing method. The terms of "the reducing method should be used for excess" described in *Spiritual Pivot* (Ling Shu) refers to the reducing method in the broad sense, just the method to expel the pathogens. There are many channels to expel the pathogens, the diaphoretic, vomiting, expectorating, laxative and diuretic methods all belongs to the reducing method. It is said in *Ten Massage Methods* (An Mo Shi Fa) that, if the reinforcing method or reducing method is not clear, massage will be ineffective.

卫外祛邪，属于泻法。《灵枢 · 经脉》的"盛则泻之"，也称实则泻之，是广义的泻法，泛指祛邪外出之法。祛邪的途径多端，发汗、催吐、排痰、通便、利尿均为泻法。《按摩十法》说："补泻不明，则按摩不灵。"

Tuina therapy can effectively expel the pathogens invading into the muscles and joints. It is recorded in *ZHANG Jingyue's Complete Compendium* (Jing Yue Quan Shu) that "the guiding technique can expel the pathogenic factor out of the joints, and massage can expel them out of the muscles". For pathogens in the joints, the passive guiding technique can be used, i. e. the manual techniques for moving the joints. For pathogens in the skin and muscles, the commonly used pushing method, rubbing method, chafing method, grasping method and patting method can be adopted. Paste massage is also an effective method. The reducing method in

推拿能有效祛除侵入肌肉、关节之邪。《景岳全书》记载："导引可逐客邪于关节，按摩可驱浮淫于肌肉。"针对关节之邪，可用被动导引之法，即运动关节类手法治疗。针对皮肤、肌肉之邪，常用的推法、摩法、擦法、拿法、拍打均可采用。膏摩法也是有效的方法。推拿之泻法，包含在汗法、散法、清法等治法中。

tuina therapy is included in the diaphoretic method, dispersing method, and clarifying method.

The effects of tuina therapy in expelling the pathogens inside the body are realized by many channels of the expectorating, laxative and diuretic method.

推拿对于祛除体内之邪,则通过排痰、通便、利尿等多种途径实现。

For instance, the laxative method is supposed to promote bowel movement by strengthening the peristalsis of the stomach and intestines. It is said in Su Wen that "the reducing method should be used for full sensation in the abdomen". The laxative method is usually used for accumulation of excessive heat in the stomach and intestines, retention of dry stool, constipation, abdominal lumps, abdominal pain, and fatty body, having the effects to dredge the hollow organs, remove the retention, and reduce body weight. Clinically, tuina is given on the abdomen, for directly irritating the stomach and intestines, by rubbing and kneading the abdomen clockwise in predominance, giving pressure on the sigmoid colon, and by stimulating the acupoints with the effects to dredge the hollow organs and promote bowel movement, such as Zusanli (ST 36), Zhigou (TE 6), Tianshu (ST 25), Shangliao (BL 31), Ciliao (BL 32), Zhonglliao (BL 33), Xialiao (BL 34), and Dachangshu (BL 25), for strengthening the peristalsis of the stomach and intestine by the meridian system.

如通便法。主要通过增强肠蠕动,促进大便排出。《素问·阴阳应象大论》篇云"中满者,泻之于内"。通便法针对胃肠实热积滞,燥屎内结,便秘不通,腹内结块,腹中疼痛,形体肥胖等里实之证,有通腑导滞,泄热排毒、减肥瘦身等的功效。推拿临床一是在腹部操作,直接刺激胃肠道,以顺时针方向摩揉腹部为主,重点在乙状结肠部加压;一是刺激有通腑排便作用的腧穴,如足三里、支沟、天枢、八髎、大肠俞等,通过经络系统增强胃肠道的蠕动功能。

As for the diuretic method, diuresis can be promoted by the manual technique. The diuretic method is used for difficult urination and retention of urine. For instance, for retention of urine in children, post-operative and postpartum retention of urine, urination can be promoted to expel pathogens

又如利尿法。通过手法刺激可促进排尿。利尿法针对小便不畅、小便不通之证,如小儿癃闭、手术后或产后尿潴留等,可通过促进小便而祛邪排毒。推拿临床一是

and discharge toxin. Clinically, tuina will be given on the lower abdomen, by kneading and rubbing the lower abdomen, pressing Guanyuan (CV 4), Zhongji (CV 3), Shuidao (ST 28), and Guilai (ST 29), and pushing and pressing the abdominal midline downward, and also on the sacral region, by pressing and kneading the lumbosacral angle, and pressing and kneading Shangliao (BL 31), Ciliao (BL 32), Zhonglliao (BL 33), Xialiao (BL 34), Xiaochangshu (BL 27), Pangguangshu (BL 28), and Zhonglushu (BL 29), and by pressing and kneading the adductor muscles of the thigh on one hand, and by irritating Sanyinjiao (SP 6), Yinlingquan (SP 9) and Kunlun (BL 60) by the manual techniques on the other hand, for strengthening the urinary functions via the meridian system.

在下腹部操作，揉摩小腹、按压关元、中极、水道、归来，从上往下推压腹部中线；一是在骶部操作，按揉腰骶角，按揉八髎、小肠俞、膀胱俞、中膂俞；一是按揉股内收肌群；一是手法刺激三阴交、阴陵泉、昆仑等腧穴，通过经络系统增强泌尿功能。

Section 2 Therapeutic principles of tuina therapy

第2节 推拿的治疗原则

The therapeutic principles of tuina therapy belong to the outline and general rules of common significance, stipulated based upon the features of tuina therapy, with the guidance of basic Chinese medical theory.

推拿的治疗原则，是在中医基础理论指导下，针对推拿疗法的特点而制定的具有普遍意义的大纲和总则。

1 Treat diseases for seeking the causative reason

It means to look for the fundamental reason of the diseases, in order to design the targeted treatment. It is said in Su Wen that "necessary to seek the original reason in the treatment of diseases".

1 治病求本

治病求本，就是寻求疾病的根本原因，而作针对性的治疗。《素问·阴阳应象大论》篇所说的"治病必求于

This is the most basic therapeutic principle for treatment based upon pattern identification in Chinese medicine and tuina therapy. “Root” and “branch” belong to a pair of relative concept. In terms of the anti-pathogenic ability and pathogenic factor, the anti-pathogenic ability is a root and the pathogenic factor is a branch. In terms of the causative factor, symptoms and signs, the causative factor is a root, and the symptoms and signs belong to a branch. In terms of priority of diseases, the primary diseases and old diseases are a root, and the secondary diseases and new diseases belong to a branch. The symptoms and signs are the external manifestations of the diseases, but do not exactly reflect their intrinsic quality, and even false phenomena. The root is the source of diseases and the branch is just the changes of diseases. Therefore, it is necessary to collect the key information about the diseases as much as possible, and to find out the “root” of diseases by comprehensive analysis and by seeing the essentials through appearance, in order to define the corresponding therapeutic methods.

本”，是中医和中医推拿辨证施治最基本的治疗原则。“本”与“标”是一对相对的概念。如从正气与邪气来看，正为本，邪为标；从病因与症状、体征来看，病因为本，症状、体征为标；从疾病的先后来看，原发病、旧病为本，继发病、新病为标。症状和体征是疾病的外在表现，但是并不一定能反映其本质，有的甚至是假象。本为病之源，标为病之变。应该尽可能充分地提取疾病的关键信息，通过综合分析，透过现象看到本质，找到病“本”之所在，以确定相应的治疗方法。

For instance, in the treatment of soft tissue pain by massage therapy, if focus of primary pain can be located and treated, the double results can be obtained by half the effort. If the secondary painful area or conductive painful region are misunderstood as the primary focus, concentrating on the trifles and neglecting the essentials, just treating the head for headache or foot for foot pain, it would be difficult to achieve the therapeutic effects or eradicate the problem. For instance, if the pathogenesis is understood about acute lumbar pain induced by incarceration of the synovial membrane of the lumbar

如推拿治疗软组织疼痛，若能找到原发性疼痛病灶而治之，往往事半功倍。假如将继发性疼痛部位或传导性疼痛区域误作原发病灶，舍本求末，简单地头痛医头、脚痛医脚，则很难取效或根治。又如腰椎滑膜嵌顿性急性腰痛，如果了解了发病机制，找到了合适的治疗体位和针对性的治疗手法，往往几分钟内就能见效。但如

vertebras, and the proper therapeutic position and targeted therapeutic techniques are found, the therapeutic effect can be achieved in several minutes. But, if treated just by the method for ordinary lumbar pain, actually no effect can be obtained by efforts, and even the pathological situation will be aggravated and linger for several days.

果按照普通的急性腰扭伤方法处理，则不仅劳而无功，甚至可能加重病情，数天不愈。

In the treatment of acute diseases by massage therapy, it is necessary to be in adaptability of "treating the branch for acute condition" in following the principle of "looking for the root in the treatment of diseases". At this moment, the attention focused on the branch is just a temporary measure in emergent situation, or just an expedient measure to create a condition for dealing with the root. For instance, if acute biliary colic occurs in travel, when acute cholecystitis or cholelithiasis cannot be confirmed, and no medical condition for emergency is available, it is advisable to press Dannangxue (Extra) or tender spot at the corresponding segment of the right back to alleviate pain, in order to save time for other treatments.

在推拿治疗急性病症时，贯彻"治病求本"的原则还应有一定的"急则治其标"的变通性。这时的治标只是在应急情况下的临时措施，或是为治本创造条件的权宜之计。如在旅游途中突发急性胆绞痛，在一时无法确诊是急性胆囊炎还是胆石症，且没有其他急救医疗条件时，可临时采用按压胆囊穴或右侧背部相应节段压痛点以镇痛，为其他治疗争取时间。

2 Support the constitution and expel pathogens

2 扶正祛邪

The major therapeutic method of "the sedative method for excess and reinforcing method for deficiency" was mentioned in Su Wen. To correct deficiency (support the constitution) and purge excess (expel pathogens) is a basic concept in the internal therapies and external therapies of Chinese medicine. Diseases are no more than deficient pattern caused by insufficiency of the constitutional energy or excessive pattern due to preponderance of pathogenic factors. The key in the treatment of diseases

《素问·至真要大论》篇提出了"盛者泻之，虚者补之"的治疗大法，补虚（扶正）泻实（祛邪）是中医内治法和外治法的基本理念。疾病不外是正气不足的虚证或邪气亢盛的实证。治疗疾病的实质，就是运用各种方法扶助正气，祛除邪气，改变邪正双方的力量对比，使之朝着有

is supposed to support the constitutional energy and expel pathogens by any possible methods, and change the force ratio between the pathogenic factor and anti-pathogenic ability, so as to help conversion beneficial to the recovery and rehabilitation. The basic contents in the therapeutic method to support the constitution and expel pathogens are supposed to correct deficiency and purge excess. The principle to correct deficiency and purge excess, mentioned in Nei Jing, is generally appropriate for all clinical departments of Chinese medicine. But, the reinforcing method and sedating method are different between the external therapies and the internal therapies of Chinese medicine.

利于痊愈和康复的方向转化。扶正祛邪法则的基本内容,是补虚与泻实。《内经》提出的补虚泻实的原则,普遍适用于所有的中医临床各科。但是,包括推拿在内的中医外治法的补泻与中医内治法的补泻,是有所区别的。

2.1 Support the constitution

It refers to the therapeutic principle to support the constitutional energy, strengthen body constitution, and enhance the anti-pathogenic ability of the body and natural repairing ability, appropriate for deficient patterns with deficiency of the constitutional energy as the main contradiction. In supporting the constitution and correcting deficiency by tuina therapy, no flesh and blood products enter the human body, and then how does it correct deficiency?

2.1 扶正

扶正是指扶助正气,增强体质,提高机体抗病能力和自然修复能力的治疗法则。适用于以正气虚为主要矛盾的虚证。推拿扶正补虚,并无血肉有情之品进入体内,那么,它是如何补虚的呢?

(1) Correct deficiency by circulating qi and blood　To correct deficiency by tuina therapy is focused to activate blood and circulate qi. It is said in Su Wen that "when pathogenic cold invades the meridian of Back-Shu acupoint, the meridian will be in disorder. Disorder in meridian will lead to blood deficiency. Blood deficiency induces pain. Because its acupoint is related to the heart, there will be radiating pain. If pressed, heat sensation will arrive.

(1) 通过流通气血而补虚　推拿补虚,重在活血行气。《素问·举痛论》篇曰:"寒气客于背俞之脉则脉泣,脉泣则血虚,血虚则痛,其俞注于心,故相引而痛,按之则热气至,热气至则痛止矣。"通过按压背部心俞而活血补血,达到治疗血虚疼痛的效

Pain will be stopped when heat sensation arrives". By pressing Xinshu (BL 15) of the back for activating blood and reinforcing blood, the therapeutic effect can be realized to treat pain due to blood deficiency. Take commonly seen dizziness due to blood deficiency for example, clinically it is understood to be caused by insufficient blood supply in the brain. By relaxing the soft tissues in the neck by the relaxing technique and pulling-stretching method for the cervical vertebras, it is possible to increase blood supply in the brain effectively. Although blood volume is not increased in the whole body, when blood deficiency is corrected in the brain, the purpose to "reinforce blood" still can be realized.

果。以常见的血虚眩晕来说,临床常责之于脑部供血不足,通过颈项部软组织放松手法和颈椎拔伸手法,可有效增加脑部的血液供应,虽然没有增加全身的血容量,但由于改善了脑部的缺血状态,同样达到了"补血"的目的。

(2) Correct deficiency by the specific areas Because of the specificity of the acupoints and areas in correcting deficiency, tuina therapy can play the role in supporting the constitution and correcting deficiency by stimulating those acupoitns or areas. The commonly used acupoints for correcting deficiency are Guanyuan (CV 4), Qihai (CV 6), Mingmen (GV 4), Shenshu (BL 23) and Gaohuang (BL 43), and the commonly used areas are lower abdomen and lower back.

(2) 通过特殊部位而补虚 由于一些腧穴和部位的补虚特异性,推拿可以通过刺激这些腧穴或部位发挥扶正补虚作用。常用的补虚腧穴如关元、气海、命门、肾俞、膏肓俞等,部位有丹田、腰部等。

(3) Correct deficiency by topical application of medicinal stuffs The oral administration of the medicinal stuffs for correcting deficiency can play a role in correcting deficiency by transdermal absorption of paste massage therapy. For instance, in *Han's Medical Rules* (Han Shi Yi Tong), "Deer Marrow Pills" were used to "chafe and rub Shenshu (BL 23) for greatly reinforcing primary yang. Its effect is magic for joint pain due to deficiency and cold". Also, in *Savior General Compendium* (Sheng

(3) 借助药物外用而补虚 内服的补虚药物可以通过膏摩法经皮吸收而发挥补虚作用。如《韩氏医通》用"外鹿髓丸""以擦摩肾俞,大补元阳。凡骨节痛,属虚寒者,其效如神"。又如《圣济总录》用"大补益摩膏"摩腰补肾。明清流行的朱丹溪摩腰膏,也是常用的补虚膏摩

Ji Zong Lu), "Great Tonic Massage Paste" was used to rub the lower back for reinforcing the kidney. ZHU Danxi's Low Back-Rubbing Paste prevailing in the Ming and Qing Dynasties was also a commonly used paste massage formula for correcting deficiency.

方。

(4) Correct deficiency by self massage or training　To support the constitution and correct deficiency by guiding the patient self massage and self training is a specific feature in tuina therapy. Self massage methods are supposed to press Gaohuang (BL 43), chafe Shenshu (BL 23), rub the lower abdomen, and chafe Yongquan (KI 1). The internal-works tuina school usually guides the patients to train Shaolin internal art (Shao Lin Nei Gong) to strengthen the body, for treating the intractable diseases of pulmonary tuberculosis in combination of internal-works massage therapy.

（4）辅以自我按摩或练功而补虚　通过指导病人自我按摩或自我练功来扶正补虚，是中医推拿的一大特色。自我按摩操作法有运膏肓、擦肾俞、摩丹田、擦涌泉等。内功推拿流派更通过指导病人练习少林内功而强壮身体，配合内功推拿以治疗肺痨等顽疾。

2.2　Expel pathogens

It refers to the therapeutic principle to expel and eliminate the pathogenic factors, appropriate for excessive patterns with the preponderant pathogens as the main contradiction. The pathogenic factors can come from the exogenous wind, cold, summer-heat, dampness, dryness and fire, and also can come from the internally-produced turbid phlegm, blood stasis, retained food, and accumulated qi. In expelling the pathogens, it is necessary to "provide a way-out", i. e. the channels for the pathogens to go out. In terms of the channels to expel the pathogens, there is no more than defecation, urination, expectoration, perspiration or respiration, forming various therapeutic methods of defection, diruresis, expectoration and perspiration, etc. For the above

2.2　祛邪

祛邪，是指祛除病邪，消除致病因素的治疗法则。适用于以邪气盛为主要矛盾的实证。邪气，可以是自外而入的风、寒、暑、湿、燥、火，也可以是由内而生的痰浊、瘀血、宿食、郁气等。祛邪要注意"给出路"，就是说要提供把病邪排出体外的途径。祛邪外出的途径，无非通过大便、小便、痰液、汗液和呼吸。因此就形成了通便、利尿、排痰、发汗等各种治法。推拿对于通过上述途径的排毒祛邪，均有直接或间接的作用。

channels to release toxin and expel pathogens, tuina therapy has the direct and indirect effects. tuina therapy for expelling the pathogens can supplement herbal therapy, and can achieve some effects that the internal therapy by herbal drugs cannot realize. For instance, in the treatment of obstructive pulmonary diseases, or accumulation of abundant heat in the pulmonary system, manifested by deep yellow and tenacious sputum, and difficult expectoration, simple and large dose of antibiotics or oral administration of herbal drugs cannot reach the focus of the lung to bring into fully effect. At this moment, if the patting method and vibrating method are selected and applied on the back and sternum, it will be beneficial to dilution and discharge of sputum by the ciliary movement, and will assist Chinese and western medications to bring into the fully effects.

推拿祛邪,可以弥补药物疗法的不足,有些作用甚至是药物内治法无法达到的。例如,阻塞性肺部疾病,或肺系邪热壅盛,痰色深黄而黏稠,咳痰不出,单纯用大剂量抗生素或中药内服可能因药力无法到达肺部病灶而不能发挥作用。此时如果能选择运用拍法、振法在上背部和胸骨部操作,通过促进气道内的纤毛运动,将有助于稀释和排出痰液,协助中西药物更好地发挥作用。

3 Regulate yin and yang

Imbalance of yin and yang is the pathological developing process and final result of all diseases. Imbalance of yin and yang is a disorder in the mutual relationship of Zangfu organs, meridians and collaterals, qi and blood, and Ying-nutrient and Wei-defensive qi, and a generalization of disorder in the upflow, downflow, outflow and inflow of qi dynamics and the internal foundation of the occurrence, development and prognosis of diseases. Yin and yang belong to the general outline of pattern identification in Chinese medicine. It is mentioned in Su Wen "necessary to observe the condition of yin and yang and regulate them, in order to normalize them". Therefore, to regulate yin and yang is regarded as one of the fundamental rules in the treat-

3 调整阴阳

阴阳失衡是一切疾病的病理发展过程和最终归宿。阴阳失衡是人体脏腑、经络、气血、营卫等相互关系失调,以及气机升降出入失常的概括,是疾病发生、发展和转归的内在依据。阴阳是中医辨证的总纲。《素问·至真要大论》篇提出"谨察阴阳所在而调之,以平为期",将调整阴阳作为中医防治疾病的根本法则之一。调整阴阳的治疗原则针对疾病过程中阴阳失衡的病理状态,损其偏盛,补其偏衰,使之恢复相对平

ment and prevention of diseases by Chinese medicine. The therapeutic principle in regulating yin and yang is aimed to the pathological state of imbalance between yin and yang during the process of disease, in order to suppress its preponderance and supplement its insufficiency, so as to restore the relative balance and "maintain balance between yin and yang for maintaining welling being" (Su Wen).

衡，达到"阴平阳秘，精神乃治"(《素问·生气通天论》)。

To regulate yin and yang is also the basic principle in tuina therapy. In his annotation to "the treatment should be given by massage with medicated paste" in Su Wen, WANG Bing said: "massage is to remove obstruction and guide yin and yang." QIAN Ruming said in his preface to *Confidential Instruction of Tuina Secrets* (Mi Chuan Tui Na Miao Jue): "once yin and yang are in good order, all diseases will be gone. If the reinforcing method or reducing method can be used, the constitution is not injured." tuina therapy for regulating yin and yang can regulate imbalance of yin and yang of Zangfu organs, and can regulate the imbalance of yin and yang in the joints, meridians and tendons, too. The body trunk is maintained in bilateral symmetrical balance with the spine as an axis. Due to errors in the life habits, in body posture, and over fatigue and chronic strain, etc, the injury of soft tissues can be induced and yin and yang can be imbalanced in the spine and skeletal muscles, manifested by chronic pain in the low back and thigh, nodes, spasm and even tenderness in the skeletal muscles of the lumbosacral region, buttocks and thigh, and lateral curvature of the spine, migration of the pelvis, rugged shoulders, unequal length in the two legs, asymmetrical functions in the articular activities, and further

调整阴阳，同样也是推拿治疗的基本原则。王冰在注释《素问·血气形志》篇"治之以按摩醪药"时说："夫按摩者，所以开通闭塞，导引阴阳。"《秘传推拿妙诀》钱汝明序云："阴阳调则诸病自去，补泻寓而本原不伤。"推拿调整阴阳，既可以调整五脏六腑的阴阳失衡，更可以调整骨节经筋的阴阳失衡。人的躯干，以脊柱为轴而左右对称平衡，如因错误的生活习惯、不良的身体姿势、过度疲劳等慢性劳损因素，可造成软组织损害，引起脊柱、骨骼肌的阴阳失衡。症见慢性腰腿痛，腰骶、臀、股等骨骼肌出现硬节、痉挛、压痛点以及脊柱侧凸，骨盆旋移，两肩高低，双下肢不等长，左右关节活动功能不对称等，进一步还可以出现头痛、眩晕、腹泻、痛经、月经不调等内科、妇科征象。推拿可运用点按、拔伸、旋转复位等手法

internal and gynecological signs of headache, dizziness, diarrhea, amenorrhea, and irregular menstruation. tuina therapy can be used to regulate them by the point-pressing method, pulling-stretching method and reduction by rotation.

调整之。

4 Take measures in accordance with the time, circumstances and person

4 因时、因地、因人制宜

4.1 Take measures in accordance with the time

It means to design or adjust tuina therapeutic plan in accordance with the season, climate, and time period.

The humans correspond to the heaven and earth. The physiological and pathological activities of the human body would change correspondingly with the different time of the natural world. Generally speaking, in the spring and summer, yang qi tends to rise and spread, and the skin striation of the human body is loose and open. Even in infection of exogenous wind and cold, it is not advisable to use the manual technique and herbal drugs in spicy, warm and dispersing property, in order to awoid cosuming body fluid and damaging yin. In autumn and winter, yang qi is restrained, if not a pattern of strong heat, it is neccessary to use the cooling technique and herbal drugs carefully, in order to avoid consuming qi and damaging yang. There is such a saying of "massage must be done by seasonal climate" in Tendon-changing Exercises (Yi Jin Jing). Tuina treatment should be given in accordance with the condition of qi and blood, and opening and closing situation of the acupoints of the human body in the twelve time periods in a day. The tuina methods of "massage by midnight time and noon time" and

4.1 因时制宜

即根据季节、气候、时辰等因素,制定或调整推拿治疗方案。

人与天地相应。人的生理、病理活动会因自然界不同的时间而产生相应的变化。一般而言,春夏季节,阳气升发,人的腠理疏松开泄,即使患有外感风寒,也不宜使用辛温发散的手法和药物,以免耗津伤阴;秋冬之际,阳气内敛,此时若非大热之证,当慎用寒凉手法和药物,以防耗气伤阳。《易筋经》有"揉有节候"之说。根据一日十二时辰人体气血的盛衰、气穴的开阖来推拿,古代有"子午按摩法""十二时辰点穴法"等顺时而治的推拿法可供借鉴。气温偏低时,推拿操作中和操作后要注意保暖防风。

"acupoint-pressing method in twelve time periods" based upon the time in the ancient times can be used for reference. When the temperature is too low, it is necessary to keep warm and stay away from wind during and after tuina treatment.

2.2 Take measures in accordance with circumstances

It means to give tuina treatment in accordance with the natural environment and geological features. Differences in the geological environment lead to differences in the life habits and in disease spectrum in different regions. The therapeutic methods and operating modes in tuina therapy should also be different. For instance, high altitude myocardial ischemia is common in Tibet plateau. Hypertension, diabetes and gout are common in the economically developed regions. Asians are not used to expose the skin for tuina. Western people like to expose the skin for oil massage. Japanese are used to enjoy Shiatsu on the bedding or lower massage table. Western people like massage on a high massage table. It is also necessary to consider the regional features in the tuina clinical service.

2.3 Take measures in accordance with the person

It means to take the different therapeutic measures for the patients in accordance with their differences in age, gender, body constitution, occupation and life habits. In terms of intensity of stimulation of the manual techniques, the manual technique can be strong for those with strong body constitution, and should be light for those with weak body constitution. The manual techniques should be light for those who accept tuina treatment for the first time, and can be gradually strong for those treated by

2.2 因地制宜

即根据自然环境和地理特点来实施推拿治疗。地理环境的差异导致了不同地域人群生活习惯的不同和疾病谱的差异，推拿治疗方法和操作方式也应当有所区别。如西藏高原多发高原性心肌缺氧；经济发达地区多高血压、糖尿病、痛风；亚洲人不习惯暴露皮肤推拿，而西方人较喜欢裸露肌肤的油性按摩，日本人习惯于在草垫上或很低的按摩床上指压，西方按摩则喜欢在较高的按摩床上操作，推拿临证应该考虑到地域的特点。

2.3 因人制宜

即根据病人的年龄、性别、体质、职业、生活习惯的不同，采取不同的推拿治疗措施。以手法刺激强弱而言：体质强壮者手法可稍重，身体柔弱者手法宜稍轻。初次接受推拿治疗的病人手法宜轻，长期反复推拿的患者手法可逐渐加重。小儿气血未充，肌肤娇嫩，推拿时可使

tuina for long time. Because qi and blood are not sufficient and the skin is delicately tender in the children, it is advisable to use lubricating creams, and tuina with light force and short time. In accordance with the physiological features of menstruation, leukorrhea, pregnancy and delivery, it is necessary to select the proper manual techniques and stimulation intensity during the treatment. Because the elders are mostly in osteoporosis and in smaller motion range, it is necessary to use the pulling method for motion of the joints carefully, to have light tuina on the head, face, chest and abdomen, and strong tuina on the buttocks and thighs with thick muscles. The manual techniques should be light for those with problems in the shallow position of the skin, and should be strong for those with problems in the deep position of the tendons and joints. The manual techniques should be light for those with chronic sub-health problem and should be strong for those with acute pain. The manual techniques can be comparatively strong for the Asians, because of their high tolerance to pain, and should be light and gentle for the westerners, because of their lower pain threshold.

用润滑介质,且力量要轻,时间宜短。妇女有经、带、胎、产的生理特点,推拿时应酌情选用合适的手法和刺激量。老年人多骨质疏松,关节活动度较小,应当慎用扳法等运动关节类手法。头面胸腹之处手法宜轻,臀股等肌肉丰厚之处手法宜重。病在皮部等病位较浅者手法宜稍轻,病在筋骨关节等病位较深者手法宜稍重。慢性亚健康疾病手法宜轻柔,急性痛证病人手法可稍重。亚洲人较为耐痛,手法可偏重;欧美人一般痛阈较低,手法宜轻柔。

5 Treat unformed diseases

It is mentioned in Ling Shu that, the top medical practitioners treat the unformed diseases and do not treated formed diseases. It is also mentioned in Su Wen: "the top medical practitioners deal with the problem while it is still in embryonic stage, and the poor medical practitioners deal with the problem while it is already formed." Since Nei Jing, to treat the unformed diseases has been always the guiding

5 治未病

《灵枢・逆顺》提出"上工治未病,不治已病"。《素问・八正神明论》篇也指出:"上工救其萌芽……下工救其已成。"从《内经》始,治未病一直是中医防治疾病的指导思想。《金匮要略》明确将按摩作为治未病的外治法之

thought in the treatment and prevention of diseases. It is clearly pointed out in *Essential Prescriptions of the Golden Coffer* (Jin Kui Yao lue) that massage was one of the external therapies for treating the unformed diseases, and the best moment for massage treatment of the unformed diseases was when the exogenous pathogens attack the meridians but not involve Zangfu organs. It is pointed out in *Thousand Ducat Prescriptions for Emergencies* (Qian Jin Yao Fang) about the importance of self massage for prevention of diseases: "it is necessary to regulate qi for reinforcement and reduction every day, and massage and guiding technique are the best. It is necessary not to think the health is an absolute certainty. It is needed to remember risk in peace and prevent various diseases."

一，并且提出了按摩治未病的最佳时机是在外邪侵犯经络而未深入脏腑之时。《千金方》指出了自我按摩预防疾病的重要性："每日须调气补泻，按摩导引为佳。勿以康健便为常然。常须安不忘危，预防诸病也。"

5.1 Prevent first before disease is formed

In carrying out the thought to prevent first before the disease is formed, tuina therapy is mainly reflected in the two aspects of healthcare tuina and self-guiding massage.

Chinese healthcare tuina is a preventive and healthcare tuina guided with Chinese medical theory, and is not just an ordinary massage for relaxation of the limbs. By Chinese medical holistic concept, theory of meridians, theory of the internal organs and theory of qi and blood, it is able to comprehensively regulate the functions of Zangfu organs and meridians and able to stop the development from sub-health state to the pathological state for the subjects.

Self-guiding massage is a tuina method of traditional guiding or life preservation by self operation, with the guidance of Chinese life-preservation

5.1　未病先防

推拿疗法贯彻未病先防的思想，主要体现在保健推拿和自我导引按摩法两个方面。

中医保健推拿，是在中医理论指导下的预防保健性的推拿，决非一般的肢体放松按摩。它运用了中医的整体观念、经络学说、藏象学说、气血学说，通过全面调整脏腑经络机能，阻止受术者由亚健康状态向疾病状态发展。

自我导引按摩，是在中医养生思想指导下，运用自行操作的传统导引或养生按

thought, so as to realize the purposes to strengthen the body and prevent diseases. It is pointed out in *Real Instruction of Life and Longevity* (Shou Shi Chuan Zhen): "massage and guiding technique are the first choice for longevity and elimination of diseases." It is pointed out in *Experience on Cultivation of Longevity* (Xiu Kun Lun Zheng Yan) that self "kneading method" "not only could treat your own problems but also treat disease before it occurs". The traditional self massage and guiding art includes the methods applied on the various body parts, such as rub the face, chafe the nose, strike the heavenly drum, flex the knee and lift the leg, and dry bath, and also includes the training exercises summarized over several thousand years. The typical self massage and guiding exercises include "Eight-Section Exercises" (Ba Duan Jin), "Twelve-Section Exercises" (Shi Er Duan Jin), "Ten Massage Techniques" (An no Shi Shu), "Eight Methods for Eradicating Diseases" (Que Bing Ba Ze), "Twelve-Section Moving Exercises" (Shi Er Duan Dong Gong) and "Nine Rotating Methods for Longevity" (Yan Nian Jiu Zhuan Fa).

摩法,达到强身健体、预防疾病的目的。《寿世传真》指出:"延年却病,以按摩导引为先。"《修昆仑证验》指出自我"揉法""非但可以自治已病,并可以治病之未生"。传统自我按摩导引术,既有在全身各部位的分部操作之法,如摩面、擦鼻、鸣天鼓、洒腿、干浴等,也有千百年来总结出的套路练习法。经典的自我按摩导引套路有"八段锦""十二段锦""按摩十术""却病八则""十二段动功""延年九转法"等。

5.2 Treat before problem occurs

It means that in foreseeing the occurrence of some diseases, or that the diseases with periodic attack would attack, it is advisable to give certain targeted tuina interference to prevent its occurrence. For instance, in the treatment of dysmenorrheal by massage therapy, the treatment can be given several days prior to the menstruation.

5.2 欲病先治

指在预见到某些疾病将要发生,或有周期性发作规律的疾病即将发作,可在发病之前,予以针对性的推拿干预以预防其发病。如推拿治疗痛经,可在月经来潮前数日就开始治疗。

5.3 Prevent transmission after problem is formed

After the problem is formed, in addition to the

5.3 既病防变

已经得病之后,除了针

targeted prompt treatment, it is also necessary to foresee the possible development and transmission and take the preventive therapeutic measures positively to block the channel of its transmission, in order to avoid further aggravation. In the treatment of diseases by massage therapy, it is also necessary to prevent complications and sequelae at the same time. For instance, in the treatment of apoplectic patients by massage therapy, it is advisable to pat the back to prevent hypostatic pneumonia complicated from long-term immobilization. The rotating method and pulling method for ankle joint can be used to prevent atrophy of the heel tendon. The rotating method for the hip joint can be used to prevent deformity in the outward rotation of the hip joint.

对性地及时治疗以外，还应预见到疾病可能的发展转移方向，积极采取预防性治疗措施，截断其传变途径，避免其加重恶化。推拿治病，同样应重视预防并发症和后遗症问题。如推拿治疗中风患者，可用背部拍法预防因长期卧床不起可能并发的坠积性肺炎；用踝关节摇法和扳法预防跟腱挛缩；用髋关节摇法预防髋关节外旋畸形等。

5.4 Prevent recurrence after recovery

There is a transitional period from the preliminary cure to complete recovery of disease. If the patients in this period of time are not appropriately taken care of, old problem would have the chance to reoccur or have new diseases, such as recurrence of apoplexy after the preliminary recovery of apoplexy. In the treatment by tuina therapy, it is necessary not to be just satisfied with relief of symptoms, and necessary to treat the primary cause of the disease. This is a fundamental reason to prevent recurrence after recovery. After the preliminary effects are achieved in the treatment, it is needed to continue massage treatment for one course, in order to “make up a missed lesson” for consolidating the therapeutic effect. It is the traditional feature of tuina therapy to guide the patients to train the self-guiding therapy or self massage, and to guide the

5.4 瘥后防复

从疾病初愈到完全康复有一个过渡时期。处于这一阶段的患者，如果调养不当，往往导致旧病复起，或滋生新疾。如中风初愈之后的复中。推拿治病，不应满足于减轻症状，而应致力于治疗引起疾病的原发因素，这是预防瘥后复病的根本。治疗初见成效之后，往往还需继续推拿一个疗程，细心地“补课”以巩固疗效。指导患者配合练习自我导引疗法或自我按摩，指导患者养成良好的生活习惯，是中医推拿的传统特色，也有助于瘥后防复。

patients to build up good life habits, for it is beneficial to the prevention of recurrence after recovery.

Section 3 Indications and contraindications of tuina therapy

第3节 推拿的适应证与禁忌证

1 Indications of tuina therapy

The indications of tuina therapy include diseases in various clinics. All diseases in the orthopedic, internal, gynecological, neurological, pediatric and ENT clinic, if their certain pathological process can be altered and the symptoms can be relieved, belong to the indications of tuina therapy. tuina therapy is the major therapy and is an auxiliary treatment for some diseases. The indications of tuina therapy also include headache, insomnia, dizziness, common cold, cough, asthma, epigastric pain, diarrhea, constipation, retention of urine, edema, apoplexy sequelae, facial paralysis, neck pain, scapulohumeral periarthritis, cervical spondylopathy, lumbar disc herniation, acute lumbar sprain, tennis elbow, ankle sprain, irregular menstruation, dysmenorrhea, hysteroptosis, mastitis, perimenopausal syndrome, simple obesity, toothache, hiccups in adults, and diarrhea, anorexia, muscular tortiollis, cerebral paralysis, enuresis, constipation, indigestion, fever, night crying, and subluxation of the radial head in infants.

1 推拿的适应证

推拿的适应证涵盖了临床各科。骨科、内科、妇科、神经科、儿科、五官科等各科疾病中，凡是手法能改善其某些病理过程、缓解症状的，都是推拿的适应证。推拿的作用，有的是主治，有的是辅助治疗。推拿的适应证包括：头痛、失眠、眩晕、感冒、咳嗽、哮喘、胃脘痛、腹泻、便秘、尿潴留、水肿、中风后遗症、面瘫、落枕、漏肩风、颈椎病、腰椎间盘突出症、急性腰扭伤、网球肘、踝关节扭伤、月经不调、痛经、子宫下垂、乳痈、围绝经期综合征、单纯性肥胖、牙痛、呃逆等成人病症，及腹泻、厌食症、肌性斜颈、脑性瘫痪、遗尿、便秘、疳积、发热、夜啼、桡骨头半脱位等儿科病症等。

2 Contraindications of tuina therapy

Although tuina therapy is a natural therapy, without toxic and side effect from medications, it is

2 推拿的禁忌证

尽管推拿作为一种自然疗法，没有药物的毒副作用，

still necessary to pay attention to its contraindications.

但是仍应注意其禁忌证。

2.1 Some situations massage therapy should be used carefully

2.1 慎用推拿的几种情况

The manual techniques of tuina therapy should be used carefully or conditionally in the following situations: ① Hunger, because blood sugar is low in hungry state, tuina in this moment can cause shock. ② Within one hour after meal or abdominal distension. ③ Massage should be given for those after serious sports and with extreme fatigue, after rest for a period of time. ④ Pregnant women, the manual techniques should be used carefully in the abdominal and lumbosacral region for pregnant women. Some acupoints, such as Hegu (LI 4), Jianjing (GB 21), and Sanyinjiao (SP 6), should not be used, for it was reported in the literature that abortion might be induced. The manual techniques with strong stimulation are also not appropriate in other parts. ⑤ Intoxicated person.

下列情况应该慎用或有条件地使用推拿手法:①饥饿时,饥饿时血糖较低,此时推拿可能导致休克。②饭后1小时内,或腹胀时。③剧烈运动后和极度疲劳者,应休息一段时间后再考虑按摩。④孕妇,孕妇的腹部、腰骶部慎用手法;某些腧穴如合谷、肩井、三阴交据文献记载可能引起流产,也不宜使用;其他部位不宜使用重刺激手法。⑤酒醉者。

2.2 Strict contraindications of tuina therapy

2.2 推拿的严格禁忌证

The following diseases should be listed in the scope of strict contraindications of tuina therapy: ① high fever; ② acute infectious diseases, such as acute infectious hepatitis, active pulmonary tuberculosis, etc. ③ skin lesions, skin infection, or serious dermal diseases, local and focal areas of skin lesions; ④ bone fracture, but except fracture sequelae or recovery stage; ⑤ bone and joint tuberculosis; ⑥ acute stage of hemorrhagic cerebrovascular accidents; ⑦ hemorrhagic diseases or bleeding areas, such as gastrointestinal ulcer bleeding, thrombocytopenia, pernicious anemia, leukemia; ⑧ serious heart diseases; ⑨ locations of malignant tumors or

下列病症应列入推拿的严格禁忌范围:①高热者。②急性传染病患者,如急性传染性肝炎、活动性肺结核等。③皮肤有破损、感染,或有严重的皮肤病患者,其病损局部和病灶部位禁止推拿。④骨折部位,但骨折后遗症或骨折康复期除外。⑤骨与关节结核患者。⑥出血性脑血管意外的急性期。⑦出血性疾病或正在出血的部位,如胃肠溃疡性出血、血

locations of bone metastasis, and ⑩ instable stage of mental disorders or unconsciousness after intoxication.

小板减少、恶性贫血、白血病等。⑧严重的心脏病患者。⑨恶性肿瘤部位及其骨转移部位。⑩精神病情绪不稳定者和酒后神志不清者。

WHO Guidelines on Basic Training and Safety in Chiropractic was promulgated by World Health Organization in 2005 and its Chinese edition was published in 2008. The detailed descriptions about the contraindications of the spinal techniques are given and can be used for reference.

世界卫生组织于 2005 年发布了《世界卫生组织脊骨神经医学基础培训和安全性指南》,2008 年出版了中文版。书中对脊柱手法的禁忌证作了详细描述,可供参考。

Section 4 Management of abnormal situations of tuina therapy

第 4 节 推拿异常情况的处理

Tuina therapy is a safe, effective and side effect-free external therapy. But, if the manual techniques are not used properly, or used by violent force, or used with improper body position of the patient, or used in serious nervousness, there will be some abnormal situations. tuina practitioners must quickly make a correct judgment and correct management.

推拿疗法是一种安全有效而很少有副作用的外治法,但若手法应用不当,或用力过猛,或病人体位不当,或精神过于紧张,也会出现一些异常情况。推拿医务工作者必须迅速做出正确的判断,并及时作出正确的处理。

1 Fainting

1 晕厥

It is mostly caused by the patient's nervousness or extreme weak body constitution or over fatigue, hunger, or strong manual technique from the practitioners. During the treatment, the patient may present sudden dizziness, blurred vision, palpitation and shortness of breathing, stuffy sensation in the chest, nausea, and extreme cold sensation in the

多由于患者精神紧张或体质特别虚弱或过度劳累、饥饿,或施术者手法过重,患者在接受推拿治疗的过程中,可能突然出现头晕目眩、心慌气短、胸闷欲吐,严重者四肢厥冷、出冷汗,甚至昏倒

four limbs, cold sweating and even coma in serious cases. After the accident occurs, it is necessary to stop treatment immediately, and let the patient lie down in a position of lower head. The patient in mild condition may recover after rest for a while or drinking warm water or sugar water. For the patients with severe condition, it is necessary to press Renzhong (GV 26), Shixuan (Extra), and grasp Jianjing (GB 21) and Hegu (LI 4), to seek other first-aid measures.

等现象。发生后应立即中止手法，将患者取头稍低位平卧，轻者静卧片刻或给服温开水或糖水后即可恢复，重者可配合掐人中、十宣，拿肩井、合谷，必要时配合其他急救措施。

2　Subcutaneous bleeding

Because of strong manual techniques, or too-long treatment, or thrombocytopenia in the patient, increased capillary fragility in the elders, or long-term administration of aspirin or warfarin, ecchymosis may appear in the massaged areas. After it occurs, it is necessary to stop tuina in the local part and no management is needed usually. For serious bruises in the local areas, it is necessary to be immobile and apply cold compress. After bleeding is stopped, it is advisable to diminish swelling and disperse blood stasis by the wet hot compress or slow massage method.

2　皮下出血

由于手法过重，或时间过长，或患者有血小板减少症，或老年性毛细血管脆性增加，或长期口服阿司匹林、华法林等药物，在受术部位可出现瘀斑。发生后局部应停止施用手法，一般不必处理。局部青紫严重者，可先制动、冷敷，待出血停止后可用湿热敷或缓摩法以消肿散瘀。

3　Bone fracture

If bone fracture is caused by improper manual techniques or violent practice, it is necessary to stop treatment, maintain immobility and deal with bone fracture immediately by reduction and fixation.

3　骨折

由于手法不当或过于粗暴引起患者骨折时应立即停止手法，制动，按骨折处理，及时整复固定。

4　Skin lesions

During the treatment, the patient may present the local red color, pain and skin lesions in the local skin. If it occurs, it is necessary to stop the treatment immediately, and at the same time to disinfect

4　破皮

患者在接受治疗的过程局部出现皮肤发红、疼痛、皮肤破损等现象。发生后应立即停止手法治疗，同时做好

and protect the skin, for avoiding infection.

皮肤的消毒和保护,防止感染。

5 Burns

If blisters appear in the local areas, leading to local burns, due to improper application of wet and heat compress, it is necessary to stop wet and hot compress immediately. It is advisable to apply some oil preparations, such as guaiazulenum ointment or burns aerosol, for mild cases, and to suck out fluid from blisters (not necessary to cut off epidermis) with a syringe for severe cases and then apply some gentian violet and band it up, in order to avoid infection.

5 烫伤

由于湿热敷不当,局部出现水泡而发生局部烫伤,应立即停止湿热敷,轻者涂抹某些油剂如蓝油烃或使用灼伤气雾剂,重者用无菌注射器抽出水泡内的液体(不必剪去表皮),再涂上龙胆紫并加压包扎以免感染。

Chapter 6 Specific introduction of tuina therapy

第6章 推拿治疗各论

Section 1 Orthopedic and traumatic diseases

第1节 骨伤科疾病

Stiff neck

Clinically, it is divided into two types: subacute onset and acute onset. Subacute onset is manifested by the neck and shoulder muscles in over traction and stressful state for long time and often is related to improper sleeping posture, pillow too high or too low, lowering head for too long time or falling into asleep in watching TV on the bed. Acute onset is induced by turning the head suddenly. The above situation can lead to the static traction injury or acute sprain in some muscles of the neck and shoulder, and further the protective spasm of the relevant muscles, motor limitation and pain in the neck and shoulder. The involved muscles are mainly the sternocleidomastoid muscle, trapezius muscle and scapular elevator muscle, mostly the previous two muscles.

Diagnostic Essentials

The neck is limited in its motion and even takes

落枕

又名失枕。临床常呈两种类型：一是亚急性发病。一侧颈肩部肌肉较长时间处于过度牵拉、紧张状态。往往与睡觉姿势不当，枕头过高、过低，或靠在床上看电视低头过久甚至睡着有关。二是急性发病。有突然的转颈动作。上述情况将导致颈肩部某些肌肉的静力性牵拉伤或急性扭伤，进一步引起相关肌肉的保护性痉挛、活动受限及颈肩部疼痛。受累肌肉主要为胸锁乳突肌、斜方肌和肩胛提肌，而以前两者多见。

诊断要点

颈部活动受限，甚至转

the body truck to move in turning the neck. Neck pain is aggravated in motion and relieved in the resting state, more obvious in turning to the sick side. In severe condition, neck pain can involve the shoulder and back. The patient's head inclines to the sick side. In touching the sternocleidomastoid muscle and trapezius muscle, the elevated muscular tension and spasm and even cord-like and lump-like stuffs are palpable. Tender spots are distributed differently based upon the involved muscles: at the side and attached point of the sternocleidomastoid muscle, at 1/3 part lateral to the clavicle, area of Jianjing (GB 21), upper border of the scapula, medial border of the scapula, and lateral to the spinous process of the upper cervical vertebras and at the superior angle of the scapula.

颈时连带躯干一起转动。颈项疼痛,活动时加剧,静止时减轻,尤以向患侧旋转更为明显。严重者疼痛可牵引至肩背部,病人头向患侧偏斜。用手触摸胸锁乳突肌或斜方肌等肌肉可感觉肌张力增高、痉挛,甚至可触及条索状、块状物。压痛点根据受累肌肉不同而分布于:胸锁乳突肌沿线和附着点;锁骨外 1/3 处、肩井部、肩胛冈上缘、肩胛骨内侧缘;上位颈椎棘突旁和肩胛骨上角。

Basic Therapeutic Method

基本治法

Therapeutic principle: To soothe the tendons, relieve spasm, activate blood and dredge the collaterals.

治则:舒筋缓急,活血通络。

The patient takes a sitting position.

患者取坐位。

1 Type of the sternocleidomastoid spasm

1 胸锁乳突肌痉挛型

(1) Press Hegu (LI 4), Waiguan (TE 5), Fengchi (GB 20), Yifeng (TE 17), Tianding (LI 17), Qishe (ST 11), Quepen (ST 12), the attached spot of the sternocleidomastoid muscle in predominance, for totally two minutes.

(1) 点按合谷、外关、风池、翳风、天鼎、气舍、缺盆穴,以胸锁乳突肌的附着点为重点,共 2 分钟。

(2) Push (or press and knead) the sternocleidomastoid muscle with one thumb, for two minutes.

(2) 一指禅推(或按揉)胸锁乳突肌,2 分钟。

(3) Roll the nape and shoulder, together with passive movement of lateral flexion of the head and neck rotation, for two minutes.

(3) 㨰项肩部,配合头部侧屈与转颈被动运动,2 分钟。

(4) Grasp the sternocleidomastoid muscle, together with the plucking method, for one minute.

(4) 拿胸锁乳突肌,结合弹拨,1 分钟。

(5) Apply the traction with rotation for the cervical vertebras and the rotating method for the cervical vertebras, for one minute.

(5) 颈椎旋转牵引法和颈椎摇法,1分钟。

2 Type of the trapezius spasm

2 斜方肌痉挛型

(1) Press Houxi (SI 3), Waiguan (TE 5), Fengchi (GB 20), Fengfu (GV 16), Dazhu (BL 11), Fengmen (BL 12), Feishu (BL 13), Cervical and Thoracic Huatuo Jiaji points (Extra), Jianjing (GB 21), Tianliao (TE 15), Jugu (LI 16), Bingfeng (SI 12), Tianzong (SI 11), attached spot of the trapezius muscle in predominance, for two minutes.

(1) 点按后溪、外关、风池、风府、大杼、风门、肺俞、颈胸夹脊穴、肩井、天髎、巨骨、秉风、天宗穴,以斜方肌的附着点为重点,共2分钟。

(2) Push (or press and knead) Cervical and Thoracic Huatuo Jiaji points (Extra) and the supraspinous fossa with one thumb, for two minutes.

(2) 一指禅推(或按揉)颈胸夹脊穴和冈上窝,2分钟。

(3) Roll the shoulder and upper back, together with flexion and extension of the nape and rotation of the neck, for two minutes.

(3) 㨰肩背部,配合颈部屈伸与转颈,2分钟。

(4) Push the left and right trapezius muscle with the two thumbs divergently, along the muscular fibers, for one minute.

(4) 两拇指分推左右斜方肌,顺其肌纤维走向,1分钟。

(5) Apply the traction with rotation for the cervical vertebras and the rotating method for the cervical vertebras, for one minute.

(5) 颈椎旋转牵引法和颈椎摇法,1分钟。

3 Type of the scapular elevator spasm

3 肩胛提肌痉挛型

(1) Press Tianliao (TE 15), Quheng (SI 13), Jianwaishu (SI 14), Fufen (BL 41), Upper Cervical Huatuo Jiaji points (Extra), the attached spot of the superior angle of the scapular elevator muscle in predominance, for two minutes.

(1) 点按天髎、曲垣、肩外俞、附分、风池、上颈段夹脊穴,以肩胛提肌的上角附着部为重点,共2分钟。

(2) Push (or press and knead) Cervical Huatuo Jiaji points (Extra) with one thumb, together with the plucking method, for two minutes.

(2) 一指禅推(或按揉)颈夹脊穴,结合弹拨,2分钟。

(3) Roll the medial and superior part of the

(3) 㨰肩胛骨内上方,配

scapula, together with the flexion and extension of the neck, for two minutes.

合颈部屈伸,2 分钟。

(4) Push the medial border of the scapula with the two thumbs divergently, for one minute.

(4) 二拇指分推肩胛骨内缘,1 分钟。

(5) Apply the traction with rotation for the cervical vertebras and the rotating method for the cervical vertebras.

(5) 颈椎旋转牵引法和颈椎摇法。

All of the above three steps are finished by grasping Jianjing (GB 21), rubbing the shoulder and back, and striking (or patting) the shoulder and back.

以上三型均以拿肩井、搓肩背部和叩击(或拍)肩背部结束。

Precautions

注意事项

(1) For neck pain due to muscular spasm, the traction method by rotation is mainly used to extend the muscles to relieve spasm. It is not advisable to use the pulling method and violent force. For disturbance of the posterior cervical vertebra joints, it is advisable to select the repositioning method by rotation for the cervical vertebras accordingly.

(1) 对于肌痉挛性落枕,旋转牵引法主要起拉伸肌肉以解痉的作用,不作扳法,不可滥施暴力。对有颈椎后关节紊乱者,方可酌情选用颈椎旋转复位法。

(2) It is necessary to operate the rotating method for the cervical vertebras slowly, with increasing amplitude.

(2) 颈椎摇法应缓缓操作,幅度逐渐加大。

(3) It is needed to tell the patient to have a pillow in proper height for sleep.

(3) 嘱患者睡眠时注意枕头高低适中。

Cervical spondylopathy

颈椎病

It refers to the chronic degenerative disease occurring in the cervical spine and is a common and frequent disease in the middle-aged and old people. It is believed in modern medicine that it is mostly related to the degenerative hyperosteogeny of the cervical vertebras, degenerative change of the cervical intervertebral disc, sequela of acute injury or

颈椎病是发生在颈段脊柱的慢性退行性疾病,是中、老年人的常见病、多发病。现代医学认为多与颈椎退行性骨质增生、颈椎间盘退行性变化、颈部软组织的急性损伤后遗症或慢性劳损有

chronic strain of the neck soft tissues, involving the nerves and blood vessels of the neck, irritating the local soft tissues and forming a series of clinical symptoms of aseptic inflammation. It is believed in Chinese medicine that this problem is mostly related to the high age, weak constitution, insufficiency of the kidney qi, plus invasion of pathogenic wind, cold and dampness, or injury due to repeated strain, and obstruction of phlegm and dampness in the meridians and collaterals of the spine.

关,累及颈部神经、血管或刺激局部软组织形成无菌性炎症而产生一系列临床症状,又称为颈椎综合征。中医认为本病多由于年老体虚,肾气不足,复因风寒湿邪所侵,或反复积劳成损,痰湿瘀阻脊柱经络,发为本病。

Diagnostic Essentials

This disease is mostly seen in the group over 40, manifested clinically by numbness and pain in the head, neck, shoulder and arm in mild condition, and by soreness and weakness in the limbs, and even dizziness, palpitation, incontinence of urine and feces, and flaccidity in severe condition. In the specific examinations, top-knocking test, intervertebral foramen-crushing test and brachial plexus traction test can be positive.

诊断要点

本病多见于 40 岁以后的人群,临床常见症状是:轻者头、颈、肩、臂麻木疼痛;重者可见肢体酸软无力,甚至头晕、心慌、大小便失禁、瘫软等。特殊功能检查可见叩顶试验、椎间孔挤压试验、臂丛神经牵拉试验等阳性。

Basic Therapeutic Methods

Therapeutic principle: Soothe the tendons, dredge the collaterals, activate blood and disperse blood stasis.

基本治法

治则:舒筋通络,活血化瘀。

The patient takes a sitting position or bending sitting position (please refer to section two of chapter one). The patient with weak constitution should take a prone position, with the pillow under the chest.

患者坐位或伏坐位(见第 1 章第 2 节)。体弱者可取俯卧位,胸前垫枕。

(1) Push the lines of cervical Huantuo Jiaji points (Extra) with one thumb from Fengchi (GB 20) to Dazhu (BL 11) bilaterally, for two to three minutes.

(1) 一指禅推颈夹脊线,从风池到大杼穴水平,双侧,2～3 分钟。

(2) Press and knead the second lateral line of

(2) 拇指按揉颈椎膀胱

the bladder meridian of the cervical vertebras with the thumb: Starting with the tip of the thumb transversely from the border of the trapezius muscle at the level of the seventh cervical vertebra of the sick side, separate the trapezius muscle backward with the nail, and then press and knead with the cushion of the finger toward the posterior vertebral joint forcefully upward to Fengchi (GB 20), for twice. This method can be done with the two hands on the bilateral sides at the same time.

经第二侧线：以拇指指端从患侧第7颈椎水平的斜方肌边缘横向切入，以指甲将斜方肌向后分开，然后指腹朝着颈椎后关节用力，边按揉，边向上移动至风池，2遍。此法可双手同时操作两侧。

(3) Spring and pluck the lateral line of the neck: Starting with the thumb from the spinous process of the second cervical vertebra inferior to the mastoid process of the sick side, pluck and move downward to the level of the spinous process of the seventh cervical vertebra, for twice.

(3) 弹拨颈部侧线：以拇指从患侧乳突下方的第2颈椎横突开始，边由前向后弹拨边向下移动至第7颈椎横突水平，2遍。

(4) Roll the nape and shoulder, for two minutes.

(4) 㨰项肩部，2分钟。

(5) Roll the nape and shoulder together with the passive movement of the neck: ① roll the back side of the nape upward and downward, together with the passive movement of forward flexion and backward extension of the cervical vertebras. ② roll the lateral side of the nape upward and downward, together with the passive movement of the lateral flexion of the cervical vertebras. ③ adhere and roll the lateral side of the seventh cervical vertebra and first thoracic vertebra, together with the horizontal rotation of the cervical vertebras, for totally two to four minutes.

(5) 㨰项肩部配合颈部被动运动：①㨰项部后面并上下移动，配合颈椎前屈后伸被动运动；②㨰颈部侧面并上下移动，配合颈椎左右侧屈被动运动；③吸定㨰第7颈椎和第1胸椎结合部的侧面，配合颈椎水平旋转，共2～4分钟。

(6) Pull and extend the cervical vertebras in the sitting position, for one to three minutes. The supine position should be taken for the patients with high age and weak constitution.

(6) 坐位拔伸颈椎，1～3分钟。年老体弱者可采用仰卧位颈椎拔伸法。

Modification by Symptoms

(1) For those with the radiating pain and numb and electric sensation in the upper limb, in addition to the basic therapeutic methods, Press and knead Quepen (ST 12): Press and knead lightly with the thumb or index finger the attached spot of the anterior scalene muscle and middle scalene muscle at the upper border of the first rib in the supraclavicular fossa, for one minute.

(2) For those with serious dizziness, in addition to the basic therapeutic methods, Press with the thumb the nuchal plane of the connecting line of the two mastoid processes, on Fengchi (GB 20) and Fengfu (GV 16) in predominance, for totally two minutes.

(3) For those with disturbance of the posterior cervical vertebra joint, it is advisable to select the pulling method by positioning and rotation for the cervical vertebras accordingly.

随证加减

（1）有上肢放射痛和麻木触电感者，基本治法加按揉缺盆，以拇指或食指轻轻按揉患侧锁骨上窝中第一肋骨上缘的前斜角肌、中斜角肌附着点，1 分钟。

（2）眩晕严重者，基本治法加拇指点按两侧乳突连线的项平面，以风池、风府穴为重点，共 2 分钟。

（3）有颈椎后关节紊乱者，可酌情选用颈椎定位旋转扳法。

Scapulohumeral periarthritis

Because this disease often occurs around the age of 50, it is also termed "fifty year old shoulder". It is also nicknamed by "frozen shoulder", due to obvious functional disturbance. It is mostly seen in the teachers, housewives, computer operators, and accountants. It is believed in modern medicine that this problem is mostly related to the endocrine dysfunction, traumatic injury, strain and chronic degenerative change of the soft tissues around the shoulder, involving aseptic inflammation of the tendons, tendon sheaths, ligaments and bursa of the shoulder. It is believed in Chinese medicine that this

漏肩风

又名肩周炎、肩关节周围炎。因发病年龄多在 50 岁左右，故又称“五十肩”。其功能障碍突出者又有“肩凝症”“冻结肩”之称。以教师、家庭妇女、电脑录入员、会计等人员多见。现代医学认为本病的发生多与人体内分泌功能紊乱、外伤、劳损以及肩周组织的慢性退行性变等因素有关，进而引起肩部的肌腱、腱鞘、韧带、滑囊的

problem is often caused by overwork and injury of the shoulder, deficiency of qi and blood, plus invasion of pathogenic wind, cold and dampness.

无菌性炎症而致病。中医认为本病常因肩部积劳损伤、气血亏虚,复受风寒湿邪侵袭而致。

Diagnostic Essentials

诊断要点

This problem is mainly manifested by shoulder pain in the early stage and functional disturbance of the shoulder joint in the later stage.

早期以肩部疼痛为主;后期以肩关节功能障碍为主。

(1) Pain: Resting pain (relieved in the daytime and aggravated at night, and even waken up by pain at midnight, relieved by a little movement in the morning), vague pain (no obvious painful spot, extensive tenderness in the shoulder, involving the upper limb in some cases), and serious pain by the specific movement of the shoulder joint.

(1) 疼痛:静止痛(昼轻夜重,甚则半夜痛醒;晨起略作活动后减轻);模糊痛(无明确痛点,肩部广泛压痛,有的牵涉到上肢)。后期在肩关节作特定动作时痛剧。

(2) Functional disturbance: Because the shoulder functions are limited by adhesion of the joint capsule and tendon, muscular weakness due to disuse, and atrophy of the coracohumeral ligament, the functional disturbance is mostly seen in abduction and backward extension. The patients are often unable to have the hands at the back, comb the hair, fasten the belt and put on clothes.

(2) 功能障碍:因关节囊及肌腱的粘连、废用性肌力降低、喙肱韧带挛缩等因素引起肩关节功能受限,以外展、后伸功能障碍多见。病人常不能做背手、梳头、系腰带、穿衣等动作。

Basic Therapeutic Methods

基本治法

Therapeutic principle: Dredge the meridians and collaterals, activate blood and stop pain in predominance in the early stage, by the gentle and moderate techniques, and relax adhesion and lubricate the joints, mainly by the manual techniques for the passive movement of the joint in the later stage. During tuina treatment, it is necessary to guide the patient to do functional training correctly.

治则:初期以疏经通络、活血止痛为主,手法宜轻柔缓和;后期重在松解粘连、滑利关节,手法以关节被动运动为主。推拿治疗期间应指导病人正确地进行功能锻炼。

The patient takes a sitting position or lying position.

患者取坐位或卧位。

(1) Press the acupoints: Press Hegu (LI 4), Waiguan (TE 5), Quchi (LI 11), Tianzong (SI 11), Jianzhen (SI 9), Jugu (LI 16), Jianyu (LI 15), Jianliao (TE 14), or press the tenderness spots at the lateral and inferior border of the acromion, the coracoids the supraspinatus muscle, infraspinatus muscle, and the attached part of teres minor muscle and teres major muscle, for totally two to three minutes, to circulate qi and stop pain.

(1) 点按腧穴:选取合谷、外关、曲池、天宗、肩贞、巨骨、肩髃、肩髎等穴,或查找肩峰外下方、喙突部和冈上肌、冈下肌、小圆肌、大圆肌附着处的压痛点点按之,共 2～3 分钟,以行气止痛。

(2) Roll the shoulder: First roll the anterior, middle and posterior part of the deltoid muscle, and then roll together with the passive movement of abduction, adduction and rotation of the shoulder joint, for two to three minutes.

(2) 㨰肩部:先在三角肌的前、中、后部操作,再边㨰边配合肩关节的外展、内收和旋转被动运动,2～3 分钟。

(3) Grasp the shoulder, with the two hands, for one minute.

(3) 拿肩部,双手操作,1 分钟。

(4) Uphold the elbow and rotate the shoulder: In the sitting position, rotate the shoulder with the increasing amplitude, without violent force, together with the forward flexion and backward extension of the shoulder joint, for one minute.

(4) 托肘摇肩:坐位。幅度由小到大,不可用暴力。配合肩关节的前屈、后伸运动,1 分钟。

(5) Pull the shoulder joint: After the patient takes the sitting position, apply the pulling method by abduction for the shoulder joint (Figure 3-85), the pulling method by adduction (Figure 3-86), the pulling method by forward upholding action (Figure 3-89) and the pulling method by forward rotation and adduction (Figure 3-90). It is necessary to do with proper amplitude and strength and prohibited to use violent force.

(5) 肩关节扳法:坐位。行肩关节外展扳法(图 3-85)、内收扳法(图 3-86)、前上举扳法(图 3-89)和旋前内收扳法(图 3-90)。幅度和力量不可过大,勿用爆发力。

(6) Rub the upper limb: After the patient takes the sitting position, the medical practitioner lowers down body and holds the sick shoulder with the two palms, slightly upwards with circular rubbing and

(6) 搓上肢:坐位。医者下蹲以调整高度,用双掌抱住患肩,在略向上夹持的同时,作环形搓揉,随即过渡到

kneading action, and then holds the upper arm with the two palms to rub and knead slowly downward to the wrist joint, for repeatedly three to four times.

以双手掌面夹持上臂，一面搓揉，一面缓缓向腕部移动。由上而下反复 3～4 次。

(7) Shake the upper limb: Hold the patient's wrist with the two hands, and abduct the sick arm for about 60°, and then shake the sick arm upward and downward, and send the shaking wave to the shoulder necessarily.

（7）抖上肢：以双手扣住患者腕部，外展患肢 60°左右，作患肢的上下抖动，务必将抖动波送至肩部。

(8) Strike the shoulder, for one minute.

（9）叩击肩部，1 分钟。

Modification by Symptoms

随证加减

(1) For those with serious pain in the anterior shoulder in the backward extension of the shoulder joint, in addition to the basic therapeutic methods, ① In the supine position, knead the anterior shoulder with the palm, for one minute, ② push (or press and knead) the coracoids, for one minute, and ③ vibrate the anterior shoulder with the palm, for one minute.

（1）肩关节后伸时肩前部疼痛严重者，基本治法加：①仰卧位，掌揉肩前部，1 分钟；②一指禅推（或按揉）喙突部，1 分钟；③掌振肩前部，1 分钟。

(2) For those with obvious dysfunction in abduction, in addition to the basic therapeutic methods, ① pluck the lateral border of the scapula and the attached spot of the teres minor muscle and teres major muscle, for half a minute, ② push (or press and knead) with one thumb the infraglenoid tubercle of the scapula, for one minute, and ③ roll the infraspinatus fossa of the scapula, for half a minute.

（2）肩关节外展功能障碍明显者，基本治法加：①弹拨肩胛骨外侧缘的小圆肌、大圆肌附着点，半分钟；②一指禅推（或按揉）肩胛骨盂下结节部，一分钟；③擦肩胛骨冈下窝，半分钟。

(3) For those with serious dysfunction of the shoulder joint in the later stage, in addition to the basic therapeutic methods, apply the method to pull the arm and uphold the shoulder: after the patient takes a sitting position, the medical practitioner stands a little bit behind the sick side of the patient, holds and pulls down the wrist of the sick limb with

（3）后期肩关节功能障碍严重者，基本治法加拉臂端肩法：患者坐位，医者站在患者的患侧稍后方。一手握住患肢腕部向下牵拉，一手屈肘以前臂勾住患肢腋窝向上端提，两手相对用力牵拉

one hand, and hooks and upholds the armpit of the sick limb with the forearm by flexing the other hand, by the opposite force in the two hands, for three to four times.

3～4次。

Precautions

It is necessary to instruct the patient to do the following functional trainings.

(1) Swing the arm with heavy weight: The patient bends the body forward, with the sick limb dropping downward, and holds a light dumbbell or sand bag to swing forward and backward first, and leftward and rightward, and then circularly, for two to three minutes.

(2) Pull the arm over the head: The upper limb of the healthy side goes over the head to clasp with the five fingers of the upper limb of the sick side, with the vertex as a fulcrum, to pull the sick limb to the vertex in a small amplitude, till slight pain appears, for 20 to 30 times.

The above two methods are appropriate for the patients with the serious dysfunction of the shoulder joint. After the mobility of the shoulder joint is improved, it is advisable to do the circular training of the shoulder joint in a large amplitude.

注意事项

应指导患者作下列功能锻炼。

(1) 负重摆臂法。患者上身前屈,患肢下垂,手握一较轻的哑铃或沙袋,先作前后、左右方向的摆动;再作画圈运动,2～3 分钟。

(2) 过顶拉臂法。健侧上肢经过头顶与患侧上肢五指交叉相扣,以头顶为支点,将患肢向头顶方向作小幅度拉动,以感觉有轻度疼痛为度,20～30 次。

以上两法适用于肩关节功能障碍严重者的康复锻炼。待肩关节活动度改善后,方可进一步作肩关节的大幅度环转锻炼(摇膀子)。

Acute lumbar sprain

It refers to the acute injury of the muscles, fascias, ligaments, zygapophysial joints, and lumbosacral joints of the lumbar region, mostly induced by sudden attack of indirect external force, one of the most common lumbar pains. It mostly occurs in the young and middle-aged laborers, and groups in the stoop position for long time or lack of sport in the

急性腰扭伤

急性腰扭伤是指腰部肌肉、筋膜、韧带、关节突关节、腰骶关节的急性损伤,多因突然遭受间接外力所致,俗称闪腰、岔气,是腰痛病症中最常见的一种。多发于青壮年体力劳动者、长期弯腰工

ordinary time. Over weight, too fast or too violent action in the lumbar region, or improper posture and improper force in the lumbar mobility, or falls and sprain would induce serious traction and torsion of the lumbar muscles, fascias and ligaments, resulting in injury. Acute lumbar sprain mostly occurs in the spinal erectors and lumbosacral joints.

作或平时缺乏锻炼的人群。腰部若过度负重,动作过快或过猛;或腰部活动姿势不正确,用力不当;或跌仆闪挫,使腰部的肌肉、筋膜、韧带受到强烈的牵拉、扭转而致损伤。急性腰扭伤绝大多数发生在竖脊肌和腰骶关节等处。

Diagnostic Essentials

(1) Lumbar pain occurs immediately after the injury of the lumbar region. Pain is generally characterized by serious and continuous nature with fixed location. The patient usually is able to point out the painful spot precisely. The mild patient can walk barely. The severe patient is completely unable to move, turn, and get up from the bed, with pain seriously aggravated by cough and deep respiration.

(2) Obvious tenderness is palpable in the injured area. Some patients can be accompanied by pulling pain in the lower limb. Most patients can have lumbar spasm on one side or two sides, mostly in the spinal erectors and gluteus maximus. Or the protective spasm could be seen, leading to lateral curvature in varying degrees. The imageological examination can exclude osseous changes such as fracture of the lumbar vertebras and tumors.

诊断要点

(1) 腰部受伤后即出现典型的腰痛,疼痛一般较剧烈,呈持续性,部位局限固定,患者一般能准确指出疼痛部位。轻者能勉强行走,重者则完全不能活动,甚至不能翻身、起床,咳嗽、深呼吸时疼痛加剧。

(2) 损伤局部可触及明显的压痛点,部分患者可伴有下肢牵涉痛。多数患者有一侧或双侧腰肌痉挛,多位于竖脊肌、臀大肌等处。或者可见保护性的肌肉痉挛,造成不同程度的脊柱侧弯。影像学检查排除腰椎骨折和肿瘤等骨性病变。

Basic Therapeutic Methods

Therapeutic principle: Soothe the tendons, dredge the collaterals, circulate qi and stop pain.

The patient takes a prone position.

(1) Press the acupoints: Principle of acupoint selection is to select the lower acupoints for upper problem, select the right acupoints for the left

基本治法

治则:舒筋通络,行气止痛。

患者俯卧位。

(1) 点按腧穴:取穴原则为上病下取,左病右取,由外围到中央。点按委中(或屈

problem, and select the acupoints centripetally. Press Weizhong (BL 40) (or pluck Weizhong (BL 40) with the knee flexed), Yanglingquan (GB 34), opposite spot of tenderness on the healthy side, and around tenderness, for two minutes.

膝弹拨委中)、阳陵泉、压痛点的健侧对称点、压痛点周围,2 分钟。

(2) Roll the lumbar region: First roll the lumbar region for two to three minutes, and then roll with backward extension of the lumbar region and abduction of the hip joint, for one minute.

(2) 滚腰部:先滚腰部 2～3 分钟,再边滚边配合腰部后伸和髋关节外展活动,1 分钟。

(3) Press and knead the lumbus and back: Operate by the two hands by piling up the palms, for one to two minutes.

(3) 按揉腰背部,双手叠掌操作,1～2 分钟。

(4) Pull and extend the lumbus: After the patient holds the treatment table with the two hands, the medical practitioner uplifts the patient's two knees above the table by pulling his two legs, continuously for one minute, and finishes it by shaking the low back leftward and rightward.

(4) 拔伸腰部:患者双手拉住治疗床,术者拉其双腿使其膝部略离开床面,持续牵引 1 分钟,以左右晃腰动作结束。

(5) Pull the lumbus obliquely: The patient takes a lateral recumbent position on the healthy side. It is not necessary to seek the cracking sound in the joint.

(5) 斜扳腰部:患者健侧卧位。不要追求关节弹响。

(6) Chafe the lumbus: Chafe the bilateral spinal erectors with the hypothenar, for one minute. The oil medium, such as evergreen ointment, can be applied on the body surface.

(6) 擦腰部:以小鱼际擦腰部棘突两侧竖脊肌,1 分钟。体表可涂以冬青膏等油性介质。

Modification by Symptoms

随证加减

(1) If acute lumbar sprain is accompanied by subluxation of the posterior lumbar vertebral joint, in addition to the above oblique pulling method in the lateral recumbent position, it is advisable to select the pulling method by positioning and rotation for the lumbar vertebras in the sitting position.

(1) 如急性腰扭伤伴腰椎后关节半脱位,除了上述侧卧斜扳法外,还可选用坐位腰椎定位旋转扳法。

(2) If the patient is unable to stand up after

(2) 患者弯腰不能直立,

bending down, or unable to straighten the lower limbs in the supine position, it may be related to the injury of the iliopsoas muscle. After the patient takes the lateral recumbent position on the sick side, after the hip joint of the healthy side is extremely flexed, it is advisable to pluck the tendon of the iliopsoas muscle superior to the lesser trochanter of femur.

或仰卧时下肢不能伸直者，可能是髂腰肌损伤。可患侧卧位，在极度屈曲健侧髋关节后，弹拨股骨小转子上方的髂腰肌肌腱。

(3) If the patient comes to seek medical treatment by supporting the two knees with the two hands, unable to stand up completely, with sharp pricking pain in the lower back, it is necessary to doubt the possibility of synovial incarceration in the posterior lumbar vertebral joints. In tuina treatment, it is necessary to take the sitting position (not the prone position), and give the targeted treatment with the pulling method for the lumbar vertebras in the sitting position, by pulling continuously for one to two minutes. As soon as the synovial incarceration is removed, the patient can stand up immediately.

(3) 若患者双手撑住双膝弯腰前来就诊，上身完全不能直立，且腰部有尖锐刺痛者，应怀疑有腰椎后关节滑膜嵌顿可能。推拿治疗应取坐位（不可俯卧位操作），以坐位腰椎拔伸法作针对性治疗，持续拔伸 1～2 分钟。一旦滑膜嵌顿解除，即可直立。

Chronic lumbar pain

慢性腰痛

It is one of the commonly seen symptoms and is a syndrome induced by many diseases. Lumbar pain is mostly induced by aseptic inflammation in the soft tissues of the muscles, ligaments and fascias of the lumbar region and lower limbs, irritating the nerve endings in the focus. Injury of the lumbar spine, congenital lumbosacral deformity, and serious lumbar disc herniation may aggravate the aseptic inflammation of the soft tissues. The pain induced by aseptic inflammation of the soft tissues can further

慢性腰痛是临床常见病症之一，是一种可由多种疾病引起的证候群。腰痛的发生大多是腰部和下肢部的肌肉、韧带、筋膜等软组织的无菌性炎症，刺激病灶区的神经末梢，而引起疼痛。腰脊柱的损伤、先天性腰骶椎畸形、严重的腰椎间盘突出，都可能加重软组织的无菌性炎

induce the protective spasm of the soft tissues. Pain and spasm are interacted, forming a vicious circle. Chronic lumbar pain caused by the pathological change of the internal organs, such as kidney and urinary bladder, is not discussed in this section. It is believed in Chinese medicine that in addition to the close relationship with the functional change of the kidney, invasion of exogenous pathogenic wind, cold and dampness, sequela of acute injury from falls and sprains, or chronic strain may induce the spasm of the tendons in the lumbar region, leading to stagnation of qi and blood and hence pain.

症。软组织的无菌性炎症造成的疼痛可进一步引起肌肉等软组织的保护性痉挛，疼痛与痉挛互为因果，形成恶性循环。肾、膀胱等内在脏器的病变造成的慢性腰痛，不在本节范围之内。中医认为，腰痛除与肾脏的功能改变密切相关外，风、寒、湿等外邪的侵袭，跌仆闪挫等急性损伤的后遗症，或慢性劳损的形成，都可导致腰部经筋拘挛，气血瘀滞，进而产生疼痛。

Diagnostic Essentials

If chronic lumbar pain is accompanied by radiating pain in the lower limb, it is necessary to exclude lumbar pain caused by the pathological changes of visceral problems or spinal occupation, by the experimental examination. Generally, there are two major types of lumbar pain due to strain, and lumbar pain due to deficiency and cold.

(1) Lumbar pain due to strain　It is mostly related to history of acute injury of lower back, or occupation, types of job resulting in chronic lumbar pain, such as driver, long-term sitting workers, or mother giving birth to child, those catching cold from long-term sleeping in the humid area, chronic cough patients, or athletes often bending to picking up heavy objects or playing balls, and those in lack of outdoors activities. It is mostly seen in the middle-aged and young adults. In the attack, there will be lumbar pain, or lumbar pain accompanied by pain in the lower limb of one side, radiating pain in

诊断要点

慢性腰痛或伴下肢传导痛，结合实验室的检查，排除内脏疾病、脊髓占位性病变所致的腰痛。主要有劳损腰痛和虚寒腰痛两大类。

(1) 劳损腰痛　多有腰部急性损伤既往史，或职业、工种与导致腰部慢性劳损有关，如司机、长期坐位工作者，或生过孩子的母亲，长期睡卧湿地及受寒冷者，慢性咳嗽者，经常弯腰捡重物或打球的运动员，缺乏户外活动者。中、青年多见。发作时有腰痛，或腰痛伴有单侧下肢痛，咳嗽时牵涉下肢痛。可见腰椎侧凸，腰椎活动受

the lower limb by cough, noticeable lateral protrusion of the lumbar vertebras and limited activity of the lumbar vertebras. The tenderness spots are regularly distributed at the bilateral sides of the lumbar vertebras, superior border of the iliac crest, medial border of the posterior superior iliac spine, gluteus maximus, gluteus medium, gluteus minimus, iliac attachment of the tensor fasciae latae muscle, pubic attachment of the adductors of the femur, and lower border of the knee cap. The straight leg-raising test in the supine position is positive, manifested by the tense or traction sensation in the posterior aspect of the lower limb. The tenderness at the bilateral sides of the lumbar vertebras are alleviated after putting a pillow under the chest and aggravated by putting a pillow under the abdomen. There can be weakness in the extensor and flexor muscles of the big toe, abnormality in the knee and ankle reflex or sensory change in the lower limb, but without ankle spasm. X-ray examination, CT examination and MRI examination can show the imaging changes such as protrusion of nucleus pulposus of lumbar intervertebral disc, lateral curvature, and osteophyma of lumbar vertebras, but without specificity. The attack of lumbar pain is often related to fatigue and climate change.

限。压痛点多有规律地分布于腰椎两侧、髂嵴上缘、髂后上棘内侧缘，臀大肌、臀中肌、臀小肌、阔筋膜张肌的髂骨附着点，股内收肌群的耻骨附着点，髌骨下缘等处。仰卧直腿抬高试验阳性，抬高时下肢后部绷紧或有牵拉感。腰椎两侧的压痛在胸部垫枕后减轻，而在腹部垫枕后加重。踇趾伸屈肌力减弱。可有膝、踝反射异常或下肢感觉改变。无踝阵挛。X 线检查、CT 检查和 MRI 检查，可有腰椎间盘髓核突出、脊柱侧弯、腰椎骨赘等影像学改变，但非特异性。腰痛发作可与劳累、气候变化有关。

(2) Lumbar pain due to deficiency and cold It is mostly seen in the middle-aged and old people. Lumbar pain is insidious, or accompanied by aching pain in the two lower limbs, extensive tenderness, preference of warmth and dislike of cold in the low back and lower limb, weakness in the low back and feet, muscular atrophy in the quadriceps muscle of the thigh or leg, lustrousless complexion, pale

(2) 虚寒腰痛　中老年人多见。腰痛绵绵，或伴有双侧下肢酸痛，压痛较为广泛，腰部和下肢喜暖怕寒，腰脚无力，股四头肌或小腿可有肌萎缩。面色不华，舌淡苔白，脉弱。

tongue, white tongue coating, and feeble pulse.

Basic Therapeutic Methods

Therapeutic principle: Circulate qi, activate blood, soothe the tendons and stop pain.

The patient takes a prone position.

(1) Roll the lumbus and back: Roll the Muscle Meridian of Foot Taiyang at the bilateral sides of the back, from the top to the bottom to the superior border of the iliac crest, bilaterally for three times respectively.

(2) Roll the lumbus and back, together with backward extension of the lumbosacral part: Roll the lumbosacral part with one hand, and raise the patient's one leg with the other hand, for a passive movement of backward extension of the lumbar vertebras, for one to two minutes.

(3) Press and knead Huantiao (GB 30), Weizhong (BL 40), Yanglingquan (GB 34) and Kunlun (BL 60), for one minute respectively.

(4) Pull and stretch the lumbus: The practitioner holds the patient's two ankles, to pull and stretch the lumbus stably, for one to three minutes.

Modification by Symptoms

(1) Lumbar pain due to strain　In addition to the basic therapeutic methods, ① press the tenderness spots: detect the tenderness spots and press with the tip of the thumb the bilateral sides of the lumbar vertebras, superior border of the iliac crest, medial border of the posterior superior iliac spine, gluteus maximus, gluteus medium, gluteus minimus, iliac attachment of the tensor fasciae latae muscle, pubic attachment of the adductors of the femur, and tenderness spot at the lower border of the knee cap, for totally five to seven minutes, ② chafe the blad-

基本治法

治则：行气活血，舒筋止痛。

患者俯卧位。

（1）㨰腰背部：㨰腰背部两侧的足太阳经筋，从上往下至髂嵴上缘，左右各 3 遍。

（2）㨰腰背部配合腰骶后伸：一手㨰腰骶部，另一手同时将患者一侧下肢抬起，作腰椎后伸被动运动，1～2 分钟。

（3）按揉环跳、委中、阳陵泉、昆仑穴，各 1 分钟。

（4）拔伸腰部：术者握住患者两踝，平稳拔伸腰部，1～3 分钟。

随证加减

（1）劳损腰痛　基本治法加：①点按压痛点：探寻压痛点，并以拇指指端点按腰椎两侧、髂嵴上缘、髂后上棘内侧缘，臀大肌、臀中肌、臀小肌、阔筋膜张肌的髂骨附着点，股内收肌群的耻骨附着点，髌骨下缘等处的压痛点，共 5～7 分钟；②纵擦腰背部膀胱经，沿竖脊肌肌纤维方向掌擦腰部，以透热为

der meridian at the lumbar region vertically, along the muscular fibers of the spinal erectors, till the heat sensation penetrates, and ③ select the oblique pulling method for the lumbar vertebras accordingly, with the patient in a lateral recumbent position on the healthy side.

佳;③酌情选用腰椎斜扳法,患者取健侧卧位。

(2) Lumbar pain due to deficiency and cold In addition to the basic therapeutic methods, ① chafe the lumbosacral region transversely, ② chafe the three yin muscle tendons of the foot, and chafe the medial aspect of the leg and thigh with the hand part between the thumb and index finger, till the heat sensation penetrates, ③ rotate and pull the lumbar muscles: After the patient takes a lateral recumbent position, do the similar preparatory movements of the oblique pulling method for the lumbar vertebras, to rotate the patient's lumbar vertebras to the limited position, for one minute (without the pulling method), for stretching the lumbar muscles bilaterally, ④ Apply hot compress on the lumbosacral region.

(2) 虚寒腰痛 基本治法加:①横擦腰骶部;②擦足三阴经筋,以虎口擦小腿和大腿内侧,以透热为佳;③旋转牵引腰部肌肉:患者侧卧位,作类似于腰椎斜扳法的准备动作,将患者腰椎旋转到限制位后,保持该体位1分钟(但不作扳法),以拉伸腰部肌肉。左右双侧操作;④热敷腰骶部。

Tennis Elbow

Soft tissue pain in the lateral side of the elbow is a common clinical symptom. It is termed "tennis elbow", because it is related to the backhand stroke in playing tennis in the early observation. It is also termed "external humeral epicondylitis", because pain mainly appears at the attachment of the extensor tendon of the forearm on the external humeral epicondyle. Some people believe that traumatic injury of the neurovascular bundle goring through the common extensor tendon is the pathogenic factor of tennis elbow. Some people think the primary patho-

网球肘

肘部外侧软组织痛,是临床常见症状。因早期观察到与打网球反手击球有关而被称为"网球肘"。又其疼痛部位主要在前臂伸肌腱肱骨外上髁附着处而被称为"肱骨外上髁炎"。有人认为穿出伸肌总腱的血管神经束创伤性炎症是网球肘的病因,有人提出网球肘的首要病理变化是伸肌总腱起始部损

logical change of tennis elbow is injury of the staring part of the common extensor tendon and is also related to the traumatic inflammation and degeneration of the annular ligaments.

伤，也与环状韧带创伤性炎症、变性有关。

Diagnostic Essentials

It mostly occurs in the occupations or jobs using the wrist or forearm repeatedly, or due to the repeated rotation of the forearm before the onset, forceful extension of the wrist or backhand motion, leading to gradual or sudden pain at the lateral side of the elbow. Pain is mostly seen in the three spots of the external humeral epicondyle, humeroradial joint and articualr circumference. Pain can radiate to the middle and upper part of the extensor muscle of the forearm, and will be aggravated in clenching the fist and extending the wrist, leading to disability to hold objects. In severe condition, it will be difficult to dry up the towel, sweep the floor and hold water bottle. Tennis elbow test (Mill's syndrome) is positive. Anti-resistance backward extension test of the extensor muscles of the forearm is positive.

诊断要点

多发生于反复使用手腕或前臂的职业或工种，或发病前有反复旋转前臂、用力伸腕或反手运动史，逐渐或突然出现肘外侧疼痛。疼痛多见于肱骨外上髁、肱桡关节和桡骨头环状关节面 3 处，疼痛可放射至前臂伸肌中上部，在用力握拳、伸腕时加重，以致不能持物。严重时绞毛巾、扫地和提水瓶均感困难。网球肘试验(Mill's 征)阳性，前臂伸肌群抗阻力背伸试验阳性。

Basic Therapeutic Methods

Therapeutic principle: Activate blood and soothe the tendons.

The patient takes a sitting position or supine position.

Operation:

(1) Press and knead Hegu (LI 4) and Neiguan (PC 6), for about one minute.

(2) Roll the extensor muscles of the forearm, for one to two minutes.

(3) Push the extensor muscles of the forearm with one thumb, or press and knead with one thumb, mainly around the tenderness, for about

基本治法

治则：活血舒筋。

患者坐位或仰卧位。

操作：

(1) 按揉合谷、内关穴，约 1 分钟。

(2) 㨰前臂伸肌群，1～2 分钟。

(3) 一指禅推前臂伸肌群，或代之以拇指按揉法，重点针对压痛点周围，约 2 分

two minutes.

钟。

(4) Grasp the extensor muscles of the forearm, for about half a minute.

(4) 拿前臂伸肌群，约半分钟。

(5) Push the forearm divergently: Push with the thumbs of the two hands from the middle part of the extensor muscles of the forearm to the two sides divergently, along the extensor muscles, from the elbow to the wrist, for two times.

(5) 分推前臂：以双手拇指，从前臂伸肌群的中间向两侧横向分推，并沿着伸肌走向从肘向腕移动，2 遍。

(6) Pluck the extensor muscles of the forearm: Pluck the upper 1/3 part of the extensor muscles of the forearm with the thumb transversely, for about half a minute.

(6) 弹拨前臂伸肌群：以拇指横向弹拨前臂伸肌上1/3部，约半分钟。

(7) Rotate the elbow forward: In a position of the flexed elbow, rotate the elbow of the forearm backward to its extension position, for eight to ten times.

(7) 旋前摇肘：从屈肘位，将前臂旋后摇肘至伸肘位，8～10 次。

(8) Rotate the elbow backward: In the position of flexed elbow and flexed wrist, rotate the elbow of the forearm forward to its extension position, for eight to ten times.

(8) 旋后摇肘：从屈肘屈腕位，将前臂旋前摇肘至伸肘位，8～10 次。

(9) Rub and knead the forearm.

(9) 搓揉前臂。

(10) Chafe the extensor muscles of the forearm: Chafe the sick area with evergreen oil, for 30 times.

(10) 擦前臂伸肌群：以冬青油等介质擦患部，30 次。

(11) Finally, apply wet hot compress on the sick area, for five minutes.

(11) 最后可配合湿热敷患部，5 分钟。

Precautions

注意事项

For acute stage or serious pain, it is necessary to limit the activity of the wrist joint and middle finger.

急性期或疼痛剧烈者，需限制腕关节和中指的活动。

Ankle joint sprain

踝关节扭伤

It refers to the sudden forced introversion of

踝关节扭伤是指踝关节

the ankle joint, with the ankle joint in plantar flexion, leading to injury of the lateral collateral ligament of the ankle. It is mostly caused by walking or running on uneven ground, slipping down from the stairs or slope, or falling down from riding a bicycle, playing a ball, leading to over introversion of the ankle. In injury of introversion in the plantar flexion of the ankle joint, the anterior talofibular ligament of the lateral collateral ligament is easily injured. In severe condition, the calcaneofibular ligament can also be split. But, the posterior talofibular ligament is comparatively tough and the injury will seldom take place. After the ligament is injured, there will be local bleeding, effusion of tissue fluid, pain and dysfunction in activities. The injury of foot extroversion is seldom and will not be discussed in this book.

在跖屈位时，足踝突然强力内翻，而致踝部外侧副韧带损伤。多见于行走或跑步时因地面不平，或下楼梯、下坡时不慎失足，或骑自行车、踢球等运动中不慎跌倒，使足踝过度内翻所致。踝关节跖屈内翻损伤时，容易损伤外侧副韧带中的腓距前韧带，严重者，腓跟韧带亦可撕裂。而腓距后韧带较为坚强，极少发生损伤。韧带损伤后，局部出血，组织液渗出，引起疼痛和活动功能障碍。足外翻扭伤的情况较少见，本书省略。

Diagnostic Essentials

诊断要点

(1) There is a history of traumatic injury or ankle joint sprain, obvious pain and swelling in the ankle, local subcutaneous bruises, functional disturbance of the ankle activities, worse in flexion and introversion, and difficult walking. In sprain of the external malleolus, swelling mainly appears anterior and inferior to the external malleolus. If pricking pain in the foot is accompanied by deformity or abnormal activity of the ankle joint, it is necessary to consider image and detailed examination, due to the possibility of avulsion fracture of the external malleolus or complete avulsion of the ligament.

（1）有外伤史或踝关节扭伤史，踝部明显疼痛，肿胀，局部皮下淤血，踝关节活动功能障碍，以屈伸和内翻活动为甚，步行困难。外踝扭伤时，肿胀主要在外踝前下方。足部刺痛伴踝关节畸形或异常活动时，应考虑外踝撕脱性骨折或韧带完全撕裂，需摄片及详细检查。

(2) X-ray anteroposterior and lateral film of the ankle joint can help to exclude the avulsion fracture of both the internal and external malleolus. If injury is serious, it is necessary to film the forced

（2）踝关节 X 线正侧位片，可以帮助排除内外踝的撕脱性骨折，若损伤较重者，应作强力内翻、外翻位摄片，

introversion and extroversion, in order to see the enlarged angle of talar tilt, and even displacement phenomenon.

可见到距骨倾斜的角度增大,甚至可见到移位的现象。

Basic Therapeutic Methods

The basic principle is supposed to increase pain threshold of local tissues, promote the absorption of stagnant blood and tissue fluid, benefit the repair of injured tissues, and restore the activity of the ankle joint.

Take injury of the lateral collateral ligament as an example.

基本治法

以增加局部组织痛阈,促进淤血及组织液吸收,利于损伤组织的修复,恢复踝关节的活动为基本原则。

以外侧副韧带损伤为例。

1 Acute state (within 48 hours)

Therapeutic principle: Stop bleeding, diminish swelling, relieve spasm and alleviate pain.

The patient takes a prone position with the knees flexed or lying position on the healthy side.

(1) Press Zusanli (ST 36), Yanglingquan (GB 34) and Juegu (GB 39), for one minute.

(2) Grasp Chengshan (BL 57), for half a minute.

(3) Palm-vibrating method by pressure: Put the palm on the injured part of the lateral collateral ligament, with the part of the thumb and index opposite to the external malleolus and vibrate for with the palm, for three minutes. This method is effective in alleviating pain and stopping bleeding. Or, it is advisable to apply the thumb-pressing method instead, to slightly press the sick area (equal to Qiuxu (GB 40)) with the cushion of the thumb for five minutes.

(4) If hematoma already appears, it is advisable to push the leg centripetally with the hand, in order to promote reflux of stagnant blood for diminishing swelling, for two minutes. After tuina treat-

1 急性期(48 小时之内)

治则:止血消肿、解痉镇痛。

患者取俯卧屈膝位,或健侧卧位。

(1) 点按足三里、阳陵泉、绝骨,1 分钟。

(2) 拿承山,半分钟。

(3) 加压掌振法:以掌心置于外侧副韧带的损伤处,虎口相对外踝,行掌振法 3 分钟。本法镇痛效果很好,且有压迫止血之功。或代之以拇指按压法,以拇指指腹轻压患部(相当于丘墟穴)5 分钟。

(4) 如已出现血肿,可以虎口部向心性直推小腿,促进淤血回流以消肿,2 分钟。推拿后以弹性绷带加压包

ment, elastic bandage is tightly fastened. The patient should take a supine position to rest with the knee flexed and leg raised.

扎。患者应取仰卧屈膝高抬腿体位休息。

2 The recovery stage (after 48 hours)

2 恢复期(48 小时以后)

Therapeutic principle: Activate blood, disperse blood stasis, diminish swelling and stop pain.

治则:活血祛瘀,消肿止痛。

The patient takes a supine position or sitting position.

患者仰卧或取坐位。

(1) Press Zusanli (ST 36), Yanglingquan (GB 34), Juegu (GB 39), Kunlun (BL 60), Qiuxu (GB 40), Jiexi (ST 41), and Taichong (LR 3), for three minutes.

（1）点按足三里、阳陵泉、绝骨、昆仑、丘墟、解溪、太冲等穴,3 分钟。

(2) Press and knead around the sick area and leg, together with the light rotating method of the ankle joint, for two minutes.

（2）按揉患部周围和小腿,可配合踝关节轻度摇法,2 分钟。

(3) Chafe the sick area with the palm till heat sensation penetrates, for one minute.

（3）患部掌擦透热,1 分钟。

(4) The pulling and rotating method for the ankle joint: The ankle joint should be rotated with proper amplitude and strength, for one minute. For old injury, it is advisable to rotate in large amplitude with strong strength.

（4）拔伸摇踝法:摇踝的幅度和力度适中,1 分钟。如为陈旧性损伤,幅度宜大,手法可较重。

Precautions

注意事项

(1) It is advisable to adopt ice cube massage method, if the condition is possible in the moment of injury. After ice cubes are put into a rubber or plastic bag, it can be used to press and knead the local area instead of the finger, for stopping bleeding and alleviating pain.

（1）损伤即刻有条件者可使用冰块按摩法。置冰块于胶袋或塑料袋内,代替手指进行局部按揉,有止血镇痛之功。

(2) It is appropriate to tuina with the static manual techniques in the acute stage, and necessary not to irritate the local focus as much as possible, and prohibited to use the rotating method of the ankle joint.

（2）急性期的推拿以静止性手法为宜,尽量不要刺激病灶局部,禁止使用踝关节摇法。

(3) It is prohibited to use wet hot compress within 48 hours of injury.

(4) In the acute stage, it is necessary to guide the patient to rest with the knee and hip flexed and leg raised in a supine position.

(3) 损伤48小时内局部禁止湿热敷。

(4) 急性期应指导患者屈膝屈髋高抬腿仰卧休息。

Section 2 Internal and gynecological diseases

第2节 内妇科疾病

Facial paralysis

It refers to a disease characterized by deviation of the eye and mouth due to paralysis of the facial nerve as the main symptom. There are central type and peripheral type. The muscles in the lower face are dominated by the opposite cerebral cortex. The muscles in the upper face are dominated by the bilateral corticonuclear tract. Central facial paralysis is induced by the cerebrovascular diseases and intracranial tumor, with paralysis only limited in the lower part of the face. Peripheral facial paralysis, also termed Bell's palsy, is caused by non-specific inflammation of the facial nerve inside the stylomastoid foramen. In this section, only peripheral facial paralysis is introduced.

Diagnostic Essentials

Acute onset, pain in the mastoid process behind the ear, inside the ear and in the face mostly in the early stage, and abnormal sensation, expression muscles in asymmetrical appearance on the two sides of the face, disappearance of frontal creases in the sick side, disability to raise the eyebrow, close the eye, bulge the cheek, expose the teeth and blow, shallow nasolabial groove, deviation of the mouth

面瘫

面瘫，是指面神经麻痹而致的以口眼歪斜为主要症状的一种病证。有中枢性和周围性之分。颜面下部的肌肉受对侧大脑皮质支配，颜面上部的肌肉受双侧大脑皮质脑干束支配。中枢性面瘫因脑血管疾病及颅内肿瘤等原因引起，瘫痪仅限于颜面下部。周围性面神经麻痹又称Bell麻痹，因茎乳孔内面神经非特异性炎症所致。本节仅介绍周围性面神经麻痹。

诊断要点

起病急，初期多有耳后乳突部、耳内及面部疼痛，感觉异常，随后出现两侧面部表情肌不对称，患侧额纹消失，不能蹙眉、闭眼、鼓腮、露齿、吹气，鼻唇沟变浅，口角偏向对侧，常有流泪、流涎等。进食时食物常滞留于患

corner to the opposite side, frequent lacrimation and salivation. In ingesting food, food stuffs are often retained between the teeth and cheek of the sick side. The taste sense decreases in the anterior 2/3 part of the tongue in the sick side, and the auditory sense becomes hyperactive. Reflex disappears in the orbicular muscle of eye in the sick side. The eyelash sign is positive (In closing the eye tightly, the eyelid of the sick side is unable to close tightly and expose the eyelash instead. It occurs in mild facial paralysis. In the patient with history of facial paralysis, the disability to maintain the eyelid closed for long time is also regarded as positive). Bell's sign is positive (In closing the eye, there are incomplete closure of the sick eye, upward motion of the eyeball, and exposure of sclera under the cornea).

侧颊齿之间，同侧舌前 2/3 部味觉减退，听觉过敏。患侧眼轮匝肌反射消失。睫毛征阳性(用力闭眼时，患侧眼睑不能闭紧而露出睫毛。轻度面瘫即有。有面瘫史者患侧眼睑往往不能持久闭合，故亦可为阳性)。Bell 氏征阳性(闭眼时，患眼闭合不全，眼球上窜，在角膜下露出巩膜带)。

Basic Therapeutic Methods

Therapeutic principle: Activate blood, expel wind, warm up the meridians and dredge the collaterals, and correct deficiency for flaccid side by the light technique, and sedate excess for spasmodic side by the heavy technique.

(1) Grasp Hegu (LI 4), on the sick side, with heavy technique, for half a minute.

(2) Press and knead the acupoints: Press and knead with the thumb or middle finger Yintang (Extra), Jingming (BL 1), Zanzhu (BL 2), Yangbai (GB 14), Sizhukong (TE 23), Chengqi (ST 1), Sibai (ST 2), Yingxiang (LI 20), Dicang (ST 4), Jiache (ST 6), Tinggong (SI 19), and Tinghui (GB 2), bilaterally for totally three minutes. The above acupoints on the flaccid side can be knocked lightly with the tip of the middle finger.

(3) Push the face with the thumb side: The

基本治法

治则：活血祛风，温经通络。弛缓侧用轻手法补其虚，痉挛侧用重手法泻其实。

(1) 拿合谷：取患侧，手法宜重，半分钟。

(2) 按揉腧穴：以拇指或中指按揉印堂、睛明、攒竹、阳白、丝竹空、承泣、四白、迎香、地仓、颊车、听宫、听会穴，双侧，共 3 分钟。弛缓侧上述腧穴可以采取中指端轻叩法。

(3) 一指禅偏锋推面部：

route is to push starting from Chengjiang (CV 24), around the lips, via Dicang (ST 4) to Shuigou (GV 26), along Yingxiang (LI 20) next to the nasal wing, upward to the lower border of the orbit, and encircling the orbit, via Taiyang (Extra), Sizhukong (TE 23) to Yintang (Extra), and then to the healthy side, against the above route downward to Chengjiang (CV 24), and then back to Jiache (ST 6), along Tinghui (GB 2), Tinggong (SI 19) and Ermen (TE 21) upward, along the hairline to Shenting (GV 24) of the forehead, and continuously to the sick side, and downward along the above route to Chengjiang (CV 24), for three to five times. This method can be replaced by the nimble finger-kneading method.

路线为,从承浆起,环唇,经地仓到水沟,绕过鼻翼迎香,上行至眶下缘,再绕行眼眶,经太阳、丝竹空至印堂;然后行向健侧,逆上述路线下行至承浆;再折向健侧颊车,沿听会、听宫、耳门上行,沿发际推至前额神庭下;再继续推向患侧,按上述路线下行至承浆,3～5 遍。本法可代之以轻巧的指揉法。

(4) Knead the face with the thenar, along the above route for two to three times.

(4) 鱼际揉面部,按上述路线操作 2～3 遍。

(5) Press Yifeng (TE 17) with the finger, on the sick side.

(5) 指按翳风,患侧。

(6) Grasp Fengchi (GB 20), for half a minute.

(6) 拿风池,半分钟。

Modification by Symptoms

随证加减

(1) Acute stage In addition to the basic therapeutic methods, add the finger-vibrating method: ① vibrate the area of the mastoid process with the finger, for one minute, in order to circulate qi and expel blood stasis, for preventing the possible adhesion inside the nerve canal, ② vibrate Yifeng (TE 17), Tinggong (SI 19) and Tinghui (GB 2) with the finger, for two minutes, in order to expel the accumulation of wind and dampness from the facial nerve trunk.

(1) 急性期 基本治法加指振法:①指振患侧乳突部,1 分钟。以行气祛瘀,防治面神经管内可能形成的粘连;②指振翳风、听宫、听会穴,2 分钟。针对面神经干,有驱散风湿性淤积物之功。

(2) Sequela stage In addition to the basic therapeutic methods, add paste massage therapy. With ointment prepared of Anti-Contracture Pow-

(2) 后遗症期 基本治法加膏摩法。以牵正散(白附子、僵蚕、全蝎)加防风、秦

der (Qian Zheng San) (Rhizoma Typhonii Gigantei (Bai Fu Zi), Bombyx Batryticatus (Jiang Can), Scorpio (Quan Xie)) plus Radix Ledebouriellae (Fang Feng), Radix Gentianae Macrophyllae (Qin Jiao), and Rhizoma Arisaematis (Tian Nan Xing), rub the face of the sick side with the finger, for three to five minutes.

艽、南星等制成软膏，以指摩法轻摩患侧面部，3～5 分钟。

Precautions

(1) This pattern belongs to flaccid paralysis. No heavy techniques should be used on the face.

(2) It is necessary to avoid pulling and stretching the paralyzed muscles too much.

(3) It is prohibited to use the heavy chafing technique on the face.

(4) Tuina treatment should be within fifteen minutes and given one to two times per day.

注意事项

(1) 本证属弛缓性麻痹，面部不宜用重手法。

(2) 应避免过度牵伸麻痹肌肉。

(3) 面部禁用重擦法。

(4) 每次推拿时间不超过 15 分钟，最好每天 1～2 次。

Apoplexy sequela

Apoplexy is also termed cerebrovascualr accident. The sequelae caused by apoplexy refers mainly to hemiplegia. Long-term immobilization or improper nursing will bring about the complications and sequelae of hypostatic pneumonia, urinary stones, bed sores, extorsion deformity of hip, talipes equinovarus or foot drop, and frozen shoulder.

Tuina treatment is uniquely effective from other therapies in promoting the rehabilitation of the limb functions and preventing and treating complications. Tuina treatment for hemiplegia should be applied as early as possible. As soon as some autonomic movement starts to recover, it is necessary to guide the patients to start the correct self-guiding

中风后遗症

中风，又称脑血管意外。中风引起的后遗症，主要指半身不遂（偏瘫）。久病卧床或护理不当，还可并发坠积性肺炎、尿路结石、褥疮、髋外旋畸形、马蹄内翻足或足下垂、冻结肩等并发症和后遗症。

推拿治疗对促进肢体功能的康复，以及并发症的防治，具有不同于其他疗法的独特效果。推拿治疗偏瘫应尽早实施。一旦肢体开始恢复部分自主运动，即应指导患者进行正确的自我导引锻

training, significantly beneficial to early rehabilitation.

Diagnostic Essentials

In modern medicine, cerebrovascular accidents are divided into the two major types of ischemic accident and bleeding accident. The former includes cerebral thrombosis and cerebral embolism. The latter includes cerebral hemorrhage and subarachnoid hemorrhage. The differential diagnosis for those four situations can be seen in Table 6-1.

炼，这对于早日康复有重要意义。

诊断要点

现代医学将脑血管意外分为缺血性和出血性两大类。前者包括脑血栓形成和脑栓塞，后者包括脑出血和蛛网膜下隙（Subarachnoid Space）出血。这 4 种情况的鉴别诊断见表 6-1。

Table 6-1 Differential Diagnosis of Cerebral Accidents

Main Points	Ischemic Apoplexy		Hemorrhagic Apoplexy	
	Cerebral Thrombosis	Cerebral Embolism	Cerebral Hemorrhage	Subarachnoid Hemorrhage
Age	Above 60	Young adults	Above 50	Young, middle and old age
Common factors	Atherosclerosis	Rheumatoid Heart Disease	Hypertension	Aneurysm, vascular malformation, atherosclerosis
Incidence	Slow onset (hour, day), in quiet state, mostly at night, mostly with premonitory symptoms of dizziness	Urgent onset (second, minute), at seizure of heart disease, with signs of the nervous system	Acute onset (minute, hour), at the activity or emotional excitement, quick development	Fairly acute onset (minute), at the activity
Headache	Seldom, mild	Seldom, mild	Common	Common
Vomiting	Seldom	Seldom	Common	Common
Blood pressure	Higher	Normal	High	Generally normal
Aphasia	Yes	Yes	Yes	No
Disturbance of consciousness	Mostly no	Mild or no	Yes	Transient

表 6-1 脑血管意外鉴别诊断

鉴别要点	缺血性中风		出血性中风	
	脑血栓形成	脑栓塞	脑出血	蛛网膜下隙出血
发病年龄	60 岁以上	青壮年	50 岁以上	青、中、老年
常见病因	动脉粥样硬化	风湿性心脏病	高血压	动脉瘤、血管畸形、动脉粥样硬化

续表

鉴别要点	缺血性中风		出血性中风	
	脑血栓形成	脑栓塞	脑出血	蛛网膜下隙出血
发病情况	起病较慢(小时、天),安静时,夜间发病较多,多有眩晕等前驱症状	发病最急(秒、分),可在心脏病发作时发病,神经系统体征迅速出现	发病急骤(分、小时),活动时或情绪激动时发病,病情迅速进展	发病较急(分),活动时发病
头　痛	少见而轻	少见而轻	常见	剧烈
呕　吐	少见	少见	常见	常见
血　压	有的较高	正常	高	一般正常
失　语	有	有	有	无
意识障碍	多无	轻或无	有	一过性

(1) This pattern is mainly characterized by paralysis and weakness of the unilateral upper and lower limb, deviation of mouth and eye, stiff tongue and aphasia. In the initial stage, the patient's limb is soft and feeble (flaccid paralysis), with slow or light tough perception, limited activity, and gradually becomes stiff and spasmodic (spastic paralysis), with change and deformity in the posture of the limb at the sick side.

(1) 本证以单侧的上下肢瘫痪无力、口眼歪斜,舌强语謇为主症。初期患者肢体软弱无力(软瘫),知觉迟钝或稍有强硬,活动功能受限;以后逐渐趋于强直挛急(硬瘫),患侧肢体姿势常发生改变和畸形等。

(2) Examinations: After the shock stage, the muscular tension of the limb at the sick side is elevated, with spastic deformity of the joint, slightly decreased sense, and basically loss of its activity, and with hyperactive reflex of the biceps tendon and triceps tendon of the arm, positive in Hoffmann's sign, hyperactive reflex of the patellar tendon and heel tendon at the sick side, normal at the healthy side. Blood pressure is slight higher in the patients with cerebral hemorrhage and cerebral thrombosis. The meningeal irritation is positive in the patients with subarachnoid hemorrhage. The signs of the nervous system may be present in the patients with

(2) 检查:脊休克期过后患侧肢体肌张力增高,关节挛缩畸形,感觉略减退,活动功能基本丧失,患侧上肢肱二头肌、肱三头肌腱反射亢进,霍夫曼征阳性,下肢膝腱和跟腱反射亢进,健侧正常。脑出血和脑血栓形成患者血压偏高,蛛网膜下隙出血的患者脑膜刺激征阳性,脑栓塞可出现神经系统体征。脑脊液检验:脑出血和蛛网膜下腔出血患者为血性;脑血

cerebral embolism. Cerebrospinal fluid examination: It is hemorrhagic in the patients with cerebral hemorrhage and subarachnoid hemorrhage, and normal in the patients with cerebral thrombosis and cerebral embolism.

栓形成和脑栓塞患者均为正常。

(3) The key for diagnosis of this disease is the history of hypertension, heart disease, headache and dizziness, plus sudden fall, unconsciousness, or gradually appearance of hemiplegia, deviation of mouth and eye, stiff tongue and aphasia in the static state.

(3) 本病诊断要点是既往有高血压、心脏病和头痛、眩晕的病史;猝然仆倒不省人事,或静止状态下逐渐出现半身不遂、口眼歪斜、舌强语涩等症者即可确诊。

Basic Therapeutic Methods

基本治法

Therapeutic principle: Activate blood, disperse blood stasis, soothe the tendons and lubricate joints, with the passive guiding techniques for the joints in predominance.

治则:活血化瘀,舒筋利节。以关节被动导引手法为主。

Operation in different body parts:

分部操作:

1 Head and face

1 头面部

Please refer to tuina treatment for "facial paralysis", and intensify the operation on the nape and increase the pressing operation on the vertex, motor zone of scalp acupuncture in particular.

参见"面瘫"的推拿治疗,加强颈项部操作,增加按压头顶部操作,以头针的运动区为主。

2 Lower limb

2 下肢部

Main goals: Help to obtain the functions to extend the hip and flex the knee and the controlling ability to extend the lower limb, in order to avoid disuse syndrome.

主要目标:帮助获得伸髋屈膝功能和下肢伸展控制能力,防止废用综合征。

Body position: Lateral recumbent position on the healthy side is best, because the muscular tension in flexion and extension is similar. It is necessary to avoid the semi-reclining position as much as possible. It is necessary to flex the knee and hip in the supine position, with the hip joint adducted and inward rotated, to avoid spasm in the extensor mus-

体位:以健侧卧位为最佳,此时屈伸肌张力大致相当。应尽量避免半卧位。仰卧位时应屈膝屈髋,且髋关节内收内旋,以避免下肢伸肌痉挛。俯卧位不适宜于老年患者。

cle of the lower limb. The prone position is not appropriate for the old patients.

Lateral recumbent position on the healthy side:

健侧卧位。

(1) Press and knead Taichong (LR 3), Jiexi (ST 41), Zusanli (ST 36) and Fenglong (ST 40) of the sick side, for two minutes.

（1）按揉患侧太冲、解溪、足三里、丰隆穴，2 分钟。

(2) Pluck Weizhong (BL 40) and Huantiao (GB 34), for one minute.

（2）弹拨委中、环跳，1 分钟。

(3) Roll the buttocks, lateral, anterior and posterior side of the thigh, and lateral side of the leg, for three minutes.

（3）㨰臀部、大腿外侧、前后侧、小腿外侧，3 分钟。

(4) Grasp the muscle groups of the thigh and leg, for one minute.

（4）拿大腿、小腿肌群，1 分钟。

(5) Passive guiding technique: Apply the method for knee flexion and hip flexion, the method for knee flexion and hip extension, for two minutes.

（5）被动导引法：屈膝屈髋法，屈膝伸髋法，2 分钟。

Supine position with knee flexion:

屈膝仰卧位。

(1) Flex the knee and rotate the hip: Flex the knee toward the healthy side, to make a circular rotation for the hip joint, for one minute.

（1）屈膝摇髋法：屈膝，膝关节倒向健侧，作髋关节环转摇法，1 分钟。

(2) Flex the knee and rotate the ankle: Flex the knee, flex the ankle and rotate the ankle, and maintain the ankle joint in dorsal flexion and extroversion as much as possible, for one minute.

（2）屈膝摇踝法：屈膝，作屈踝、转踝动作，尽量使踝关节保持背屈外翻位，1 分钟。

3　Upper limb

3　上肢部

Goals: Prevent and treat spasm in the flexor muscle of the upper limb, and promote the natural restoration of the upper limb.

目标：防治上肢屈肌痉挛，促进上肢自然恢复。

Body position: Lateral recumbent position on the healthy side or supine position. The sitting position and semi-reclining position tend to increase the spasm of the flexor muscle of the upper limb.

体位：取健侧卧位或仰卧位。坐位和半卧位有增加上肢屈肌痉挛的倾向。

(1) Press and knead Hegu (LI 4), Neiguan (PC 6), Quchi (LI 11), Jianyu (LI 15) and Jianliao (TE

（1）按揉合谷、内关、曲池、肩髃、肩髎穴，2 分钟。

14), for two minutes.

(2) Grasp Jianjing (GB 21) and Jiquan (HT 1), for one minute.

(2) 拿肩井、极泉穴,1分钟。

(3) Extend the finger and wrist: The medical practitioner crisscrosses and holds the five fingers of one hand with the five fingers of the patient externally, to help to extend the patient's metacarpophalangeal joints and wrist joint backward. It is necessary not to touch the palm of the sick limb, in order to avoid inducing spasm of the flexor muscle, for one minute.

(3) 伸指伸腕法:术者一手五指与患者五指外相叉而握,帮助患者的掌指关节和腕关节背伸。注意避免触及患肢掌心,以免诱发屈肌痉挛,1分钟。

(4) Extend the wrist and elbow: In extending the wrist and fingers, slowly straighten the elbow joint, for one minute.

(4) 伸腕伸肘法:在伸腕和伸指的同时将肘关节缓慢伸直,1分钟。

(5) Straighten the arm and raise the shoulder: Extend and raise the elbow of the sick limb passively, over 90°, for one minute.

(5) 直臂举肩法:患肢伸肘被动前举,超过90°,1分钟。

(6) Straighten the arm and stretch the shoulder: Extend and abduct the elbow of the sick limb, for one minute.

(6) 直臂展肩法:患肢伸肘外展,1分钟。

(7) Straighten the arm and rotate the shoulder: In extending the elbow, passively uphold, abduct and rotate the shoulder joint backward, for one minute.

(7) 直臂摇肩法:在伸肘状态下作肩关节的被动前举、外展和旋后复合动作,1分钟。

4 Abdomen

4 腹部

Body position: Supine position with knee flexed.

体位:屈膝仰卧位。

(1) Press and knead Qihai (CV 6), Guanyuan (CV 4) and Zhongwan (CV 12), for two minutes, to benefit qi and consolidate the kidney.

(1) 按揉气海、关元、中脘穴,2分钟。以益气固元。

(2) Rub the abdomen, for two minutes, to strengthen the spleen and harmonize the center.

(2) 摩腹,2分钟。以健脾和中。

5 Back and lumbosacral region

5 背部和腰骶部

Body position: Prone position. Lateral recum-

体位:俯卧位。老人、过

bent position on the healthy side is appropriate for the elderly, over obesity, stiff joint and deficiency of qi and blood.

度肥胖者、关节僵硬者及气血两虚者改健侧卧位。

(1) Press and knead or push the bilateral bladder meridian at the back with the thumb, Feishu (BL 13), Xinshu (BL 15), Shenshu (BL 23), Shangliao (BL 31), Ciliao (BL 32), Zhongliao (BL 33) and Xialiao (BL 34) in particular, for two minutes.

（1）按揉或一指禅推背部两侧膀胱经，以肺俞、心俞、肾俞、八髎穴为重点，2分钟。

(2) Pat the upper back: Pat the upper back with a loose palm, upward & inward, to promote the lung for expectoration, for one minute.

（2）拍上背部：以虚掌拍上背部，方向由下而上，由外而内，功能宣肺豁痰，1分钟。

Modification by Symptoms

随证加减

Prevent the main complications and sequelae:

主要并发症及后遗症的预防：

(1) Hypostatic pneumonia: In the lateral recumbent position, pat the back with the palm, for two minutes. It is necessary to avoid supine position for long time.

（1）坠积性肺炎：侧卧位掌拍背部，2分钟。避免长时间仰卧位。

(2) Osteoporosis and urinary stones: It is necessary for the paralyzed patient to maintain a straight sitting position for a certain period of time, in order to maintain the normal force line of the skeleton, and prevent decalcification due to the rearrangement of the force line of the bone trabecula from causing further urinary stones.

（2）骨质疏松及尿路结石：瘫痪病人应尽可能维持一定时间的直立位，保持骨骼正常的力线，防止因骨小梁力线的重新排列而脱钙，并进一步导致尿路结石。

(3) Bed sores: It is necessary to help the paralyzed patient to change the body position frequently, in order to avoid long-term compression of the condyle areas. It is needed to press and knead those areas frequently, and to apply safflower oil or alcohol on those areas in the initial stage of swelling.

（3）褥疮：应帮助瘫痪病人经常变换体位，避免骨突部位长时间受压。经常按揉这些部位，在红肿初起时可用红花油或酒精擦法。

(4) Extorsion deformity of hip: By box foot plate, rotate the hip joint inward, for one minute, for several times per day.

（4）髋外旋畸形：使用箱形足夹板。并作髋关节内旋摇法，1分钟。每天数次。

(5) Talipes equinovarus or foot drop: By box foot plate, rotate and pull the ankle joint, for one minute, for several times per day.

(6) Frozen shoulder: Rotate the shoulder joint, and abduct and pull the shoulder joint, for two minutes, for several times per day.

(5) 马蹄内翻足或足下垂：使用箱形足夹板。踝关节摇法及扳法，1 分钟。每天数次。

(6) 冻结肩：肩关节摇法及外展扳法，2 分钟。每天数次。

Headache

It is one of the commonly seen symptoms clinically and is divided into the functional type and organic type. The causative factors of headache are complicated and numerous. The pathological changes of cerebrovascular dilation and intracranial occupation can induce headache. In particular, headache induced by muscular tension in the occipital and nuchal region and vertebrabasilar ischemia is most common. It is believed in Chinese medicine that headache is related to six exogenous pathogenic factors and seven emotional factors. Namely, the invasion of the pathogenic wind and heat into the brain, blockage of the brain by phlegm and dampness, hyperactivity of the liver fire, failure of the essence and blood in nourishing the brain due to kidney deficiency can all induce headache. Massage therapy is precisely effective for headache due to muscular tension and poor blood supply in the vertebrabasilar artery.

头痛

头痛是临床常见症状之一，分为功能性与器质性两类。头痛的病因复杂多端。脑血管扩张和颅内占位性病变等皆可引起头痛，尤以枕部和项部肌肉紧张和椎基底动脉缺血引起的头痛较为常见。中医学认为头痛的发生与外感六淫之邪及内伤七情有关，即风寒、风热侵扰清窍，痰湿上蒙清窍，肝火上炎，肾虚精血不能上荣于脑，均可导致头痛。推拿对肌紧张性头痛和椎基底动脉供血不足引起的头痛疗效确切。

Diagnostic Essentials

The common symptoms of headache are headache with dizziness and heavy sensation, fixed or non-fixed location, accompanied by nasal obstruction, aversion to cold, fever, flushed cheeks, red ears, or pale complexion, etc.

诊断要点

头痛证的临床常见症状是：头痛昏重，痛有定处或无定处。兼症可见鼻塞、畏寒、发热、面红耳赤或面色苍白等。

Basic Therapeutic Methods

Therapeutic principle: Soothe the tendons, activate blood, tranquilize the heart and calm down the mind, by the relaxing method and pulling method for the nuchal region and the mind-calming method for the head and face in predominance.

Usually the patient takes a supine position or sitting position.

1 Nuchal region

(1) Uphold and knead cervical Huatuo Jiaji (Extra): Uphold and knead the bilateral sides of the nape with the index, middle and ring finger of the two hands by force in opposition, for one minute.

(2) Hook and knead Fengchi (GB 20): Use the force with the middle fingers of the two hands, for half a minute.

(3) Pull and extend the cervical vertebras: Hold the occipital region with one hand, and hold the chin with the othar hand, to pull and extend the cervical vertebras vertically, for one minute.

(4) Grasp Jianjing (GB 21): Operate with the two hands, for half a minute.

The sitting position is also advisable for operation on the nuchal region. The pushing method with one thumb or pressing-kneading method with the thumb can be used alternatively for upholding and kneading the nuchal region. To hook and knead Fengchi (GB 20) can be altered to grasp Fengchi (GB 20). The pulling method by upholding the elbow in the sitting position can be used to pull and extend the cervical vertebras, and the grasping method for the nuchal region can be added.

2 Head and face

(1) Open the heavenly gate: Push with the

基本治法

治则:舒筋活血、宁心安神。手法以颈项部放松手法、拔伸手法和头面部安神手法为主。

患者一般取仰卧位,亦可取坐位。

1 颈项部

(1) 托揉颈夹脊:双手食、中、无名指对称用力,托揉项部两侧,1 分钟。

(2) 勾揉风池:双手中指用力,半分钟。

(3) 拔伸颈椎:一手托住枕部,一手勾住下颌,沿颈椎纵轴拔伸,1 分钟。

(4) 拿肩井:双手操作,半分钟。

颈项部也可坐位操作。托揉项部改一指禅推法或拇指按揉法;勾揉风池改拿风池;颈椎拔伸取坐位肘托拔伸法;并可增加项部拿法。

2 头面部

(1) 开天门:以双手拇指

thumbs of the two hands from Yintang (Extra) to Shenting (GV 24) alternatively, for about twenty times.

从印堂交替推至神庭，约20次。

(2) Push the supraorbital ridge divergently: Push with the thumbs of the two hands from Yintang (Extra) divergently along the eyebrow to the end of the eyebrow, for about ten times.

(2) 分推眉弓：以双手拇指从印堂起沿眉毛分推至眉梢，约10次。

(3) Push the forehead divergently: Push with the thumbs of the two hands from the midline of the forehead to the bilateral Taiyang (Extra), and move downward from Shenting (GV 24) slowly to Yintang (Extra) repeatedly, for four to five times.

(3) 分推前额：双手拇指从前额正中线分推至两侧太阳穴，并从神庭向印堂慢慢上下往返移动，4～5遍。

(4) Press and knead Taiyang (Extra): Knead Taiyang (Extra) with the thumbs of the two hands or the cushions of the middle fingers, for half a minute.

(4) 按揉太阳：以双手拇指或中指指腹揉太阳穴，半分钟。

(5) Press Shangxing (GV 23) and Baihui (GV 20) with the finger, for half a minute.

(5) 指按上星、百会穴，半分钟。

(6) Push the orbit with one thumb: Push the two orbits with the side of the thumb in a route of "8", for one to two minutes.

(6) 一指禅推眼眶：以一指禅偏锋推法沿两眼眶作横"8"字运行，1～2分钟。

(7) Knead the forehead with the thenar: Knead the forehead with the thenar, from Taiyang (Extra) on one side to Taiyang (Extra) on the other side, repeatedly for several times.

(7) 鱼际揉前额：以鱼际肌揉前额，从一侧太阳穴到另一侧太阳穴，往返数次。

(8) Sweep the temple: Sweep the bilateral temples with the five fingers of the two hands backward and downward lightly in curve, for about twenty times.

(8) 扫散颞部：以双手五指从头两侧颞部向后下方轻快地弧形推动，约20次。

(9) Hit the vertex with the joined palms, for ten to twenty times.

(9) 合掌击头顶，10～20次。

Modification by Symptoms

随证加减

(1) Headache due to wind and cold Additionally chafe the bilateral bladder meridian at the back

(1) 风寒头痛 加擦背部两侧膀胱经透热。

till heat sensation penetrates.

(2) Headache due to wind and heat　Additionally grasp the five meridians (stretch the five fingers, with the middle finger on Shenting (GV 24), and grasp the vertex forcefully and backward), for three to five times.

(2) 风热头痛　加抓五经(五指张开,中指置于神庭穴,用力抓拿头顶,并从前向后移动),3～5 遍。

(3) Headache due to phlegm and dampness　Additionally rub the abdomen clockwise, for three minutes, together with the passive movement of the four limbs for those with heavy sensation in the four limbs.

(3) 痰湿头痛　加顺时针摩腹,3 分钟;四肢困重者加四肢被动运动。

(4) Headache due to liver fire　Additionally press and knead Neiting (ST 44) and Taichong (LR 3), for one minute, and chafe Yongquan (KI 1), for one minute.

(4) 肝火头痛　加按揉内庭、太冲,1 分钟;擦涌泉,1 分钟。

(5) Headache due to kidney deficiency　Additionally rub Yongquan (KI 1), for one minute, and vibrate the lower abdomen with the palm, for one to three minutes.

(5) 肾虚头痛　加摩涌泉,1 分钟,掌振丹田,1～3 分钟。

Appendix: Migraine

附:偏头痛

Therapeutic principle: Balance the liver and expel wind in the seizure stage in predominance.

治则:发作期以平肝祛风为主。

The patient takes a sitting position. The treatment is mainly applied on the sick side.

患者取坐位。重点治疗患侧。

(1) Basic therapeutic methods of the head, face and nuchal region for headache.

(1) 头面部和颈项部的头痛基本操作法。

(2) Press Hegu (LI 4), Lieque (LU 7), Fengchi (GB 20), Fengfu (GV 16), Taiyang (Extra), and Xiaxi (GB 43), for two minutes.

(2) 重按合谷、列缺、风池、风府、太阳、侠溪穴,2 分钟。

(3) Chafe Yongquan (KI 1), for two minutes.

(3) 擦涌泉,2 分钟。

Modification by Symptoms: For nausea and vomiting, press and knead Neiguan (PC 6) and Zusanli (ST

辨证加减:有恶心呕吐者加按揉内关、足三里,2 分

36) additionally for two minutes. For pain around the eye, press and knead Zanzhu (BL 2), Yangbai (GB 14), Fengchi (GB 20), and Hegu (LI 4) additionally for two minutes. For vertex pain, press and knead Baihui (GV 20), Shangxing (GV 23), and Taichong (LR 3) additionally for two minutes.

钟;眼区疼痛者加按揉攒竹、阳白、风池、合谷穴,2 分钟;巅顶疼痛者按揉百会、上星、太冲穴,2 分钟。

When it appears in the prodromal stage of the premonitory symptoms, such as visual disorder, it is necessary to start massage treatment as early as possible, by pushing and grasping the neck to activate blood and disperse blood stasis. In the remission stage it is also advisable to massage the neck in predominance, together with the manual technique to support the body constitution.

本证在出现视觉障碍等先兆症状的前驱期就应及早推拿治疗,可重点推拿颈项部以活血通络。缓解期亦以颈项部推拿为主,佐以扶正手法。

Vertigo

眩晕

It refers to blurred vision and dizziness, which can appear alone or together. It is believed in modern medicine that vertigo is a disturbance of the directional sense and static sense of the human body in the spatial relationship, is a common symptom of many diseases, is mostly commonly seen in anemia, hypertension, arteriosclerosis, and neurosis, etc. There is another type of vertigo, accompanied by tinnitus and fluctuating hearing loss, termed Meniere's disease. It is believed in Chinese medicine that pathogenic wind, phlegm, deficiency and fire can all cause vertigo. Pathologically, it is manifested by deficient pattern and excessive pattern. The deficient pattern is related to deficiency of the heart and spleen, insufficiency of qi and blood, or deficiency of yin essence in the liver and kidney, failing to nourish the brain upward. The excessive pattern

眩晕即目眩、头晕的简称。可单独出现,也可同时出现。现代医学认为眩晕是人体对于空间关系的定向感觉障碍或平衡感觉障碍,是多种疾病的一种常见症状,最常见于贫血、高血压、动脉硬化、神经官能症等。还有一种眩晕,伴有耳鸣和波动性听力下降,称为梅尼埃病。中医认为风、痰、虚、火均可导致眩晕发病。病理表现有虚实两个方面:虚证为心脾亏虚,气血不足,或肝肾阴精亏损,不能上荣于脑;实证为肝阳上亢或痰浊中阻,清阳不升,清窍闭塞等。枕项部

is induced by hyperactivity of the liver yang or obstruction of phlegm and in the Middle Energizer, failing to send the clear yang and blocking the brain. The soft tissue spasm in the occipital region is a common reason to induce vertigo. There is another type of vertigo appearing with the position of the head, termed "Benign Paroxysmal Positional Vertigo" (BPPV), also nicknamed "Otolith Disease". The instant effect can be achieved by a specific method for reposition of otolith. But, it will not be discussed in this section.

软组织痉挛是导致眩晕的常见原因。还有一种随头部体位改变而出现的眩晕，称为"良性阵发性位置性眩晕"(BPPV)，俗称"耳石症"，实施一种特殊的耳石复位手法常可立竿见影，本节不赘述。

Diagnostic Essentials

The common symptoms of vertigo are dizziness with rotation sense, darkness in the eyes, nausea, and even falling sensation due to dizziness, like sitting on a boat.

(1) Pattern of liver yang hyperactivity　Vertigo, tinnitus, dizziness and distending pain in the head, poor sleep, dreamful sleep, irritability and easy anger, numb sensation in the four limbs, fleshed cheeks, stuffy sensation in the chest, red tongue, yellow tongue coating, wiry pulse.

(2) Pattern of qi and blood deficiency　Vertigo aggravated by motion, seizure by fatigue, pale complexion, lustrousless lips and nails, palpitation, insomnia, low spirit, reluctance in speaking, poor appetite, pale tongue, thready and feeble pulse.

(3) Pattern of phlegm blocking the brain　Vertigo with blurred and heavy sensation in the head and eyes, stuffy sensation in the chest, nausea, poor appetite, somnolence, white and greasy tongue coating, soft and rolling pulse.

诊断要点

眩晕的常见症状有：头晕旋转，两目昏黑，泛泛欲吐，甚至昏眩欲仆，如坐舟船之中。

(1) 肝阳上亢型　眩晕耳鸣，头昏胀痛，少寐多梦，急躁易怒，四肢麻木，面赤胸闷，舌质红，苔黄，脉弦。

(2) 气血亏虚型　眩晕动则加剧，劳累即发，面色㿠白，唇甲不华，心悸，失眠，神疲懒言，饮食不馨，舌质淡，脉细弱。

(3) 痰蒙清窍型　眩晕时头目昏重，胸闷恶心，少食多寐，舌苔白腻，脉濡滑。

Basic Therapeutic Methods

The therapeutic principle of massage therapy is

基本治法

推拿治疗眩晕的原则是

to soothe the tendons, activate blood, and wake up the brain.

舒筋活血,醒脑开窍。

1 Prone position

1 俯卧位

(1) Roll the muscles of the lower back, for three minutes. Roll the lumbosacral region from the top to the bottom, forcefully toward the upper border of the iliac crest.

(1) 擦腰背部肌群,3 分钟。擦腰骶部时须从上往下,朝着髂嵴上缘方向用力。

(2) Knead the lower back with the piled palms, for two minutes.

(2) 叠掌揉腰背部,2 分钟。

(3) Push the two sides of the nape with one thumb, for one minute.

(3) 一指禅推项部两侧,2 分钟。

(4) Press the two sides of the nape, for one minute.

(4) 按揉项部两侧,1 分钟。

(5) Press Fengchi (GB 20) and Fengfu (GV 16), with the finger cushion upward, forcefully in the finger tip, toward the vertex forcefully, for one minute.

(5) 点按风池、风府。指腹向上,指端着力,朝着头顶方向用力,1 分钟。

2 Supine position

2 仰卧位

(1) Knead the forehead with the thenar, for one minute.

(1) 鱼际揉前额,1 分钟。

(2) Knead Yintang (Extra) with the middle finger, for one minute.

(2) 中指揉印堂,1 分钟。

(3) Push the orbit with the side of the thumb, for two minutes.

(3) 一指禅偏锋推眼眶,2 分钟。

(4) Pull the cervical vertebras in the supine position, for over one minute.

(4) 仰卧位拔伸颈椎,1 分钟以上。

Modification by Symptoms

随证加减

(1) Pattern of liver yang hyperactivity In addition to the basic therapeutic methods, ① in the sitting position, press and knead bilateral Taiyang (Extra) for one minute, ② sweep the temples for half a minute, ③ grasp the five meridians (grasp the vertex) for half a minute, ④ chafe the chest and ribs, respectively for one to two minutes, and

(1) 肝阳上亢型 基本治法再加:①坐位,按揉双侧太阳穴,1 分钟;②扫散颞部,半分钟;③抓五经(抓头顶),半分钟;④擦胸胁部,各 1~2 分钟;⑤仰卧位:揉按阳陵泉、太冲、足临泣穴,各 1 分

⑤ in the supine position, knead and press Yanglingquan (GB 34), Taichong (LR 3) and Zulinqi (GB 41), respectively for one minute.

钟。

(2) Pattern of qi and blood deficiency　In addition to the basic therapeutic methods, ① chafe the bladder meridian at the back with the palm, for one minute, ② push with one thumb or knead Guanyuan (CV 4) and Qihai (CV 6) respectively for one minute, ③ rub the abdomen for three to five minutes, and ④ vibrate the lower abdomen with the palm for three minutes.

(2) 气血亏虚型　基本治法再加:①掌擦背部膀胱经,1 分钟;②一指禅推或揉关元、气海穴各 1 分钟;③摩腹 3～5 分钟;④掌振小腹部,3 分钟。

(3) Pattern of phlegm blocking the brain　In addition to the basic therapeutic methods, ① knead the abdomen with the palm for two minutes, ② push the abdomen divergently for one minute, ③ press Zhongwan (CV 12) and Tianshu (ST 25) for one minute, ④ press Zusanli (ST 36) and Fenglong (ST 40) for one minute, and ⑤ press and knead Pishu (BL 20) and Weishu (BL 21) for one minute.

(3) 痰蒙清窍型　基本治法再加:①掌揉腹部,2 分钟;②分推腹部,1 分钟;③点按中脘、天枢穴,1 分钟;④点按足三里、丰隆穴,1 分钟;⑤按揉脾俞、胃俞穴,1 分钟。

Insomnia

Insomnia is a disease of insufficient sleep or shallow sleep due to many factors and is often seen in dysfunction of the nervous system, such as neurosis. It is believed in Chinese medicine that insomnia is caused by many reasons. Deficient pattern is mostly induced by over fatigue, deficiency of the heart and spleen, or fire hyperactivity due to yin deficiency, and malnourishment of the mind. Excessive pattern is mostly related to internal disturbance of phlegm and heat or emotional factors, and transformation of fire by liver qi stagnation, and also related to improper food ingestion, leading to in-

失眠

失眠是一种源于多种因素而致睡眠不足或睡眠不深的病证。常见于神经系统的功能失调,如神经衰弱。中医认为导致失眠的原因很多,虚证多属劳倦太过、心脾两虚或阴虚火旺、神失所养,实证多由于痰热内扰或情志所伤、肝郁化火所致,亦有因饮食不节,肠胃受伤,胃气不和引起。

jury in the stomach and intestine and disharmony in the stomach qi.

Diagnostic Essentials

(1) Deficient pattern: Dreamful sleep, easy waking, palpitation, poor memory, low spirit, lassitude, lustrousless complexion, pale tongue, thin tongue coating, thready and feeble pulse.

(2) Excessive pattern: Difficulty to fall into asleep, irritability, easy anger, stuffy sensation in the epigastric region, belching, discomfort in the abdomen, constipation, greasy and turbid tongue coating, rolling and rapid pulse.

Basic Therapeutic Methods

The therapeutic principle: Strengthen the spleen and tranquilize the mind in predominance, plus clear away heat and dissolve phlegm for excessive pattern, and nourish yin and nourish blood for deficient pattern.

1 Prone position

(1) Operation on the four limbs: Relax the muscles of the lower limbs, upper limbs and two shoulders by the grasping method with the two hands, for ten minutes.

(2) Operation on the back: ① knead the back with the piled palms: knead the muscles at the two sides of the spine with the palm from the top to the bottom, for two minutes, ② push the back with one thumb: push the bilateral lines of thoracic and lumbar Huatuo Jiaji (Extra) and the first and second lateral lines of the bladder meridian with one thumb, for five minutes.

2 Supine position

(1) Operation on the four limbs: Grasp the anterior aspect of the thigh and upper limb, for five

诊断要点

（1）虚证：多梦易醒，心悸健忘，神疲乏力，面色少华，舌质淡，苔薄，脉细弱。

（2）实证：不易入睡，烦躁易怒，脘闷嗳气，腹中不舒，大便干结，苔腻浊，脉滑数。

基本治法

治则：健脾安神为主。实证佐以清热化痰；虚证辅以滋阴养血。

1 俯卧位

（1）四肢操作：以双手拿法分别放松下肢、上肢和两肩的肌肉，10 分钟。

（2）背部操作：①叠掌揉背部：从上而下掌揉脊柱两侧肌群，2 分钟；②一指禅推背部：一指禅推法推双侧胸腰夹脊线和膀胱经第一、第二侧线，5 分钟。

2 仰卧位

（1）四肢操作：拿大腿前部、上肢，5 分钟。

minutes.

(2) Operation on the abdomen: ① rub the abdomen clockwise for about five minutes, by the light manual techniques, ② vibrate the lower abdomen with the palm, for three minutes, with the pressure decreased to the minimum, and with penetration of heat sensation.

(2) 腹部操作:①顺时针摩腹,约 5 分钟,手法宜轻;②掌振丹田,3 分钟。压力减小到最小程度,应有热感渗入。

(3) Operation on the head and face: After the patient closes the eyes, the medical practitioner stands behind the patient. ① open the heavenly gate: Push from Yintang (Extra) to Shenting (GV 24) with the two thumbs alternatively, for about ten times, ② push the forehead divergently: push from the forehead to Taiyang (Extra) divergently with the two thumbs, for about ten times, ③ wipe the orbit divergently: wipe the upper and lower orbit with the two thumbs transversely from the root of the nose to Taiyang (Extra), for respectively four to five times, ④ knead Taiyang (Extra) with the finger: press and knead bilateral Taiyang (Extra) with the thumb or middle finger, for two minutes, and ⑤ push the orbit with side of the thumb: push the two orbits with the side of the thumb in a route of "8", for about five minutes.

(3) 头面部操作:患者闭眼。医者最好坐于患者头后。①开天门:以双拇指交替从印堂直推至神庭,约 10 次;②分推前额:双拇指分推前额至太阳穴,约 10 次;③分抹眼眶:以双拇指从山根至太阳穴横抹上下眼眶,各 4～5 次;④指揉太阳:以拇指或中指按揉两侧太阳穴,2 分钟;⑤一指禅偏锋推眼眶:以一指禅推法沿两眼眼眶作横"8"字操作,约 5 分钟。

Modification by Symptoms

随证加减

(1) Deficiency of heart and spleen: Additionally press and knead Xinshu (BL 15), Jueyinshu (BL 14), Pishu (BL 20) and Zusanli (ST 36), for two minutes, and prolong the time for rubbing the abdomen.

(1) 心脾两虚:加按揉心俞、厥阴穴、脾俞、足三里,2 分钟;延长摩腹时间。

(2) Fire hyperactivity due to yin deficiency: Additionally chafe Yongquan (KI 1) for one minute. To vibrate the lower abdomen with the palm as the last step, and prolong its therapeutic time.

(2) 阴虚火旺:加擦涌泉穴,1 分钟。将掌振丹田改为最后操作,并延长其治疗时间。

(3) Internal disturbance of phlegm and heat: Additionally press and knead Pishu (BL 20), Weishu (BL 21), and Xinshu (BL 15), for two minutes. In rubbing the abdomen, press Zhongwan (CV 12) and Qihai (CV 6) together, and press and knead Zusanli (ST 36), Fenglong (ST 40), and Neiguan (PC 6), for two minutes.

(3) 痰热内扰:加按揉脾俞、胃俞、心俞,2分钟。在摩腹时配合揉中脘、气海,并按揉足三里、丰隆、内关,2分钟。

(4) Transformation of fire by liver qi stagnation: Additionally press and knead Ganshu (BL 18), Danshu (BL 19), Yanglingquan (GB 34), and Taichong (LR 3) for two minutes, and push Taiyang (Extra) heavily for one minute.

(4) 肝郁化火:加按揉肝俞、胆俞、阳陵泉、太冲,2分钟;重推太阳穴,1分钟。

Constipation

便秘

It refers to a symptom manifested constipation, prolonged defecation or difficult defecation due to dry stool. It can be seen in many diseases. It is believed in modern medicine that it is related to lack of defecation power (weakness in the diaphragm and abdominal muscles), insufficient mechanical or chemical irritation of the intestinal contents to the intestinal wall of the large intestine and rectum, and weakened stress of the intestinal mucosa (pathological change of intestinal mucosa), and it is caused by long-term retention of feces inside the intestine, leading to absorption of water and hence dry and hard stool. It is believed in Chinese medicine that injury of body fluid in febrile disease, emotional disorder, over ingestion of spicy food, high age, weak constitution, deficiency of qi and blood, and yang deficiency in the spleen and kidney could bring about dysfunctions in the spleen, stomach, small intestine, and large intestine in their transformation

便秘指大便秘结不通,排便时间延长,或虽有便意而粪便干燥、艰涩难解的一种症状,可见于多种疾病。现代医学认为与排便动力缺乏(膈肌、腹肌无力)、肠道内容物对大肠、直肠肠壁的机械或化学刺激不足、肠黏膜应激力减弱(肠黏膜病变)等有关,粪便在肠内停留时间过久,水分被吸收,而至粪质干燥、坚硬所致。中医认为,热病伤津,情志失调,过食辛辣,年老体弱,气血亏虚,脾肾阳虚等均可造成脾胃和大小肠运化、传导功能失常而致各种类型的便秘。

and transportation, resulting in various types of constipation.

Diagnostic Essentials

Dry stool, difficult defecation, one bowel movement every three to five days or every seven to eight days, or normal bowel movement, but dry stool, and difficult defecation, and abdominal distension, abdominal pain, poor appetite, bad temper, etc. Long-term constipation could also induce hemorrhoids or anal fissure.

(1) Constipation due to accumulation of heat: Dry stool, scanty and brown urine, flushed cheeks, feverish sensation in the body, dry mouth, vexation, red tongue, yellow or dry tongue coating, rolling and rapid pulse.

(2) Constipation due to qi stagnation: Constipation, no defecation upon desire, frequent belching, distending sensation in the abdomen and ribs poor appetite, thin and greasy tongue coating, wiry pulse.

(3) Constipation due to food retention: Dry stool, distending pain in the abdomen, putrid belching, acid regurgitation, no appetite, dry mouth, foul breath, yellow and greasy tongue coating, rolling and rapid pulse.

(4) Constipation due to blood deficiency: Constipation, lustrousless complexion, dizziness, blurred vision, pale tongue, thready pulse.

(5) Constipation due to qi deficiency: Difficult defecation, forced defecation stool not dry by forced defecation, perspiration after defecation, shortness of breath, pale tongue, thin tongue coating, soft pulse.

(6) Constipation due to yang deficiency: Diffi-

诊断要点

大便干燥，排便困难，经常三五天或七八天才大便一次。或大便次数正常，但粪质干燥，坚硬难解。还可见到腹胀甚至腹痛，食欲减退，脾气暴躁等。长期便秘还可引起痔疮或肛裂。

（1）热结便秘：大便干燥，小便短赤，面红身热，口干心烦，舌红苔黄或燥，脉滑数。

（2）气滞便秘：大便秘结，欲便不得，嗳气频作，胁腹痞胀，纳食减少，舌苔薄腻，脉弦。

（3）食积便秘：大便干燥，脘腹胀痛，嗳腐吞酸，不思饮食，口干口臭，舌苔黄腻，脉滑数。

（4）血虚便秘：大便秘结，面色不华，头晕目眩，唇舌淡，脉细。

（5）气虚便秘：大便不畅，临便努挣，便下并不干结，便后汗出，短气，舌淡苔薄，脉软。

（6）阳虚便秘：大便艰

cult defecation, clear and profuse urine, cold sensation in the four limbs, preference of hot temperature, aversion to cold, cold pain in the abdomen, cold sensation in the lower back, pale tongue, white tongue coating, deep and slow pulse.

涩，难以排出，小便清长，四肢欠温，喜热恶寒，腹中冷痛，腰脊酸冷，舌淡苔白，脉沉迟。

Basic Therapeutic Methods

Therapeutic principle: Dredge the hollow organs and remove retention.

基本治法

治则：通腑导滞。

1 Supine position

(1) Push Zhongwan (CV 12), Tianshu (ST 25), Qihai (CV 6), Guanyuan (CV 4), and Daheng (SP 15) with one thumb, repeatedly for eight to ten times.

(2) Rub the abdomen: Rub the abdomen with the palm clockwise, forcefully at the left lower abdomen, at the same time observe quickened borborygmus, flatus and belching, for five to seven minutes, till a desire for defecation appears.

1 仰卧位

（1）一指禅推中脘、天枢、气海、关元、大横穴，往返8～10遍。

（2）摩腹：顺时针方向掌摩腹部，摩至左下腹时手法加重。注意观察肠鸣音加快、矢气和嗳气等征象，5～7分钟，以通为度。

2 Prone position

Press and knead Pishu (BL 20), Weishu (BL 21), Dachangshu (BL 25), Shangliao (BL 31), Ciliao (BL 32), Zhongliao (BL 33), and Xialiao (BL 34), for two minutes.

2 俯卧位

按揉脾俞、胃俞、大肠俞、八髎穴，2分钟。

Modification by Symptoms

(1) Constipation due to accumulation of heat Additionally press Neiting (ST 44), Zusanli (ST 36), Shangjuxu (ST 37), grasp Hegu (LI 4), Quchi (LI 11) and Zhigou (TE 6), for three minutes.

(2) Constipation due to qi stagnation Additionally press and knead Tanzhong (CV 17), Zhangmen (LR 13), Qimen (LR 14), Ganshu (BL 18), Geshu (BL 17), for two minutes, and grasp Jianjing (GB 21) for half a minute, and chafe the ribs with the palm for one minute.

随证加减

（1）热秘：加点按内庭、足三里、上巨虚；拿合谷、曲池、支沟穴，3分钟。

（2）气秘：加按揉膻中、章门、期门、肝俞、膈俞穴，2分钟；拿肩井，半分钟；掌擦两侧胁肋，1分钟。

(3) Constipation due to food retention Prolong the time to rub the abdomen. Press and knead Zhigou (TE 6) for one minute.

(3) 食积：延长摩腹时间；按揉支沟，1分钟。

(4) Constipation due to blood deficiency Additionally press and knead Geshu (BL 17), Xinshu (BL 15), Zusanli (ST 36), and Sanyinjiao (SP 6), for two minutes.

(4) 血虚：加按揉膈俞、心俞、足三里、三阴交穴，2分钟。

(5) Constipation due to qi deficiency Additionally press and knead Feishu (BL 13), Zusanli (ST 36), and Sanyinjiao (SP 6), for two minutes, and chafe Shangliao (BL 31), Ciliao (BL 32), Zhongliao (BL 33), and Xialiao (BL 34), for one minute.

(5) 气虚：加按揉肺俞、足三里、三阴交，2分钟；擦八髎，1分钟。

(6) Constipation due to cold Additionally press and knead Taixi (KI 3) for one minute, and chafe Shenshu (BL 23), Shangliao (BL 31), Ciliao (BL 32), Zhongliao (BL 33), and Xialiao (BL 34) till heat sensation penetrates, and vibrate the lower abdomen with the palm till heat sensation penetrates.

(6) 冷秘：加按揉太溪，1分钟；擦肾俞、八髎透热；掌振丹田透热。

Precautions

注意事项

(1) It is necessary to build up the habit to defecate at the regular time.

(1) 养成定时排便习惯。

(2) It is necessary to drink one cup of low salt water in the morning after getting up.

(2) 晨起可空腹喝一杯淡盐水。

(3) It is necessary to eat more vegetables and fruits.

(3) 平时宜多吃蔬菜、水果。

(4) It is necessary to encourage the patient to rub the abdomen clockwise for five minutes by himself, in order to promote the gastrointestinal peristalsis.

(4) 鼓励患者早晚自我顺时针方向摩腹5分钟，以促进胃肠蠕动。

Epigastric pain

胃脘痛

Epigastric pain is a digestive disease mainly characterized by pain in the upper abdomen and is

胃脘痛是以上腹部疼痛为主症的消化道疾病，也是

also a common symptom clinically. It is believed in modern medicine that it is mostly caused by chemical and physical irritation, bacteria and viruses, leading to inflammatory reaction in the gastric wall, including gastric and duodenal ulcer. It is believed in Chinese medicine that it is induced by invasion of pathogenic cold into the stomach, over ingestion of uncooked and cold foodstuffs, blockage of yang qi by accumulation of cold in the center, or improper food ingestion, dysfunction of the Middle Energizer, internal accumulation of dampness and heat, and stagnation of qi dynamics, or liver qi stagnation, attacking the stomach, or long-term qi stagnation, obstruction of blood stasis, deficiency of central qi, and yang deficiency of the spleen and kidney. Clinically, it does not include various types of malignant tumor with epigastric pain as a main symptom.

临床常见的一种症状。现代医学认为本病的发生多因化学、物理刺激及细菌、病毒等因素引起胃壁的炎性反应，也包括胃及十二指溃疡等。中医学认为，寒邪犯胃，过食生冷，寒积于中，阳气被遏；或饮食不节，中焦不运，湿热内蕴，气机凝滞；或肝气郁结，横逆犯胃；气滞日久，血行瘀阻，中气虚寒，脾肾阳衰等都能引起胃脘痛。临床上不包括各种以腹痛为主要症状的恶性肿瘤。

Diagnostic Essentials

诊断要点

Epigastric pain is accompanied by putrid belching and acid regurgitation, or vomiting of clear fluid, poor appetite, loose stool or constipation. Usually, it is divided into the deficient pattern and excessive pattern.

胃脘部疼痛，伴嗳腐吞酸或冷吐清水，食欲不振，大便溏薄或便秘。一般可分虚实两大类。

(1) Excessive pattern: Gastric pain aggravated by pressure, abdominal distension and discomfort, belching, foul breath, nausea, feeble pulse, greasy tongue coating.

(1) 实证：胃痛拒按，腹胀不适，嗳气息秽，恶心嘈杂，脉弱，苔腻。

(2) Deficient pattern: Insidious gastric pain, relieved by pressure and warmth, vomiting of clear fluid, cold sensation in the hand and foot, deep and thready pulse, pale tongue and white tongue coating.

(2) 虚证：胃痛隐隐，喜按喜暖，泛吐清水，手足不温，脉沉细，苔淡白。

Basic Therapeutic Methods

基本治法

Therapeutic principle: Strengthen the spleen,

治则：健脾和胃，理气止

harmonize the stomach, regulate qi and stop pain.

痛。

1 Supine position with the knee flexed

(1) Press and knead Zusanli (ST 36), Gongsun (SP 4), and Neiguan (PC 6), for two minutes.

(2) Rub the abdomen with the palm, for three minutes.

(3) Vibrate the epigastric region with the palm, for one to three minutes.

1 仰卧屈膝位

（1）按揉足三里、公孙、内关,2 分钟。

（2）掌摩腹部,3 分钟。

（3）掌振胃脘部,1～3 分钟。

2. Prone position

(1) Roll the back for about two minutes.

(2) Press and knead Ganshu (BL 18), Danshu (BL 19), Pishu (BL 20), Weishu (BL 21), Shangliao (BL 31), Ciliao (BL 32), Zhonglliao (BL 33), Xialiao (BL 34), for two minutes.

2. 俯卧位

（1）𢶍背部,约 2 分钟。

（2）按揉肝俞、胆俞、脾俞、胃俞、八髎穴,2 分钟。

Modification by Symptoms

(1) Excessive pattern　In addition to the basic therapeutic methods, ① push the upper abdomen divergently, for five to ten times, ② chafe the left bladder meridian vertically from Ganshu (BL 18) and Sanjiaoshu (BL 22) till heat sensation appears, and ③ press and knead tenderness or sensitive spot at the lower back.

(2) Deficient pattern　In addition to the basic therapeutic methods, ① vibrate Qihai (CV 6) with the palm, for one to three minutes, and ② chafe the lumbosacral region transversely till heat sensation appears.

随证加减

（1）实证　基本治法再加:①分推上腹部,5～10 遍;②直擦左侧膀胱经,从肝俞到三焦俞,以热为度;③按揉腰背部压痛点或敏感点。

（2）虚证　基本治法再加:①掌振气海,1～3 分钟;②横擦腰骶部,以透热为度。

Precautions

It is necessary to exclude malignant tumor for the patient whose epigastric pain is not confirmed.

注意事项

对于未经确诊的胃脘痛患者,须排除恶性肿瘤。

Common cold

Its mild condition is nicknamed "injury by

感冒

感冒,轻者俗称“伤风”,

wind". Usually, it will last for several days. Severe epidemic condition should be treated with relevant medications comprehensively.

一般数天即愈。病情较重，引起流行者称为时行感冒。宜结合相关药物综合治疗。

Diagnostic Essentials

诊断要点

It is mostly manifested by nasal obstruction, running nose, cough, aversion to cold, fever, and headache, etc.

多出现鼻塞、流涕、咳嗽、畏寒、发热、头痛等症状。

(1) Wind-cold pattern Serious aversion to cold, mild fever, no sweating, headache, aching pain in the four limbs, cough, nasal obstruction, clear nasal discharge, pale tongue, thin and white tongue coating, superficial or tense pulse.

（1）风寒型 恶寒重、发热轻、无汗、头痛、四肢酸痛、咳嗽、鼻塞、流清涕、舌质淡、苔薄白、脉浮或紧。

(2) Wind-heat pattern Serious fever, slight aversion to wind or aversion to cold, sore throat, dry mouth, cough, tenacious sputum difficult to cough up, red tongue tip and margin, thin, greasy and slight yellow tongue coating, superficial pulse.

（2）风热型 发热重、微恶风或恶寒、咽红肿、口干、咳嗽、痰黏难咯、舌边尖红、苔薄腻微黄、脉浮。

Basic Therapeutic Methods

基本治法

Therapeutic principle: Expel pathogenic wind, promote perspiration and relieve the exterior.

治则：疏散风邪，发汗解表。

(1) Open the heavenly gate (push the forehead vertically): The medical practitioner pushes with the thumbs of the two hands in alternation from Yintang (Extra) to Shenting (GV 24) vertically, for one minute.

（1）开天门（直推前额）：医者以双手拇指从印堂向神庭交替直推，1 分钟。

(2) Push the forehead and orbital ridge divergently: Push with the thumbs of the two hands divergently from the forehead and Yintang (Extra) to Taiyang (Extra), for one minute.

（2）分推前额和眉弓：以双手拇指从前额和印堂向左右分推，1 分钟。

(3) Push Taiyang (Extra): Push Taiyang (Extra) vertically with the thumbs of the two hands, for one minute.

（3）推太阳：以双手拇指直推太阳穴，1 分钟。

(4) Knead the forehead with the thenar, for one minute.

（4）鱼际揉前额，1 分钟。

(5) Grasp the five meridians: Grasp the vertex with the five fingers, for half a minute.

(5) 抓五经:以五指抓拿头顶,半分钟。

(6) Press and knead Fengchi (GB 20), Fengfu (GV 16), Fengmen (BL 12), and Feishu (BL 13), for one minute.

(6) 按揉风池、风府、风门、肺俞穴,1分钟。

Modification by Symptoms

随证加减

(1) Wind-cold pattern: In addition to the basic therapeutic methods, ① sweep the temples, for one minute, ② press Fengchi (GB 20) heavily, for half a minute, and ③ chafe the bladder meridian vertically till heat sensation appears, for one minute.

(1) 风寒感冒:基本治法加:①扫散颞部,1分钟;②重按风池,半分钟;③直擦背部膀胱经透热,1分钟。

(2) Wind-heat pattern: In addition to the basic therapeutic methods, ① grasp Jianjing (GB 21), Quchi (LI 11) and Hegu (LI 4), for one minute, and ② push the bladder meridian at the back with the thumb, for two minutes.

(2) 风热感冒:基本治法加:①拿肩井、曲池、合谷,1分钟;②一指禅推背部膀胱经,2分钟。

(3) Nasal obstruction and discharge: In addition to the basic therapeutic methods, ① press Yingxiang (LI 20), Quanliao (SI 18) and Shangxing (GV 23), for two minutes.

(3) 鼻塞流涕:基本治法加:①点按迎香、颧髎、上星穴,2分钟。

(4) Sore throat: In addition to the basic therapeutic methods, ① grasp Quchi (LI 11) and Hegu (LI 4), respectively for half a minute, and ② knead the two sides of the Adam's apple lightly, for one minute.

(4) 咽喉红肿:基本治法加:①拿曲池、合谷,各半分钟;②轻揉喉结两旁,1分钟。

(5) Stiff neck: In addition to the basic therapeutic methods, ① push the nape with the thumb or grasp the nape, for two minutes, and ② rotate the cervical vertebras, for one minute.

(5) 项强:基本治法加:①一指禅推项部或拿项部,2分钟;②摇颈椎,1分钟。

(6) Aching and heavy sensation in the joints: In addition to the basic therapeutic methods, ① apply the guiding method for passive movement of the joints, and ② apply the corresponding striking method.

(6) 肢节酸楚困重:基本治法加:①关节被动导引手法;②相应部位叩击法。

Cough-panting

It mostly occurs in the cold season of the winter and spring. It is believed in modern medicine that chronic bronchitis, pulmonary emphysema and asthma belong to its scope. It is believed in Chinese medicine that the occurrence and development of this pattern is related to invasion of the exogenous pathogenic factors (wind, cold, summer-heat, dampness, dryness, fire, etc) and dysfunctions of the lung, spleen and kidney. When the exogenous pathogenic factors invade the human body, the pathogenic factors would be accumulated, leading to failure of the lung in its spreading ability, hence reverse flow of the lung qi and cough-panting. Or because of the production of phlegm due to the spleen deficiency, the lung is blocked by turbid phlegm, or because of hyperactivity of fire in the heart and liver, phlegm is burnt by the liver fire, blocking the lung qi, or because of deficiency of the kidney, the kidney fails to accept qi, hence leading to deficient panting. It is pointed out in *Collected Supplementary of Diagnosis and Treatments* (Zhen Zhi Hui Bu) by LI Yongcui of the Qing Dynasty: "panting refers to sound produced by long-term wheezing with sputum, because of internal qi stagnation, infection of external factors, and sticky phlegm in the diaphragm. Three of them are integrated to block the air passage, leading to sound and panting." Chronic obstructive respiratory diseases such as chronic bronchitis are especially characterized by a specific feature, i.e. blockage of air passage by phlegm, resulting in difficult respiration. tuina therapy is ad-

咳喘

咳喘多发于冬春严寒季节。现代医学的慢性支气管炎、肺气肿、哮喘等病证都属其范畴。中医学认为本证的发生和发展与外邪（如风、寒、暑、湿、燥、火等）的侵袭及肺、脾、肾三脏功能失调有关。当外邪侵袭人体后，邪气壅滞，肺失宣降，肺气上逆而咳喘；或因脾虚生痰、痰浊阻肺；或因心肝火旺，肝火烁痰，壅塞肺气；或因下元亏损，肾气不纳气而作虚喘。清代李用粹在《证治汇补》中指出："哮即痰喘之久而常发者，因内有壅塞之气，外有非时之感，膈有胶固之痰，三者相合，闭拒气道，搏击有声，发为哮病。"慢性支气管炎等慢性阻塞性呼吸道疾病，有一个显著的特点，就是痰阻气道，肺气不畅。推拿在化痰、排痰方面有其特长。

vantageous in dissolving phlegm and discharging phlegm.

Diagnostic Essentials

The commonly seen symptoms of cough-panting are long-term repeated cough, expectoration, accompanied by panting, shortness of breath or stuffy sensation in the chest.

(1) Phlegm-dampness type Cough with profuse sputum, white sputum easy to cough up, stuffy sensation in the chest and upper abdominal region, pale tongue, white and greasy tongue coating, soft and rolling pulse.

(2) Phlegm-heat type Cough and panting, shortness of breath, tenacious sputum in yellow color, dry throat or sore throat, hot breathing in the mouth and nose, stuffy sensation in the chest, red tongue, yellow and greasy tongue coating, rolling pulse.

(3) Deficient panting type Panting with exertion, short and hurried breathing, low and feeble voice, aversion to cold, spontaneous sweating, tiredness in the limbs, low spirit, poor appetite, pale tongue, thin tongue coating, and feeble pulse.

Basic Therapeutic Methods

Therapeutic principle: Dilate the chest, regulate qi, promote the lung in the spreading ability and dissolve phlegm.

The patient takes a sitting position.

(1) Press and knead Neiguan (PC 6), Fenglong (ST 40), Zhongfu (LU 1), Yunmen (LU 2), Tiantu (CV 22), and Tanzhong (CV 17), for three minutes.

(2) Push the bilateral bladder meridian at the back with the thumb, on Feishu (BL 13), Xinshu

诊断要点

咳喘常见症状可有长期的反复咳嗽，咯痰，伴有喘息，气短或胸闷。

(1) 痰湿型　咳嗽痰多，痰白易咯，胸脘痞闷，舌质淡，苔白腻，脉濡滑。

(2) 痰热型　咳喘气急，痰黏稠，色黄，咽干或痛，口鼻气热，胸闷不舒，舌质红，苔黄腻，脉滑。

(3) 虚喘型　动辄气喘，呼吸短促，语声低微，怯寒自汗，肢倦神疲，纳食不馨，舌淡，苔薄脉弱。

基本治法

治则：宽胸理气，宣肺化痰。

患者坐位。

(1) 按揉内关、丰隆、中府、云门、天突、膻中穴，3 分钟。

(2) 一指禅推背部两侧膀胱经：以肺俞、心俞、膈俞

(BL 15) and Geshu (BL 17) in particular, for five minutes.

穴为重点,5 分钟。

(3) Press Dingchuan (Extra), for one to two minutes.

(3) 点按定喘,1～2 分钟。

(4) Push the scapula divergently: Push with the thumbs of the two hands from the medial side of the superior angle of the bilateral scapula, along the spinal border of the scapula to the lower angle of the scapula, for eight to ten times.

(4) 分推肩胛骨:以双手拇指从两侧肩胛骨上角内缘起,沿肩胛骨的脊柱缘推到肩胛下角,8～10 次。

(5) Pat the chest and back: Pat the sternum with the four fingers, from the bottom to the top, for half a minute, and pat the back with a loose palm, centripetally and from the bottom to the top, for one minute.

(5) 拍胸背部:四指拍胸骨部,自下而上拍之,半分钟;虚掌拍背部,方向由外而内、自下而上,1 分钟。

(6) Grasp Jianjing (GB 21), with the two hands, for half a minute.

(6) 拿肩井,双手操作,半分钟。

Modification by Symptoms

随证加减

(1) Phlegm-dampness type: In addition to the basic therapeutic methods, ① press and knead Sanyinjiao (SP 6), Zusanli (ST 36), for two minutes, ② rub Zhongwan (CV 12), for two minutes, and ③ chafe the bilateral bladder meridian at the upper back, and the upper chest transversely (chafe Tanzhong (CV 17) vertically for women) till heat sensation appears.

(1) 痰湿型:基本治法加:①按揉、三阴交、足三里穴,2 分钟;②摩中脘,2 分钟;③擦上背部两侧膀胱经,横擦上胸部(女性可纵擦膻中),透热为度。

(2) Phlegm-heat type: In addition to the basic therapeutic methods, ① press and knead Dazhui (GV 14), Taodao (GV 13), Neiting (ST 44), Taichong (LR 3), for two minutes.

(2) 痰热型:基本治法加:①按揉大椎、陶道、内庭、太冲穴,2 分钟。

(3) Deficient panting type: In addition to the basic therapeutic methods, ① press and knead Pishu (BL 20), Feishu (BL 13), Shenshu (BL 23), Qihai (CV 6), Taixi (KI 3), and Sanyinjiao (SP 6), for three minutes, ② rub the abdomen for three mi-

(3) 虚喘型:基本治法加:①按揉脾俞、肺俞、肾俞、气海、气海、太溪、三阴交穴,3 分钟;②摩腹,3 分钟;③掌振肩胛间区,透热为度;④横

nutes, ③ vibrate the scapular region with the palm till heat sensation appears, and ④ chafe Shenshu (BL 23) transversely, chafe Yongquan (KI 1), respectively for one minute.

擦肾俞,擦涌泉,各 1 分钟。

Hiccup

It refers to an uncontrollable symptom induced by reverse flow of qi, with short and frequent rattling sound in the throat. Hiccup is different in occasional or persistent seizure. Occasional seizure will go away without medications and persistent seizure needs to be controlled by treatment. If this symptom occurs in some acute or chronic diseases, it is necessary to know it may be a sign of critical pathological condition.

Diagnostic Essentials

(1) Type of stomach cold　Slow and forceful hiccup, discomfort in the epigastric region, relieved by warmth and aggravated by cold, poor appetite, no thirst, white and moist tongue coating, and slow pulse.

(2) Type of stomach dryness and heat　Continuous, loud and forceful hiccup, thirst, constipation, flushed cheeks, irritability, preference of cold, aversion to heat, yellow tongue coating, and rolling and rapid pulse.

(3) Type of yang deficiency in the spleen and kidney　Low and forceless hiccup, shortness of breath, lustrousless complexion, cold sensation in the hand and foot, poor appetite, drowsiness, soreness and weakness of the low back and knee, pale tongue, white tongue coating, and deep and thready pulse.

呃逆

呃逆是指气逆上冲,喉间呃呃连声,声短而频,无法自控的一种症状。呃逆有偶发和持续发作之不同。偶然发作的多可不药自愈;持续不已者需要治疗控制。本症若在某些急慢性疾病过程中出现,则应警惕可能为病情危重之预兆。

诊断要点

(1) 胃中寒冷型　呃声沉缓有力,胃脘不舒,得热则减,得寒愈甚,食欲减少,口不渴,舌苔白润,脉迟缓。

(2) 胃中燥热型　呃逆连声,洪亮有力,口渴便秘,面赤烦躁,喜冷恶热,舌苔黄,脉象滑数。

(3) 脾肾阳虚型　呃声低沉无力,气不得续,面色不华,手足欠温,食少困倦,腰膝无力,舌淡苔白,脉象沉细。

Basic Therapeutic Methods

Therapeutic principle: Harmonize the stomach and descend the reverse flow of qi.

基本治法

治则：和胃降逆。

1 Tuina on single acupoint

Firstly, it is advisable to select one of the following single acupoints for tuina: ① Grasp the bilateral Jianjing (GB 21) in predominance, for half a minute, ② press Yifeng (TE 17), for half a minute, ③ press Tianzong (SI 11), for half a minute, and ④ press the phrenic never: press with the thumb from the midpoint of the sternocleidomastoid muscle to the transverse process of the fifth cervical vertebra, for half a minute. If the above simple tuina methods are ineffective, the following operations should be done.

1 单穴推拿

先选用以下单穴之一推拿：①重拿双侧肩井，半分钟；②点按翳风，半分钟；③点按天宗，半分钟；④按压膈神经：以拇指自胸锁乳突肌中点压向第 5 颈椎横突，半分钟。如上述简易推拿法无效，则实施以下操作。

2 Operation on the back

The patient takes a prone position. The medical practitioner takes a standing position.

Press and knead Geshu (BL 17) and Weishu (BL 21), for one minute.

2 背部操作

患者俯卧位，术者站立位。

按揉膈俞、胃俞，1 分钟。

3 Operation on the chest and abdomen

The patient takes a supine position. The medical practitioner sits at the right side.

(1) Press and knead Tiantu (CV 22), Geshu (BL 17), Pishu (BL 20), Weishu (BL 21), Neiguan (PC 6), and Zusanli (ST 36), for two minutes.

(2) Rub Tanzhong (CV 17), Zhongwan (CV 12), Qimen (LR 14), and Qihai (CV 6), for five minutes.

3 胸腹部操作

患者仰卧位。术者坐于右侧。

（1）按揉天突、膈俞、脾俞、胃俞、内关、足三里穴，2 分钟。

（2）摩膻中、中脘、期门、气海穴，5 分钟。

Modification by Symptoms

(1) Cold hiccup: In addition to the basic therapeutic methods, ① chafe the bilateral bladder meridian at the back with the palm till heat sensation appears, ② vibrate the epigastric region with the

随证加减

（1）寒呃：基本治法加：①掌擦背部两侧膀胱经透热；②掌振胃脘部透热；③拿风池，半分钟。

palm till heat sensation appears, and ③ grasp Fengchi (GB 20), for half a minute.

(2) Heat hiccup: In addition to the basic therapeutic methods, ① press and knead Taichong (LR 3), Neiting (ST 44) and Hegu (LI 4), for two minutes.

(2) 热呃:基本治法加:①按揉太冲、内庭、合谷穴,2分钟。

(3) Deficient hiccup: In addition to the basic therapeutic methods, ①chafe the bladder meridian at the back with the palm till heat sensation appears, and ② vibrate the lower abdomen with the palm, for two minutes.

(3) 虚呃:基本治法加:①掌擦背部膀胱经透热;②掌振丹田,2分钟。

Irregular menstruation

It is a common disease in women, manifested by abnormality in the cycle, volume, color and quality of menstruation, including disorder of menstrual cycle, prolonged or shortened bleeding cycle, increased or decreased bleeding volume, and even amenorrhea. It is believed in modern medicine that estrogen disorder, functional disturbance of vegetative nerve, nerve stimulation, cold temperature, fatigue, and some general diseases can induce this problem. It is believed in Chinese medicine that irregular menstruation is mainly caused by the disorders in the Thoroughfare Vessel and Conception Vessel and in production of qi, blood and body fluid, due to pathological changes in the heart, spleen, liver and kidney. Early menstruation is mostly caused by liver qi stagnation turning into fire and crazy blood circulation due to blood heat, or depletion of kidney yin, leading to blood deficiency and heat, or failure of the spleen in containing blood. Delayed menstruation is mostly induced by cold co-

月经不调

月经不调是妇女的一种常见病症,表现为月经在期、量、色、质上的异常,包括月经周期紊乱,出血期延长或缩短,出血量增多或减少,甚至月经闭止。现代医学认为体内雌激素分泌失调、植物神经功能紊乱、精神刺激、寒冷疲劳和某些全身性疾病等,均可以导致本症的发生。中医则认为月经失调,主要是由于心脾肝肾等脏腑病变引起冲任二脉气血津液生化失常。月经先期,多因肝郁化火,血热妄行或肾阴亏耗,血虚而热及脾不统血所致。月经后期,多为寒凝气滞,气血不足所致。月经愆期(先后无定期),多为肝郁气滞或肝肾亏损所致。经量过多过

agulation, qi stagnation, and insufficiency of qi and blood. Random irregular menstruation (random in advanced or delayed cycle) is mostly caused by liver qi stagnation or deficiency of the liver and kidney. Excessive volume or scanty volume is mostly related to failure of qi in containing blood, or blood heat and deficiency of the heart and spleen, leading to emptiness in sea of blood or blood stasis by cold.

少，多因气不摄血或血热及心脾亏损、血海空虚或寒凝瘀阻所致。

Diagnostic Essentials

Menstrual disorder, irregular cycle or abnormality in volume, color and quality, accompanied by various general symptoms of mental exhaustion or irritability, can be divided into different patterns of deficiency, excess, cold or heat clinically.

诊断要点

月经失调，经期不定或有量、色、质的异常，并伴有精神疲乏或烦躁不安等各种全身症状。临床有虚实寒热的不同证型。

(1) Blood heat type Early menstruation, large volume, deep red or purple color, thick quality, irritability, red tongue, yellow tongue coating, rolling, rapid and forceful pulse.

（1）血热型　月经先期、量多、色深红或紫、质浓，烦躁不安，舌红苔黄，脉滑数有力。

(2) Qi deficiency type Early menstruation or randomly early or delayed menstruation, large volume, light color, thin quality, tiredness in the limbs, pale complexion, pale tongue, feeble and forceless pulse.

（2）气虚型　月经先期或先后不定，量多、色淡红、质稀薄，肢体倦怠，面色㿠白，舌质淡，脉弱无力。

(3) Cold coagulation type Delayed menstruation, scanty volume, dark red color, pain in the lower abdomen, relieved by warm temperature, aversion to cold, cold sensation in the limbs, pale complexion, pale tongue, thin and white tongue coating, deep and tense pulse.

（3）寒凝型　月经后期、量少、色暗红，小腹疼痛，得热则减，畏寒肢冷，面色苍白，舌淡苔薄白，脉沉紧。

(4) Qi stagnation type Delayed menstruation, scanty volume, normal color or dark red color, distending pain in the lower abdomen, stuffy and uncomfortable sensation in the chest, distending sensation in the breast, pain in the hypochondriac re-

（4）气滞型　月经后期、量少、色正常或暗红，小腹胀痛，胸闷不舒，乳胀胁痛，舌质紫暗，脉弦或涩。

gion, purple dark tongue, wiry or choppy pulse.

Basic Therapeutic Methods

Therapeutic principle: Soothe the liver, regulate qi, harmonize blood and adjust menstruation.

1 Prone position

(1) Press and knead Ganshu (BL 18), Pishu (BL 20), Shenshu (BL 23), Shangliao (BL 31), Ciliao (BL 32), Zhongliao (BL 33), and Xialiao (BL 34), for two minutes.

(2) Vibrate with the palm Shangliao (BL 31), Ciliao (BL 32), Zhongliao (BL 33), and Xialiao (BL 34), for one to three minutes.

2 Supine position

(1) Press and knead Diji (SP 8), Yinlingquan (SP 9), Xuehai (SP 10), Qihai (CV 6), and Guanyuan (CV 4), for three minutes.

(2) Rub the lower abdomen with the palm, for two minutes.

(3) Chafe the medial side of the thigh till heat sensation appears.

Modification by Symptoms

(1) Early menstruation

For excessive heat, additionally press and knead Taichong (LR 3), Xingjian (LR 2), and Quchi (LI 11), for two minutes.

For deficient heat, additionally: ① press and knead Sanyinjiao (SP 6), Taixi (KI 3), for two minutes, and ② rub Yongquan (KI 1), for one minute.

(2) Delayed menstruation

For excessive cold, additionally chafe Shangliao (BL 31), Ciliao (BL 32), Zhonglliao (BL 33), and Xialiao (BL 34), till heat sensation appears.

For deficient cold, additionally chafe Shenshu

基本治法

治则：疏肝理气、和血调经。

1 俯卧位

（1）按揉肝俞、脾俞、肾俞、八髎穴，2 分钟。

（2）掌振八髎，1～3 分钟。

2 仰卧位

（1）按揉地机、阴陵泉、血海、气海、关元穴，3 分钟。

（2）掌摩丹田，2 分钟。

（3）擦大腿内侧，以热为度。

随证加减

（1）月经先期

实热者加按揉太冲、行间、曲池穴，2 分钟。

虚热者加：①按揉三阴交、太溪穴，2 分钟；②摩涌泉，1 分钟。

（2）月经后期

实寒者加擦八髎透热。

虚寒者加擦肾俞透热。

(BL 23) till heat sensation appears.

For qi stagnation, additionally: ① press and knead Ligou (LR 5), Tanzhong (CV 17), for one minute, and ② rub the hypochondriac region, for one minute.

气滞者加:①按揉蠡沟、膻中穴,1 分钟;②搓胁肋,1 分钟。

For blood deficiency, additionally: press and knead Zusanli (ST 36), Sanyinjiao (SP 6) and Gongsun (SP 4), for two minutes.

血虚者加按揉足三里、三阴交、公孙穴,2 分钟。

(3) Random irregular menstruation

(3) 月经愆期

For liver qi stagnation, additionally press and knead Neiguan (PC 6), Taichong (LR 3), Qimen (LR 14), Zhangmen (LR 13), for two minutes.

肝郁者加:按揉内关、太冲、期门、章门穴,2 分钟。

For kidney deficiency, additionally: ① press and knead Taixi (KI 3), Shuiquan (KI 5), and Jiaoxin (KI 8), for two minutes, and ② chafe Shenshu (BL 23), for one minute.

肾虚者加:①按揉太溪、水泉、交信穴,2 分钟;②擦肾俞,1 分钟。

For spleen deficiency, additionally: ① press and knead Zusanli (ST 36), Sanyinjiao (SP 6) and Gongsun (SP 4), for two minutes, and ② rub the abdomen, for one minute.

脾虚者加:①按揉足三里、三阴交、公孙穴,2 分钟;②摩腹,1 分钟。

(4) Prolonged menstruation

(4) 经期延长

For qi deficiency, additionally: press and knead Gongsun (SP 4), Sanyinjiao (SP 6), and Baihui (GV 20), for two minutes.

气虚者加:按揉公孙、三阴交、百会穴,2 分钟。

For blood stasis, additionally: ① chafe Shangliao (BL 31), Ciliao (BL 32), Zhonglliao (BL 33), and Xialiao (BL 34), for one minute, and ② vibrate the lower abdomen with the palm, for two minutes.

血瘀者加:①擦八髎,1 分钟;②掌振丹田,2 分钟。

For blood heat, additionally: press and knead Taichong (LR 3), Yinbai (SP 1), and Shuiquan (KI 5), for two minutes.

血热者加:按揉太冲、隐白、水泉穴,2 分钟。

Dysmenorrhea

It refers to lower abdominal pain present during, before and after menstruation, accompanied by the general symptoms of abdominal distension, and uncomfortable sensation in the breasts. There are two types of primary dysmenorrhea and secondary dysmenorrhea. Primary dysmenorrhea is mostly seen in the unmarried young females, caused by the prenatal factors, such as over anteversion, retroflexion, and uterine hypoplasia, etc. Secondary dysmenorrhea is mostly seen in the married women, caused by the postnatal factors, such as uterine inflammation, uterine polyp, etc.

It is believed in Chinese medicine that this problem is caused by poor circulation of qi and blood. Menstruation is transformed from blood. Blood flows with qi. If qi is sufficient, blood will be sufficient. If qi is smooth and blood is harmonious, menstruation will be smooth, without pain. If qi and blood are stagnant or blood is insufficient due to qi deficiency, menstruation will not be smooth, leading to pain due to stagnation. The reasons causing poor circulation of qi and blood are qi stagnation, blood stasis, retention of cold and dampness, and deficiency of qi and blood, etc.

Diagnostic Essentials

Dysmenorrhea is clinically characterized by lower abdominal pain during menstruation, present with the menstrual cycle. In accordance with time of pain and quality of pain, it can be identified into cold, heat, deficient or excessive pattern. Generally, pain before and during menstruation belongs to excessive pattern, and pain after menstruation belongs to

痛经

痛经是指月经来潮及行经前后出现的下腹部疼痛或伴有腹胀、乳房不适等全身症状。痛经有原发性和继发性两种。原发性痛经以未婚女青年多见，因先天因素如子宫过度前倾、后屈，子宫发育不良等造成。继发性痛经以已婚妇女为多见，多因子宫炎症、息肉等后天因素所致。

中医学认为本证乃因气血运行不畅所致。月经为血所化，血随气行，气充血沛，气顺血和，则经行通畅，自无疼痛之患。若气滞血瘀或气虚血少，则经行不畅，不通则痛。而造成气血不畅的原因，有气滞血瘀、寒湿凝滞、气血虚损等。

诊断要点

痛经临床表现的特点是行经时少腹疼痛，随月经周期而发作。根据疼痛发生的时间和疼痛的性质，可辨别其寒、热、虚、实的属性。一般以经前、经期痛者属实，经后痛者为虚。痛时拒按属

deficient pattern. Pain aggravated by pressure is excessive pattern, and pain relieved by pressure is deficient pattern. Pain relieved by heat belongs to cold nature, and pain aggravated by heat belongs to heat nature. Pain more obvious than distending sensation and relieved after discharge of blood clots is related to blood stasis. Distending sensation worse than painful sensation is related to qi stagnation. Colic and cold pain belongs to cold nature, and pricking pain belongs to heat nature. Continuous pain or insidious pain belongs to deficiency.

实,喜按属虚。得热痛减为寒,得热痛剧为热。痛甚于胀,血块排出疼痛减轻者为血瘀,胀甚于痛为气滞。绞痛、冷痛属寒,刺痛属热,绵绵作痛或隐痛为虚。

(1) Type of qi stagnation and blood stasis Lower abdominal pain during or before menstruation, scanty volume, dribbling bleeding, purple dark color with blood clots, pain relieved after discharge of blood clots, distending sensation in the chest, hypochondria and breasts, purple dark tongue, purple spots on tongue margin, deep and wiry pulse.

(1) 气滞血瘀型 经期或经前少腹胀痛,行经量少,淋漓不畅,血色紫暗有淤块,块下则疼痛减轻,胸胁乳房作胀,舌质紫暗,舌边有瘀点,脉沉弦。

(2) Type of retention of cold and dampness Cold pain in the lower abdomen before or during menstruation, radiating pain in the lower back, relieved by warmth, scanty volume, dark color with blood clots, aversion to cold, loose stool, white and greasy tongue coating, deep and tense pulse.

(2) 寒湿凝滞型 经前或经期少腹冷痛,甚则牵连腰背疼痛,得热则舒,经行量少色暗有血块,畏寒便溏,苔白腻,脉沉紧。

(3) Type of deficiency of qi and blood Continuous pain during or after menstruation, relieved by pressure, light color, clear and thin quality, pale complexion, low spirit, pale tongue, thin tongue coating, deficient and thready pulse.

(3) 气血虚弱型 经期或经净后小腹绵绵作痛,按之痛减,经色淡,质清稀,面色苍白,精神倦怠,舌淡苔薄,脉虚细。

Basic Therapeutic Methods

Therapeutic principle: Circulate qi, activate blood, and regulate the Thoroughfare Vessel and Conception Vessel.

基本治法

治则:行气活血,调摄冲任。

1 Supine position

(1) Push the Conception Vessel at the abdomen with one thumb: Push from Jiuwei (CV 15) below the xyphoid process to Qugu (CV 2) at the superior border of the pubic bone, for two to three minutes.

(2) Rub the lower abdomen with the palm, for two minutes.

(3) Chafe the lower abdomen with the palm: Put the two palms respectively and bilaterally to the umbilicus and chafe downward bilaterally, till heat sensation appears.

(4) Pinch and grasp the medial aspect of the thigh: Pinch and grasp the muscle tendon at the medial aspect of the leg and thigh from Sanyinjiao (SP 6) upward, for five to ten times.

2 Prone position

(1) Push the bilateral bladder meridians at the back with one thumb, downward to the lumbosacral region, for two to three times.

(2) Press and knead Ganshu (BL 18), Pishu (BL 20), Weishu (BL 21), Shenshu (BL 23), Qihaishu (BL 24), and Dachangshu (BL 25), for three minutes.

(3) Chafe the lumbosacral region transversely: Chafe the lumbosacral region with the hypothenar, on Shenshu (BL 23), Zhishi (BL 52), Shangliao (BL 31), Ciliao (BL 32), Zhongliao (BL 33), and Xialiao (BL 34), till heat sensation appears in the lower abdomen.

Modification by Symptoms

(1) Type of qi stagnation and blood stasis In addition to the basic therapeutic methods, ① press and knead with the finger or palm Zhangmen (LR 13), Ganshu (BL 18), Geshu (BL 17), Shangliao

1 仰卧位

（1）一指禅推腹部任脉：从剑突下的鸠尾穴推到耻骨上缘的曲骨穴，2～3 分钟。

（2）掌摩小腹，2 分钟。

（3）掌擦少腹：将双掌分放脐旁沿少腹两侧向下作擦法，以热为度。

（4）捏拿下肢内侧：从三阴交开始向上捏拿小腿和大腿内侧经筋，5～10 遍。

2 俯卧位

（1）一指禅推背部两侧膀胱经，从上往下操作至腰骶部，2～3 遍。

（2）按揉肝俞、脾俞、胃俞、肾俞、气海俞、大肠俞等穴，3 分钟。

（3）横擦腰骶部：以小鱼际横擦腰骶部，着重于肾俞、志室、八髎穴，以热透小腹为佳。

随证加减

（1）气滞血瘀型 基本治法再加：①指、掌按揉章门、肝俞、膈俞、八髎穴，各 1 分钟；②擦血海穴：患者仰

(BL 31), Ciliao (BL 32), Zhongliao (BL 33), and Xialiao (BL 34), respectively for one minute, ② roll Xuehai (SP 10): After the patient takes a supine position, with the knee flexed and hip abducted, roll forcefully toward the internal epicondyle of femur, for one minute, and ③ press Qugu (CV 2) with the finger forcefully toward the upper border of the pubic bone, for one minute.

卧,屈膝髋外展位,朝着股骨内上髁方向用力,1 分钟;③指按曲骨穴,朝着耻骨上缘用力,1 分钟。

(2) Type of retention of cold and dampness In addition to the basic therapeutic methods, ① chafe the bladder meridian at the back with the palm, and chafe the muscles bilateral to the spine vertically, till heat sensation appears, and ② press and knead Sanyinjiao (SP 6), Yinlingquan (SP 9), for two minutes.

(2) 寒湿凝滞型 基本治法再加:①掌擦背部膀胱经,直擦脊柱两旁肌肉,以热为度;②按揉三阴交、阴陵泉,2 分钟。

(3) Type of deficiency of qi and blood In addition to the basic therapeutic methods, ① press and knead Zusanli (ST 36), and Sanyinjiao (SP 6), for two minutes, and ② vibrate the lower abdomen with the palm, for one to three minutes.

(3) 气血虚弱型 基本治法再加:①按揉足三里、三阴交穴,2 分钟;②掌振小腹部,1～3 分钟。

In accordance with the regularity of the periodical seizure of dysmenorrhea, it is advisable to give tuina treatment one week before menstruation, once every day or every other day.

可根据痛经周期性发作的规律,在月经来潮前 1 周推拿治疗,每日或隔日 1 次。

Premenstrual syndrome

围绝经期综合征

It is also termed menopause syndrome. It refers to a group of symptoms characterized by dysfunctions of the autonomic nerve system, present before or after menopause due to fluctuation or decrease of sex hormones. In Chinese medicine, it is termed "premenopausal or postmenopausal patterns" or "hysteria". It mostly occurs at the age from 45 to 55 and can last for 3～5 years or longer. It is caused by disorders of qi and blood, because of progressive de-

围绝经期综合征又称更年期综合征,指妇女绝经前后出现性激素波动或减少所致的,以自主神经系统功能紊乱为主,伴有神经心理症状的一组症候群。中医称为"经断前后诸证"或"脏躁证"。多发生于 45～55 岁之间,可持续 3～5 年或更长时

cline of the kidney qi, exhaustion of sex hormones and imbalance between yin and yang.

间。是因为肾气渐衰，天癸将竭，阴阳平衡失调而引起气血逆乱的结果。

Diagnostic Essentials

The commonly seen symptoms of this problem are tidal feverish sensation, profuse sweating, irritability, easy anger, dizziness, insomnia, palpitation, irregular menstrual cycle, progressive obesity, or abnormal skin sensation, etc.

诊断要点

本病的常见症状有：潮热、多汗、烦躁、易怒、头晕、失眠、心悸、月经周期不规则、逐渐肥胖或皮肤感觉异常等。

Basic Therapeutic Methods

Therapeutic principle: Regulate qi, harmonize blood, and adjust yin and yang.

基本治法

治则：理气和血，调整阴阳。

1 Prone position

(1) Press and knead Ganshu (BL 18), Sanjiaoshu (BL 22), Shenshu (BL 23), Mingmen (GV 4), Ciliao (BL 32), respectively for one minute.

(2) Chafe the low back transversely, till heat sensation appears.

1 俯卧位

(1) 按揉肝俞、三焦俞、肾俞、命门、次髎穴，各 1 分钟。

(2) 横擦腰部，以透热为度。

2 Supine position

(1) Knead Tanzhong (CV 17) with the middle finger, for one minute.

(2) Press and knead Zusanli (ST 36), Sanyinjiao (SP 6), respectively for one minute.

(3) Rub the abdomen with the palm, for three minutes.

(4) Vibrate the lower abdomen with the palm, for one to two minutes.

(5) Chafe Yongquan (KI 1) with the hypothenar, till heat sensation appears.

2 仰卧位

(1) 中指揉膻中穴，1 分钟。

(2) 按揉足三里、三阴交穴，各 1 分钟。

(3) 掌摩腹部，3 分钟。

(4) 掌振小腹部，1～2 分钟。

(5) 小鱼际擦涌泉，以透热为度。

3 Sitting position

Rub and chafe the two hypochondriac regions with the two hands, for one minute.

3 坐位

双手搓擦两胁肋部，1 分钟。

Modification by Symptoms

(1) For vexation and insomnia, in additional to

随证加减

(1) 心烦失眠：基本治法

the basic therapeutic methods, press and knead Neiguan (PC 6), Shenmen (HT 7), and Xinshu (BL 15), for three minutes.

加按揉内关、神门、心俞穴,3分钟。

(2) For skin itching, in additional to the basic therapeutic methods, press and knead Xuehai (SP 10), Baichongwo (Extra) (one cun above Xuehai (SP 10)), for three minutes.

(2) 皮肤瘙痒:基本治法加按揉血海、百虫窝穴(血海穴上1寸),3分钟。

Section 3 Pediatric diseases

第3节 儿科疾病

Infantile diarrhea

It refers to increased number of bowel movement in infants, over three times per day, with thin and even watery feces. It is a commonly seen disease of the digestive tract in infants below 3 and often occurs in the summer and autumn. The developmental immaturity in the digestive system and poor regulatory function in the nervous system in infants, plus improper food ingestion, uneven cold and warm temperature, infection of bacteria or virus can all induce diarrhea, hence gastrointestinal dysfunction, and indigestion. It is believed in Chinese medicine that this problem is caused by invasion of pathogenic wind, cold, summer-heat or dampness, resulting in dysfunction of the spleen and stomach in transportation and transformation, and indigestion of foodstuffs and mixture of the clear and turbid in the large intestine, or by improper feeding, improper or unclean food ingestion, and food retention, damaging the spleen and stomach, failing to decompose water and grain.

小儿腹泻

小儿腹泻是指婴幼儿大便次数增多,每天3次以上,粪便稀薄甚至如水样便。它是3岁以下婴幼儿常见的一种消化道疾病,多发生于夏秋季节。婴幼儿消化系统发育不成熟,神经调节作用较差,加之饮食失调、冷暖不匀或细菌、病毒感染等因素即可导致腹泻,以致胃肠功能紊乱,消化不良。中医认为本病发生可由于感受风、寒、暑、湿之邪,致使脾胃运化失常,饮食难于消化,清、浊混走大肠而致腹泻;或由于喂养不当、饮食不节或不洁,宿食积滞,伤及脾胃,不能腐熟水谷,而腹泻不止。

Diagnostic Essentials

(1) Diarrhea due to cold and dampness　Clear, thin and foamy stool, light color, no stink, borborygmus, abdominal pain, pale complexion, no thirst, clear and profuse urine, white and greasy tongue coating, soft pulse.

(2) Diarrhea due to dampness and heat　Diarrhea immediately after abdominal pain, urgent defecation, yellow stool in hot and stink, slight feverish sensation in the body, thirst, scanty urine in brown color, yellow and greasy tongue coating, rolling and rapid pulse.

(3) Diarrhea due to improper diet　Abdominal pain, distension and fullness, crying before diarrhea, pain relieved after diarrhea, stool in large volume and stinky smell, foul breath, poor appetite, or accompanied by vomiting, acid regurgitation, thick and greasy tongue coating, and rolling pulse.

(4) Diarrhea due to spleen deficiency　Lingering diarrhea, or repeated attack, stool mixed with undigested food dregs, or diarrhea immediately after meal, pale complexion, poor appetite, lassitude, emaciated muscles, watery diarrhea in severe condition, pale tongue, thin tongue coating, soft and forceless pulse.

Basic Therapeutic Methods

Therapeutic principle: Strengthen the spleen, dry up dampness and stop diarrhea.

(1) Rub the abdomen, for five minutes.

(2) Knead the navel, for 300 times.

(3) Knead Pt. Guiwei (Extra) (coccygeal end), for 200 times.

(4) Push Pt. Qijiegu (Extra) upward (push with the thumbs of the two hands or the index and

诊断要点

(1) 寒湿泻　大便清稀多沫，色淡不臭，肠鸣腹痛，面色苍白，口不渴，小便清长，苔白腻，脉濡。

(2) 湿热泻　腹痛即泻，大便急迫，色黄热臭，身有微热，口渴，尿少色黄，苔黄腻，脉滑数。

(3) 伤食泻　腹痛胀满，泻前哭闹，泻后痛减，大便量多酸臭，口臭纳呆，或伴呕吐酸馊，苔厚腻，脉滑。

(4) 脾虚泻　久泻不愈，或经常反复发作，便稀夹有不消化食物残渣，或每于食后即泻，面色苍白，食欲不振，乏力，肌肉消瘦。严重者大便可成水样。舌淡苔薄，脉软无力。

基本治法

治则：健脾燥湿止泻。

(1) 摩腹，5 分钟。

(2) 揉脐，300 次。

(3) 揉龟尾(尾骨端)，200 次。

(4) 推上七节骨(以双手拇指或单手示中二指，从尾

middle finger of single hand from the coccyx to the spinous process of the fourth lumbar vertebra, Figure 6-1), for 200 times.

骨推到第 4 腰椎棘突，见图 6-1)，200 次。

Modification by Symptoms

(1) Diarrhea due to cold and dampness Additionally: ① push Shangliao (BL 31), Ciliao (BL 32), Zhongliao (BL 33), Xialiao (BL 34) with the thumbs of the two hands in alternation, for totally 200 times, ② push Pt. Sanguan (Extra) (with the thumb or index and middle finger, push from Taiyuan (LU 9) at the radial side of the forearm to Quchi (LI 11)), for 200 times, ③ knead Tianshu (ST 25), for 100 times, and ④ press and knead Zusanli (ST 36), for one minute.

随证加减

(1) 寒湿泻 逆时针摩腹，加：①推八髎，双手拇指左右交替推，共 200 次；②推三关(以拇指或示中二指，从前臂桡侧的太渊推到曲池)，200 次；③揉天枢，100 次；④按揉足三里，1 分钟。

(2) Diarrhea due to dampness and heat Rub the abdomen clockwise, and push Pt. Qijjiegu (Extra) downward, and additionally: ① press and knead Shangliao (BL 31), Ciliao (BL 32), Zhongliao (BL 33), Xialiao (BL 34), for one minute, ② sedate Pt. Liufu (Extra) (After the child's elbow flexed, push with the thumb from the tip of the elbow, along the ulnar side of the forearm, to Shenmen (HT 7), Figure 6-2), for 100 times, and ③ knead Tianshu (ST 25), for 200 times.

(2) 湿热泻 顺时针摩腹，七节骨改为向下推，加：①按揉八髎，1 分钟；②退六腑(将患儿屈肘，以拇指从肘尖沿前臂尺侧推到神门，见图 6-2)，100 次；③揉天枢，200 次。

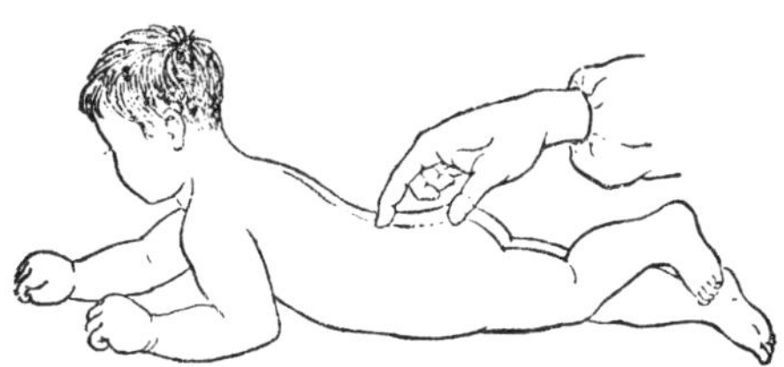

Figure 6-1 Push Pt. Qijiegu (Extra) upward
图 6-1 推上七节骨

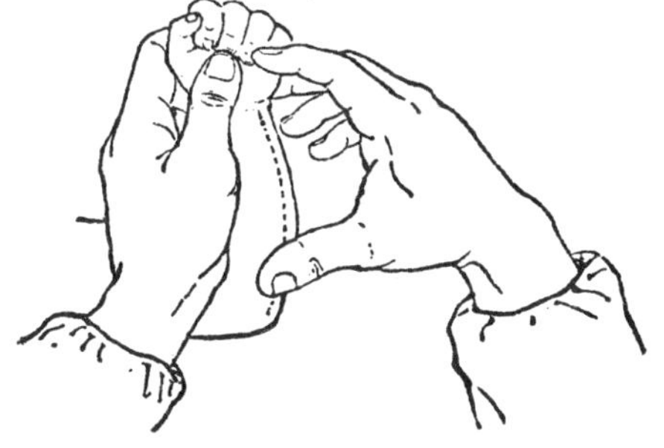

Figure 6-2 Sedate Pt. Liufu
图 6-2 退六腑

(3) Diarrhea due to improper diet　Rub the abdomen clockwise, and push Pt. Qijjiegu (Extra) downward, and additionally: ① press and knead Shangliao (BL 31), Ciliao (BL 32), Zhongliao (BL 33), Xialiao (BL 34), for one minute, ② clarify Pt. Dachang (Extra), for 100 times, ③ push Pt. Banmen (Extra) (with the thumb, push from the root of infant's thumb, along the thenar, to the transverse wrist crease, Figure 6-3), for 200 times, ④ knead Pt. Neibagua (Extra) (with the thumb, knead the infant's palm clockwise) for 100 times, and ⑤ knead Zhongwan (CV 12) for 200 times.

（3）伤食泻　顺时针摩腹，七节骨改为向下推，加：①按揉八髎，1 分钟；②清大肠，100 次；③推板门（以拇指从患儿拇指根部沿着鱼际推向腕横纹，见图 6－3），200 次；④运内八卦（以拇指在患儿掌心作顺时针方向的摩动）100 次；⑤揉中脘 200 次。

(4) Diarrhea due to spleen deficiency　Rub the abdomen counterclockwise, and additionally: ① chafe Shangliao (BL 31), Ciliao (BL 32), Zhongliao (BL 33), Xialiao (BL 34), till heat sensation appears, ② pinch up the spine (Figure 6-4), for 5 to 10 times, ③ knead Pt. Pijing (Extra) (with the thumb, knead the cushion of the last section of the infant's thumb), for 200 times, and ④ push Pt. Banmen (Extra) for 200 times, and ⑤ knead Pt. Neibagua (Extra) for 100 times.

（4）脾虚泻　逆时针摩腹，加：①擦八髎，透热为度；②捏脊（图 6－4），5～10 遍；③揉脾经（以拇指在患儿拇指末节螺纹面环旋揉动），200 次；④推板门，200 次；⑤运内八卦 100 次。

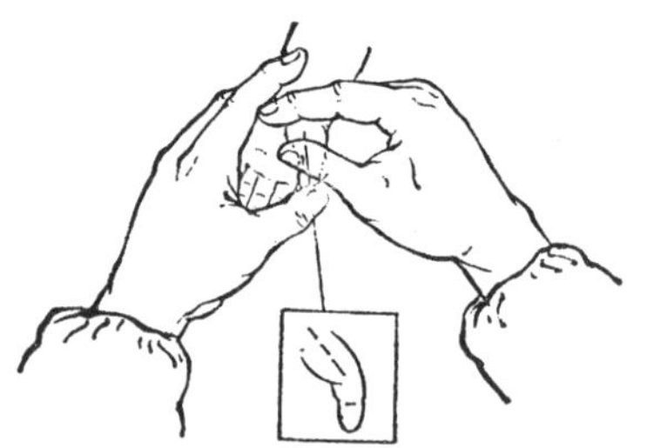

Figure 6-3　Push Pt. Banmen (Extra)
图 6-3　推板门

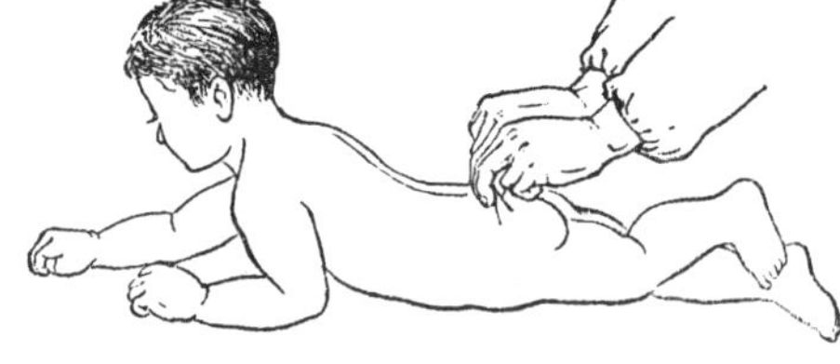

Figure 6-4　Pinch up the spine
图 6-4　捏脊

Precautions

(1) Tuina treatment is given once per day,

注意事项

（1）推拿每日 1 次，重者

twice for severe condition, with five days as one course. Three to four courses are needed for chronic diarrhea.

2次,5日为1个疗程。慢性腹泻需3～4个疗程。

(2) If the therapeutic effect is not satisfactory after several treatments or the pathological situation of the sick child becomes worse, presenting scanty urine, no urine, frequent vomiting, hollow eyes, and listlessness, etc, it is necessary to seek medications of Chinese and western medicine, including prompt intravenous infusion, correction of electrolyte balance and anti-infection, etc.

(2)如推拿治疗多次疗效不明显或发现患儿病情转重,出现少尿、无尿,呕吐频繁,眼窝凹陷,精神萎靡等症时,宜配合中、西药物治疗,包括及时静脉输液、纠正电解质平衡和抗感染等措施。

(3) For the infants during diarrhea, it is necessary to control diet, and avoid spicy and greasy food. After defecation, it is needed to clean the anus of the infant with warm water, and change diaper frequently, in order to maintain the skin clean and dry. It is necessary to feed the infant properly, at the regular time and quantity, and not to add subsidiary foodstuffs too quick and too much in variety, and necessary to pay attention to climate change for timely changing the clothes, and to dietetic hygiene for preventing intestinal diseases.

(3)对腹泻期间的小儿,应控制饮食,忌辛辣、油腻之品。患儿每次便后须用温水洗净肛门,勤换尿布,保持皮肤清洁干燥。注意合理喂养,喂食哺乳要定时定量,添加辅食不宜太快,品种不宜太多,并注意气候变化,及时增减衣服,注意饮食卫生,预防肠道疾病。

Infantile muscular torticollis

小儿肌性斜颈

It is often characterized by lateroversion of the head to the sick side, anteversion, and face turning to the healthy side. It is often seen in infants and mostly related to abnormal fetal position inside the uterus, blocking blood supply in one side of the sternocleidomastoid muscle, and hence resulting in ischemic myofibrosis, or related to malpositioon during delivery, causing the infant's sternocleidomastoid muscle compressed and injured by the birth ca-

肌性斜颈以头向患侧偏斜、前倾,颜面转向健侧为特点,常见于婴幼儿。多因胎儿在子宫内头位不正,使一侧胸锁乳突肌受压而血液供应受阻,引起该肌缺血性肌纤维变性;或因分娩时胎位不正,胎儿胸锁乳突肌受产道或产钳挤压受伤出血,血

nal or obstetric biceps, and hence hematoma organized and spasm.

肿机化形成挛缩，而导致斜颈。

Diagnostic Essentials

诊断要点

(1) After birth, the infant is found a shuttle-like lump in one side of the sternocleidomastoid muscle (lump can disappear automatically in half a year in some infants). Afterward, the sick sternocleidomastoid muscle becomes spastic and contractive, protruded like a cord.

(1) 患儿出生后，一侧胸锁乳突肌发现有梭形肿物(有的在半年后肿物可自行消退)，以后患侧的胸锁乳突肌逐渐痉挛并挛缩，突出如条索状。

(2) The sick infant's head turns to the sick side, forward, with the face turning to the healthy side.

(2) 患儿头部向患侧偏斜、前倾，颜面转向健侧。

(3) The child sick in long time can present the face asymmetrical in the two sides, bigger in the healthy side and smaller in the sick side. If not treated for long time, the cervical vertebras can bulge to the healthy side, and even the thoracic vertebras will have compensational curvature, forming strabismus or diplopia.

(3) 久病患儿可出现两侧面部不对称，健侧大而患侧小。如长期不治，颈椎可凸向健侧，甚至胸椎也可有代偿性侧弯，并形成斜视或复视。

Basic Therapeutic Methods

基本治法

Therapeutic principle: Soothe the tendons, activate blood, soften the hard and disperse the accumulation.

治则：舒筋活血，软坚散结。

The infant takes a supine position. The medical practitioner sits facing to the vertex of the sick infant.

婴儿仰卧。术者面向患儿头顶而坐。

(1) Press and knead sternocleidomastoid muscle: Hold the sick infant's occiput with one hand, press and knead sternocleidomastoid muscle with thumb, or index, middle and ring finger of the other hand, for five minutes, press and knead the lump areas of the sternocleidomastoid muscle and its upper and lower attachment spots in particular.

(1) 按揉胸锁乳突肌：一手托住患儿枕部，另一手用拇指或示、中、无名指按揉患侧胸锁乳突肌，5 分钟。按揉的重点在患侧胸锁乳突肌的肿块部位和上下附着点。

(2) Pinch, grasp and pluck the sternocleido-

(2) 捏拿、弹拨胸锁乳突

mastoid muscle: Gently pinch and grasp the sternocleidomastoid muscle of the sick side with the thumb and index finger, for one to two minutes, and then pluck it for ten to fifteen times.

肌:以拇、示指轻柔地捏拿患侧胸锁乳突肌,1～2 分钟;再弹拨 10～15 次。

(3) Rotate and pull the neck: Pull the sick infant's neck a little bit and then rotate and pull the neck to the opposite direction of spasm, i. e. pull the infant's head to the healthy side, with the face turning to the sick side, repeatedly for over ten times. In doing this technique, it is necessary to increase the strength and amplitude gradually, and not to use the sudden and violent force and go beyond the normal physiological limit.

(3) 旋转拉伸颈部:将患儿颈部略作拔伸后将头颈向痉挛的相反方向旋转拉伸,即将患儿头部扳向健侧、面部转向患侧,反复 10 余次。此法要由轻到重,幅度由小到大,切不可骤然暴力而超出正常生理限度。

(4) Press and knead to relax the neck, for two to three minutes.

(4) 按揉放松颈部,2～3 分钟。

Modification by Symptoms

随证加减

(1) For long-term torticollis, presenting different sides of the face, in addition to the basic therapeutic methods, press and knead Taiyang (Extra), Yintang (Extra), Dicang (ST 4) and Xiaguan (ST 7), for two minutes.

(1) 斜颈日久,出现颜面两侧大小不等,基本治法加按揉患侧面部太阳、印堂、地仓、下关等穴,2 分钟。

(2) If the infant sick for long time presents strabismus or diplopia, in addition to the basic therapeutic methods, press and knead Jingming (BL 1), Zanzhu (BL 2), Yangbai (GB 14), Yuyao (Extra), Taiyang (Extra), for three minutes.

(2) 如久病患儿出现斜视或复视,可在基本治法上增加按揉睛明、攒竹、阳白、鱼腰、太阳等眼区腧穴,3 分钟。

Precautions

注意事项

(1) Tuina treatment for torticollis is usually given once per day, for ten to fifteen minutes each time, with one month as one course.

(1) 推拿手法治疗斜颈,一般每日治疗 1 次,每次 10～15 分钟,1 个月为一疗程。

(2) The length of the treatment course is in positive correlation with spastic degree of the sick muscle.

(2) 推拿疗程的长短,与患侧肌肉的挛缩程度成正相关。

(3) During the treatment, it is necessary to be gentle with proper force in the manual techniques, avoid violent and rude manipulation, and use talcum as medium to protect the skin of the sick infant.

(4) It is advisable to instruct the parents to do passive movement to rotate and pull the sternocleidomastoid muscle of the sick infant.

(5) In the daily life, it is necessary to guide the sick infant to move the spastic muscle of the neck to the opposite direction, in order to correct deformity, for instance, use a pillow under the neck during sleep, and change feeding direction.

(3) 治疗时手法要刚柔相济,但忌粗暴,并用滑石粉作为介质以保护患儿皮肤。

(4) 可指导家长,每天做旋转拉伸患儿胸锁乳突肌的被动运动。

(5) 在日常生活中,应引导患儿做与颈部肌肉挛缩方向相反的动作以矫正畸形,如睡眠时的垫枕、喂奶的方向等。

Infantile enuresis

It refers to a symptom of involuntary urination during sleep in the infants above three years old. It is believed in modern medicine that dysfunctions of the cerebral cortex by various reasons can induce the voluntary urinary dysfunction of the bladder, resulting in enuresis. Enuresis due to excessive playing in the daytime in the infants below three years old or occasional enuresis in the preschool children does not belong to the pathological situation. It is believed in Chinese medicine that enuresis is mostly caused by insufficiency of the kidney qi and deficiency of the urinary bladder, failing to control the water passage, or qi deficiency in the spleen and lung after illness, failing to regulate the water passage and control the urinary bladder.

小儿遗尿

遗尿是指 3 周岁以上的小儿睡眠中不自主排尿的病证。现代医学各种原因引起的大脑皮质功能紊乱而造成膀胱随意性排尿功能失调,就会引起遗尿。3 周岁以下的小儿,或因白天嬉戏过度,或学龄前儿童夜间偶有遗尿者,不属病理现象。中医认为遗尿多因肾气不足,膀胱虚寒,不能制约水道,或病后脾肺气虚,不能通调水道,约束膀胱所致。

Diagnostic Essentials

The sick child often urinates involuntarily during sleep, once several nights in mild condition, or several times per night in severe condition. Low

诊断要点

患儿经常睡眠中不自主排尿,轻则数夜一次,重则一夜数次。遗尿日久可见患儿

spirit and cold sensation in the four limbs can be present in the children with long-term enuresis. The older children are mostly shy or nervous.

精神委顿，四肢不温。年龄较大的儿童多有怕羞或精神紧张。

(1) Deficiency cold in the urinary bladder Accompanied by pale complexion, mental retardation, cold sensation in the four limbs, clear and profuse urine.

(1) 膀胱虚寒 伴面色㿠白，智力迟钝，四肢欠温，小便清长。

(2) Qi deficiency in the lung and spleen Accompanied by shortness of breath, reluctance in speaking, tiredness in the four limbs, spontaneous or night sweating, lustrousless complexion, poor appetite, loose stool.

(2) 肺脾气虚 伴少气懒言，四肢倦怠，自汗或盗汗，面色少华，纳食不佳，便溏。

(3) Dampness and heat in the liver meridian Accompanied by quick temper, restless sleep, flushed cheeks, bitter taste in the mouth, brown urine.

(3) 肝经湿热 伴性情急躁，睡眠不宁，面赤口苦，小便黄赤。

Basic Therapeutic Methods

基本治法

Therapeutic principle: Raise yang qi, warm up and replenish the spleen and kidney.

治则：升举阳气，温补脾肾。

(1) Press and knead Baihui (GV 20), for 200 times

(1) 按揉百会，100 次。

(2) Press and knead Sanyinjiao (SP 6), for 100 times.

(2) 按揉三阴交，100 次。

(3) Knead the lower abdomen, for 100 times.

(3) 揉丹田，100 次。

(4) Press and knead Shangliao (BL 31), Ciliao (BL 32), Zhongliao (BL 33), and Xialiao (BL 34), particularly on Ciliao (BL 32), for 200 times.

(4) 按揉八髎，以次髎为重点，200 次。

Modification by Symptoms

随证加减

(1) Deficiency cold in the urinary bladder In addition to the basic therapeutic methods, ① chafe the lumbosacral region transversely, chafe Shangliao (BL 31), Ciliao (BL 32), Zhongliao (BL 33), and Xialiao (BL 34), and chafe Yongquan (KI 1), respectively for half a minute, and ② push Pt. San-

(1) 膀胱虚寒 基本治法加：①横擦腰骶部，擦八髎，擦涌泉，各半分钟；②推三关，100 次。

guan (Extra), for 100 times.

(2) Qi deficiency in the lung and spleen　In addition to the basic therapeutic methods, ① knead Pt. Pijing (Extra), knead Pt. Feijing (Extra) (knead the cushion of the last section of the ring finger of the sick child circularly with the thumb), respectively for 100 times, and ② pinch up the spine, for three to five times.

(2) 肺脾气虚　基本治法加：①揉脾经、揉肺经（以拇指在患儿无名指末节螺纹面环旋揉动），各100次；②捏脊，3～5遍。

(3) Dampness and heat in the liver meridian　In addition to the basic therapeutic methods, ① press and knead Taichong (LR 3), for 100 times, ② clarify the Pt. Ganjing (Extra) (push the cushion of the ring finger of the sick child toward the finger tip with the thumb), for 100 times, and ③ rub the ribs, for 50 times.

(3) 肝经湿热　基本治法加：①按揉太冲，100次；②清肝经（以拇指在患儿示指末节螺纹面向指尖方向直推），100次；③搓胁肋，50次。

Precautions

Tuina treatment is given once every day, with ten days as one course. It usually needs two to three or more courses.

For the sick children with enuresis, it is necessary to encourage them patiently for building up their confidence, and not make the sick children nervous, in order to avoid influencing their physiological and psychological health.

It is necessary for the sick children to build up their habits to urinate regularly, to avoid over playing in the daytime, and avoid over excitement before going to bed, and not to drink water two hours before going to bed. It is needed to wake up the sick children to urinate regularly, after they fall into asleep.

注意事项

每日推拿1次，10日为1个疗程。治疗常需2～3个疗程或更多。

对遗尿患儿应耐心鼓励，建立其自信心，勿使患儿产生紧张感，以免影响身心健康。

注意培养患儿按时排尿的习惯。白天应避免玩耍过劳；临睡前避免过度兴奋，临睡前2小时不要饮水；入睡后应定时唤醒患儿排尿。

Infantile anorexia

It refers to a disease of long-term poor appetite

小儿厌食

厌食是指小儿较长时期

and even denial of food in infants. It is believed in modern medicine that this problem is related to incomplete functions of the digestive system in infants plus improper feeding. It is believed in Chinese medicine that infants belong to immature yin and immature yang, and insufficiency in the spleen and many reasons can cause disharmony between the spleen and stomach, and disorder in transportation and transformation, and hence anorexia. Usually, the spiritual state is comparatively normal in sick infants with anorexia, but mental exhaustion and emaciation may be present in the long duration. This problem is mostly seen in children at the age of 1～6. Poor appetite due to infection of exogenous factor or some chronic diseases is not discussed in this section.

食欲不振，甚至拒食的一种病证。现代医学认为小儿消化系统功能尚未健全，加之喂养不当而导致本病的发生。中医学则认为小儿为稚阴稚阳之体，脾常不足，多种原因都可导致其脾胃不和，受纳运化失职而出现厌食。厌食患儿一般精神状态均较正常，但病程长者，也可出现精神疲惫，形体消瘦。本病多见于1～6岁儿童。若因外感或某些慢性病而出现的食欲不振者，则不属本病范围。

Diagnostic Essentials

诊断要点

Long-term loss of appetite or no desire for food is regarded as the main symptoms in the sick children.

以患儿长期食欲不振或不思饮食为主症。

(1) Poor transportation of the spleen: Pale complexion, no desire for food, or bland taste from foodstuffs, refusing food, emaciation, white or thin and greasy tongue coating, still forceful pulse.

（1）脾失健运者，面色少华，不思纳食，或食物无味，拒进饮食，形体偏瘦，舌苔白或薄腻，脉尚有力。

(2) Insufficiency of the stomach yin: Dry mouth with preference of drinks, but no desire for food, dry skin, lustrousless skin, constipation, peeled tongue coating, peeled tongue coating with scanty fluid, slight red tongue, thready pulse.

（2）胃阴不足者，口干多饮而不喜进食，皮肤干燥，缺乏润泽，大便干结，舌苔多见光剥，亦有光红少津者，舌质偏红，脉细。

(3) Qi deficiency in the spleen and stomach: Mental exhaustion, sallow complexion, anorexia, refusing food, undigested food dreg in stool, after a little food intake, or unformed stool, easy sweating, thin and white tongue coating, forceless pulse.

（3）脾胃气虚者，精神疲惫，面色萎黄，厌食、拒食，若稍进食，大便中即夹有不消化残渣，或大便不成形，易汗，舌苔薄白，脉无力。

Basic Therapeutic Methods

Therapeutic principle: Strengthen the spleen and assist transportation.

(1) Rub the abdomen, for five to ten minutes.

(2) Knead Pt. Neibagua (Extra) for 200 times.

(3) Knead Pt. Pijing (Extra), for 200 times.

(4) Knead Pt. Weijing (Extra) (press and knead the proximal cushion of the sick child's thumb with the thumb), for 200 times.

(5) Press and knead Zusanli (ST 36), Pishu (BL 20) and Weishu (BL 21), for two minutes.

Modification by Symptoms

(1) Poor transportation of the spleen: Additionally knead Zhongwan (CV 12), for three minutes.

(2) Insufficiency of the stomach yin: Additionally ① separate yin and yang (with two thumbs, push along the two sides from Daling (HT 7) in the midpoint of the transverse wrist crease of the sick child to Taiyuan (LU 9) and Shenmen (HT 7)), for 100 times, and ② press and knead Zhongwan (CV 12), Sanjiaoshu (BL 22), and Shenshu (BL 23), for two minutes.

(3) Qi deficiency in the spleen and stomach, knead Pt. Pijing (Extra) for 400 times: Additionally ① pinch up the spine, for three to five times, and ② knead the kidney meridian (press and knead the cushion of the last section of the small finger with the thumb), for 200 times.

Tuina treatment is given once per day, with ten days as one course.

Precautions

It is necessary for the sick children to build up a good dietetic habit, have no snacks before meals,

基本治法

治则:健脾助运。

(1) 摩腹,5～10 分钟。

(2) 运内八卦,200 次。

(3) 揉脾经,200 次。

(4) 揉胃经(以拇指按揉患儿拇指掌面近节指腹),200 次。

(5) 按揉足三里、脾俞、胃俞穴,2 分钟。

随证加减

(1) 脾失健运者、加摩中脘,3 分钟。

(2) 胃阴不足加:①分阴阳(两拇指从患儿腕横纹正中的大陵向两旁分推至太渊和神门),100 次;②按揉中脘、三焦俞、肾俞穴,2 分钟。

(3) 脾胃气虚者:揉脾经加至 400 次,加:①捏脊,3～5 遍;②揉肾经(以拇指按揉患儿小指末节螺纹面),200 次。

推拿每日 1 次,10 日为 1 个疗程。

注意事项

患儿要养成良好的饮食习惯。禁止饭前吃零食,平

and have less candies and deserts in the ordinary time, have meal at the regular time, and avoid carping at food.

时少吃糖果和甜食,定时进食,不偏食。

Twelve Divergent Meridians 十二经别

1.	Divergent Meridian of Bladder Meridian of Foot-Taiyand	足太阳膀胱经经别
2.	Divergent Meridian of Kidney Meridian of Foot-Shaoyin	足少阴肾经经别
3.	Divergent Meridian of Stomach Meridian of Foot-Yangming	足阳明胃经经别
4.	Divergent Meridian of Spleen Meridian of Foot-Taiyin	足太阴脾经经经别
5.	Divergent Meridian of Gallbladder Meridian of Foot-Shaoyang	足少阳胆经经别
6.	Divergent Meridian of Liver Meridian of Foot-Jueyin	足厥阴肝经经别
7.	Divergent Meridian of Small Intestine of Hand-Taiyang	手太阳小肠经经别
8.	Divergent Meridian of Heart Meridian of Hand-Sahoyin	手少阴心经经别
9.	Diergent Meridian of Large Intestine Meridian of Hand-Yangming	手阳明大肠经经别
10.	Divergent Meridian of Lung Meridian of Hand-Taiyin	手太阴肺经经别
11.	Divergent Meridian of Triple Energizer of Hand-Shaoyang	手少阳三焦经经别
12.	Divergent Meridian of Pericardium Meridian of Hand-Jueying	手厥阴心包经经别

Chapter 7 Skills of tuina therapy

第 7 章 推拿功法

The skills of tuina therapy refer to a group of the training methods for the students learning tuina therapy, which can help tuina practitioners to strengthen the body constitution for their competence in the medical job, also be beneficial to enhance their abilities of the manual techniques, at the same time can guide the patients to train those skills as the means for auxiliary treatment and rehabilitation of their diseases, and are understood as the concrete application of traditional Chinese guiding art in tuina therapy. By training the skills of tuina therapy, the medical staffs of tuina therapy can strengthen their constitutional quality and their regulatory ability of psychological and emotional activities, intensify their skills, endurance and power of the manual techniques, excite the potentials of the human body, and fully display the efficacy of tuina therapy. The common types of tuina skills include Shaoli Internal Art, and tendon-changing exercises, etc. Due to space limitation, only part of the contents will be introduced.

推拿功法是推拿医学生的一种练功方法。既能帮助推拿工作者增强体质以胜任推拿医疗工作,也有助于提高推拿手法的功力,同时也是指导病人进行功法锻炼,用于疾病的辅助治疗和康复的手段,是中国传统导引术在推拿学科中的具体应用。推拿工作者通过推拿功法锻炼,可增强身体素质和心理情绪调控能力,增强其运用手法的技巧、耐力和功力,激发人体潜能,充分发挥推拿效应。推拿功法的常用功种有少林内功、易筋经等,本书限于篇幅仅介绍部分内容。

Section 1 Features of tuina skills

第1节 推拿功法的特点

1 Train both the interior and exterior, from the exterior to the interior

It implies to train the internal Zangfu organs, qi and blood, and meridians and train the external tendons, bone, and skin and flesh simultaneously, i.e. "to train energy internally, and train tendons, bone and skin externally".

1 内外兼修,由外及内

内外兼修指对内在的脏腑、气血、经络和外在的筋骨皮肉兼顾修炼,即所谓"内练一口气,外练筋骨皮"。

2 Integrate the motion with the tranquility, and to seek the tranquility from the motion

The traditional skills are commonly characterized by integration of the motion and tranquility. On one hand, it is stressed to have a close integration between the tranquil skills and moving skills in the training method. On the other hand, it is requested to meet the requirements of "seeking the tranquility from the motion" and "contain the motion within the tranquility" in training the skills. In training the external muscles and internal qi and blood, it is necessary to maintain concentration, in a state of no distraction and mental tranquility, i.e. "to seek the tranquility from the motion", and to maintain the external limbs motionless and regulate qi and blood of Zangfu organs by integrating the internal mental activity and respiratory movement, i.e. "to contain the motion within the tranquility".

2 动静结合,动中求静

动静结合是传统功法的共同特点,一方面是指在练功方式上强调静功与动功的密切结合,另一方面是指在练功时达到"动中求静""静中含动"的要求。在外在肢体肌肉和内在气血锻炼时,保持意念集中、心无杂念、精神宁静的状态,即"动中求静";保持外在肢体不动,运用内在的意念活动与呼吸运动相结合,调节脏腑气血的运动,即"静中含动"。

3 Train strength and stress qi, for integration of form and mind

The training of the skills of tuina therapy is stressed to have the body and mind highly coordina-

3 练力重气,形神合一

推拿功法训练重视通过强壮内气来提高力量的大

ted and united by strengthening the internal energy for enhancing the power, and by regulating the allocation and releasing of the power via the activity of the internal qi dynamics, so as to realize the realm of "unity between the body and mind".

小，通过内在气机活动来调节力量的分配和释放，使形体活动和主管意念高度协调、统一，即达到"形神合一"的境界。

Section 2　Training of tuina skills

第2节　推拿练功知要

1　Basic essentials in training tuina skills

The basic essentials are supposed to regulate the body, regulate the respiration, and regulate the mind. The key in regulating the body is to "be relaxed in the body". It is requested that the body of the practitioners must be maintained in a natural relaxation, in a "relaxed but not floppy" and "gentle but not stiff" state. The key in regulating the respiration is to "have normal respiration". It means the practitioner's respiration should be natural and even. In training to the certain degree, it is necessary to haven a deep, long, even and fine respiration. The key in regulating the mind is to "be calm in the mind", i.e. concentrate the mind (intention) on the certain part of the body (or certain object), in order to gradually enter a tranquil state, and have the limbs and the internal organs successively and fully relaxed, by the integration of the mental activity and respiratory motion, so as to promote the smooth circulation of qi and blood in the whole body.

1　推拿练功基本要领

练功的基本要领即调身、调息、调心。调身的关键是"形松"，要求练功者的形体状态自然放松，处于"松而不懈，柔而不僵"的状态。调息的关键是"气平"，指练功者呼吸自然平和，练功到一定程度后，尽量做到呼吸深、长、匀、细。而调心的关键则是"心定"，即是把注意力(意念)集中到身体的某一特定部位(或某一事物)，通过意念活动与呼吸运动相结合，逐步进入入静状态，全身肢体与脏腑器官继而得到充分放松，从而促使全身气血运行通畅。

2　Requirements in training tuina skills

In training, it is requested to have the limbs in a "relaxed, tranquil and natural" state, and to have

2　推拿练功要求

推拿练功要求肢体达到"松、静、自然"，意、气、形协

the mind, qi and form in a coordinative unity. Namely, the body form, respiration and mental activity should be processed in a natural premise, in order to have the limbs and spirit in a relaxed state. Additionally, it is also necessary for the practitioners to build up their confidence, determination and persistence, and properly master their training amount in accordance with their individual condition and train progressively, so as to "yield success naturally by constant efforts".

调统一。即练功时身形、呼吸和意念活动均在自然的前提下进行，做到肢体和精神都处于放松状态。此外推拿功法要求练功者树立信心、决心和恒心，因人制宜，合理掌握好练功运动量，循序渐进，如此最终"功到自然成"。

3 Necessary instructions in training tuina skills

3 推拿练功须知

(1) In training, it is necessary to maintain warm in the room, and maintain ventilation of fresh air.

（1）练功时须室内温暖，空气流通清新。

(2) In training, it is necessary for the practitioners to wear soft, loose pants and jackets and soft shoes, to maintain the spirit and limbs naturally relaxed, and to have normal daily life in the ordinary times, and train regularly.

（2）练功者须着柔软、宽松衣裤和软底鞋；精神肢体放松自然；平时饮食起居有常，定时练功。

(3) In training, it is necessary for the practitioners to avoid exposing to wind with perspiration, avoid holding up urine and stool, avoid over fatigue and over leisure, and avoid starvation and overeating.

（3）练功者忌汗出当风、强忍溲便、劳逸失度、饥饱无常。

Section 3 Shaolin Internal Art (Shao Lin Nei Gong)

第3节 少林内功

Shao Lin Nei Gong is a training method in the school of the internal-works massage therapy. In training, it is requested to be solid in the lower body

少林内功是内功推拿流派的练功方法。在练功时，强调下实上虚，着重锻炼两

and false in the upper body, and to train the "super power" of the two lower limbs and the "internal energy" of the two upper limbs in particular. It is requested to be upright in the upper body, to be stable in the lower limbs, to step on the ground firmly with the heel, and grasp the ground with the five toes, and to be coordinative in the movements of the upper limbs, gather the force in the finger tips, to be tense externally and relaxed internally, and to breath naturally and concentrate the mind.

下肢的"霸力"和上肢的"内劲"。要求上身正直，下肢稳重，足跟踏实，五趾抓地；上肢动作协调，蓄劲指端，外紧内松；呼吸自然，意念集中。

1　Basic posture

1　基本裆势

1.1　Standing posture

1.1　站裆势

Stance: Hold the two feet together, with the tiptoes closed, drop the two hands naturally, throw out the chest and hold back the abdomen, and look straight forward.

预备姿势：两脚相靠，足尖并拢，两手自然下垂，挺胸收腹，两目平视。

(1) Walk leftward with one step, slightly wider than the shoulder, with the tiptoes turned inward, grasp the ground with the ten toes, and fill in the feet with the super strength downward (Figure 7-1).

（1）左腿向左平跨一步，略宽于肩，足尖略内收成八字，十趾抓地，运用霸力，劲由上贯下注足(图 7-1)。

(2) Throw out the chest slightly, hold back the abdomen and buttocks, extend the two arms backward, straighten the elbow and extend the wrist, close the four fingers, and stretch the thumbs outward, and tighten the shoulder and armpit. Look straight forward, do not turn the head leftward or rightward, concentrate the mind and breathe naturally (Figure 7-2).

（2）前胸微挺，收腹敛（蓄）臀，两臂后伸，挺肘伸腕，四指并拢，拇指外展，肩腋莫松；两目平视，头勿左右盼顾，精神贯注，呼吸自然(图 7-2)。

1.2　Horse Riding Posture

1.2　马裆势

Stance: As the standing posture.

预备姿势：同站裆势。

(1) Walk leftward for one step with the left foot, with the distance of the two feet about three

（1）左足向左平开一步，两脚之间的距离约为本人脚

times than the length of the foot, with the two knees and tiptoes turned inward, and stamp outward slightly with the two heels, with the tiptoes turned inward in a shape of Chinese character "Eight".

长的 3 倍，两膝和脚尖微向内扣，两脚跟微向外蹬，足尖成内"八"字形。

(2) Flex the knees, squat down, extend the two arms backward, straighten the elbow and extend the wrist, close the four fingers and stretch out the thumb (or put the two hands flat on the hips, with the part between the thumb and index inward). Throw out the chest, hold back the abdomen, with the gravity between the two legs, seemingly hold a heavy object on the head, look straight forward, and breathe naturally (Figure 7-3).

（2）屈膝下蹲，两臂后伸，挺肘伸腕，四指并拢，拇指外展（或两手平放两髂处，虎口朝内）。挺胸收腹，重心在两腿之间，头如顶物，两目平视，呼吸自然（图 7-3）。

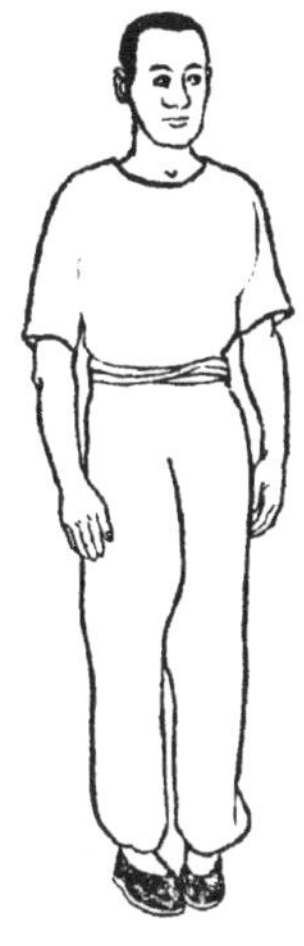

Figure 7-1
图 7-1

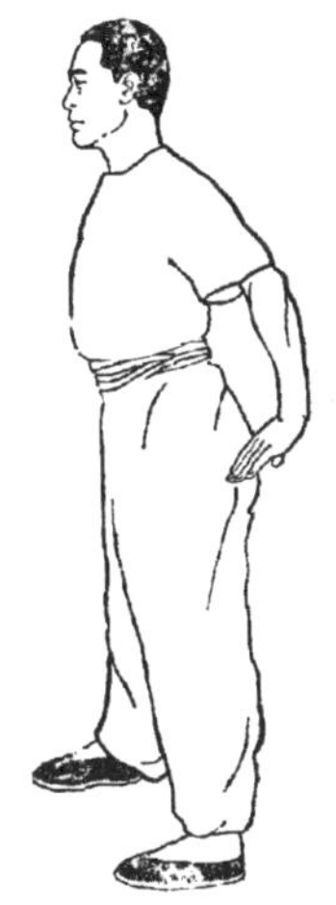

Figure 7-2
图 7-2

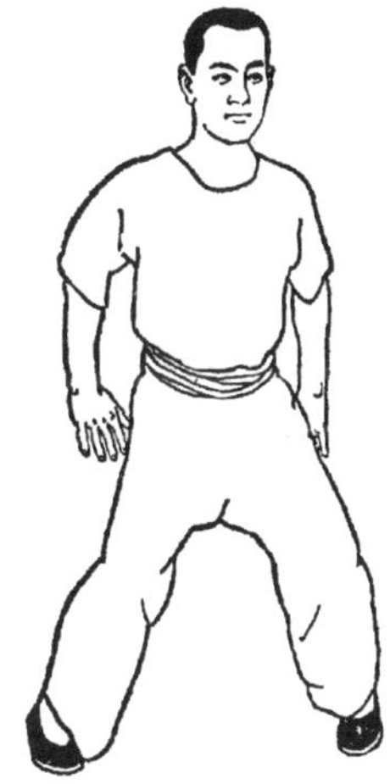

Figure 7-3
图 7-3

1.3 Bow and Arrow Posture

Stance: As the standing posture.

(1) Walk rightward and forward or rightward transversely of a big step with the right foot, turn the body rightward, and flex the knee and squat down halfway with the right leg, by the knee and foot tip on a same straight line, and then turn the

1.3 弓箭裆势

预备姿势：同站裆势。

（1）右脚向右前方或向右横跨一大步，身体右转，在前之右腿屈膝半蹲，膝与脚尖在一直线上，右足尖微向内扣；左腿在后，膝部挺直，

right foot tip inward slightly. With the left leg in the back, straighten the knee, with the left foot tip turned slightly outward, by the heel on the ground, as a posture of anterior bow and posterior arrow.

左脚尖略向外撇，脚跟必须着地，为前弓后箭之势。

(2) Bend forward slightly with the upper body, with the gravity sinking downward, and hold back the abdomen and buttocks slightly, and extend the two arms backward, straighten the elbow and extend the wrist, with the four fingers closed and the part between the thumb and index finger turned outward (or support the waist with the two hands, with the part of the thumb and index finger inward, and press Shenshu (BL 23) with the two thumbs), uplift the neck, breathe naturally and concentrate the mind (Figure 7-4).

(2) 上身略向前俯，重心下沉，腹臀微收，两臂后伸，挺肘伸腕，四指并拢，拇指外展（或两手叉腰，虎口朝内，两拇指按于肾俞穴，蓄势待发），虚领顶劲，呼吸自然，意念集中（图 7-4）。

1.4 Closed Crotch Posture

Stance: As the standing posture.

(1) Stamp outward with the two feet, with the tiptoes turned inward in a shape of Chinese character "eight", grasp the ground with the ten toes, and straighten the two knees.

(2) Extend the two arms backward, straighten the elbow and extend the wrist, with the four fingers closed and the part between the thumb and index finger turned outward, and breathe naturally and look straight forward (Figure 7-5).

1.4 并裆势

预备姿势：同站裆势。

(1) 两脚跟向外蹬，足尖靠拢成内八字，十趾抓地，两膝伸直。

(2) 两臂后伸，挺肘伸腕，四指并拢，拇指外展，呼吸自然，两目平视（图 7-5）。

1.5 Open Crotch Posture

Stance: As the standing posture.

(1) Walk leftward for a big step with the left foot (as big as possible according to the physiological condition), grasp the ground with the toes, with the tiptoes turned inward, and straighten the two knees.

1.5 大裆势

预备姿势：同站裆势。

(1) 左脚向左横跨一大步（可根据生理情况尽可能大），脚趾抓地，脚尖内扣，两膝挺直。

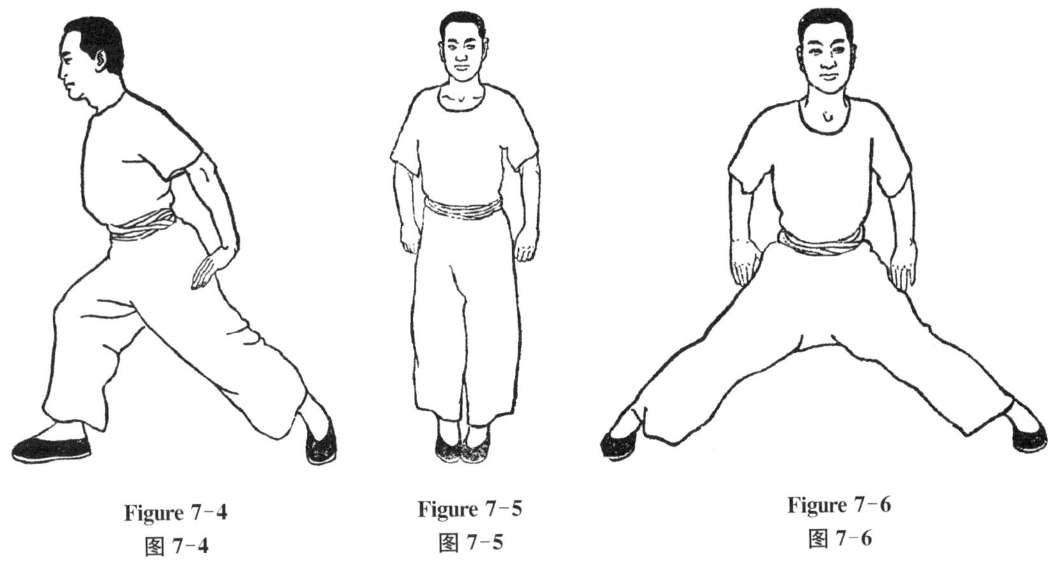

Figure 7-4
图 7-4

Figure 7-5
图 7-5

Figure 7-6
图 7-6

(2) Extend the two arms backward, with the parts of the thumb and index finger in opposition, straighten the elbow and extend the wrist, with the four fingers closed and thumb turned outward, breathe naturally and look straight forward (Figure 7-6).

(2) 两臂后伸，虎口相对，挺肘伸腕，四指并拢，拇指外展，呼吸自然，两目平视（图 7-6）。

1.6 Low Crotch Posture

Stance: As the standing posture.

(1) Flex the knee, squat down, with the toes closed, grasp the ground with the ten toes, stamp outward with the heel, sink the upper body, and sit down with the buttocks but not on the ground.

(2) Clench the fists with the two hands, uplift them forward over the head, flex the two elbows slightly, with the fist heart in opposition, and look straight forward and breathe naturally (Figure 7-7).

1.6 低档势

预备姿势：同站裆势。

（1）屈膝下蹲，足尖靠拢，十趾抓地，足跟外蹬，上身下沉，臀部后坐不可着地。

（2）两手握拳，前上举过头顶，两肘微屈，拳心相对，两目平视，呼吸自然（图 7-7）。

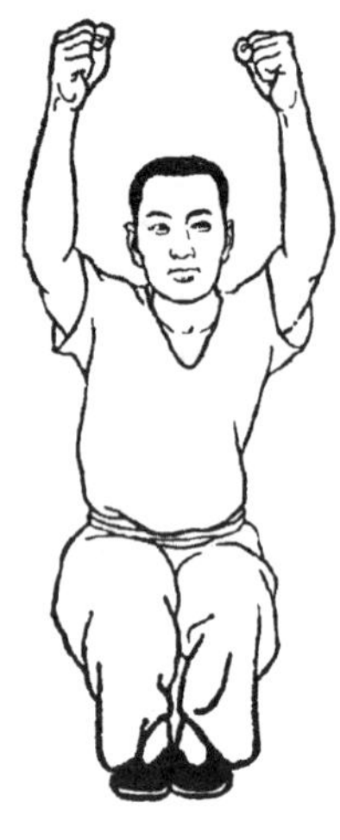

Figure 7-7
图 7-7

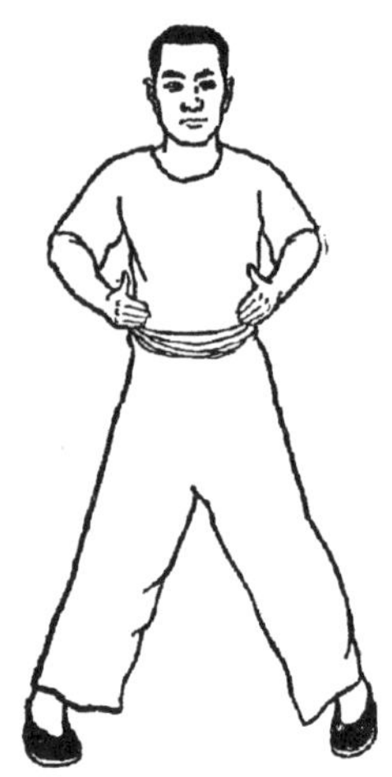

Figure 7-8
图 7-8

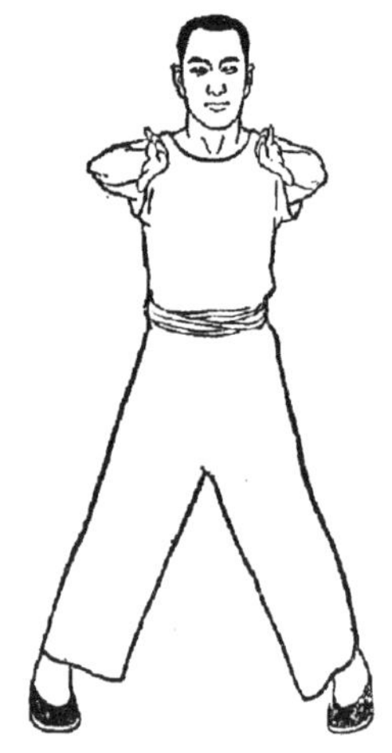

Figure 7-9
图 7-9

2 Training methods

2.1 Push eight horses forward

Training posture: Standing posture.

(1) Flex the two elbows of the two arms, with the straight palms on the two sides, with the palms in opposition, extend the thumb backward and upward, and close the four fingers forward (Figure 7-8).

(2) Gather the strength in the shoulders, arms and finger tips, push the two arms slowly forward with the force, with the shoulders and palms at the same level, and throw out the chest slightly and hold back the buttocks slightly, and look straight forward, and breathe naturally (Figure 7-9).

(3) Gather the strength in the shoulders, arms and finger tips, with the thumb upturned, by the finger tips at the same straight line of the arm as much as possible, and slowly flex the elbows to the

2 锻炼方法

2.1 前推八匹马

锻炼裆势:站裆势。

(1) 两臂屈肘,直掌于两胁待势。两掌心相对,拇指背伸向上,四指并拢向前(图 7-8)。

(2) 蓄劲于肩臂指端,使两臂徐徐运力前推,以肩与掌在同一平面上,胸微挺臀略收,两目平视,呼吸自然(图 7-9)。

(3) 蓄劲于肩臂指端,拇指上翘,指端力求与手臂成直线,慢慢屈肘,收回于两胁。

two sides.

(4) Change the straight palm slowly to a prone palm and press downward, extend the two arms backward, as the standing posture.

(4) 由直掌化俯掌下按，两臂后伸，同站裆势。

2.2 Pull nine bulls backward

2.2 倒拉九头牛

Training posture: Standing posture.

锻炼裆势：站裆势。

(1) Flex the elbows of the two arms, with the straight palms on the two sides, with the palms in opposition, extend the thumb backward and upward, and close the four fingers forward (Figure 7-10).

(1) 两臂屈肘，直掌于两胁待势。两掌心相对，拇指背伸向上，四指并拢向前(图7-10)。

(2) Push the two palms slowly form the two sides, and rotate the arms inward as well. While pushing the arms forward and straightening the elbows, turn the parts between the thumbs and index fingers of the two hands downward, close the four fingers forward, with the back of the two hands in opposition, and straighten the wrists at the level of the shoulder.

(2) 两掌从两胁缓缓前推，边推边向内旋臂，待两臂前推至肘部伸直时，两手虎口与拇指均正好向下，四指并拢向前，手背相对。腕伸直，与肩平。

(3) Flex the five fingers forcefully, change the palms into the fists like holding objects, with the strength in the fists, and flex and withdraw the elbows, and rotate the arms outward as well, till the fist eyes upward and fist centers in opposition, slowly backward to the two sides, and then slowly change the fists into the palms, and bend the body slightly forward, and hold back the buttocks (Figure 7-11).

(3) 五指用力屈收，由掌化拳如握物状，劲注拳心，屈肘收回，边收边向外旋臂，至拳眼向上，拳心相对，徐徐行至达两胁，缓缓松拳变掌。身微前倾，臀部微收(图7-11)。

(4) Turn the straight palms into the prone palms and press downward, extend the two arms backward, as the standing posture.

(4) 由直掌化俯掌下按，两臂后伸，同站裆势。

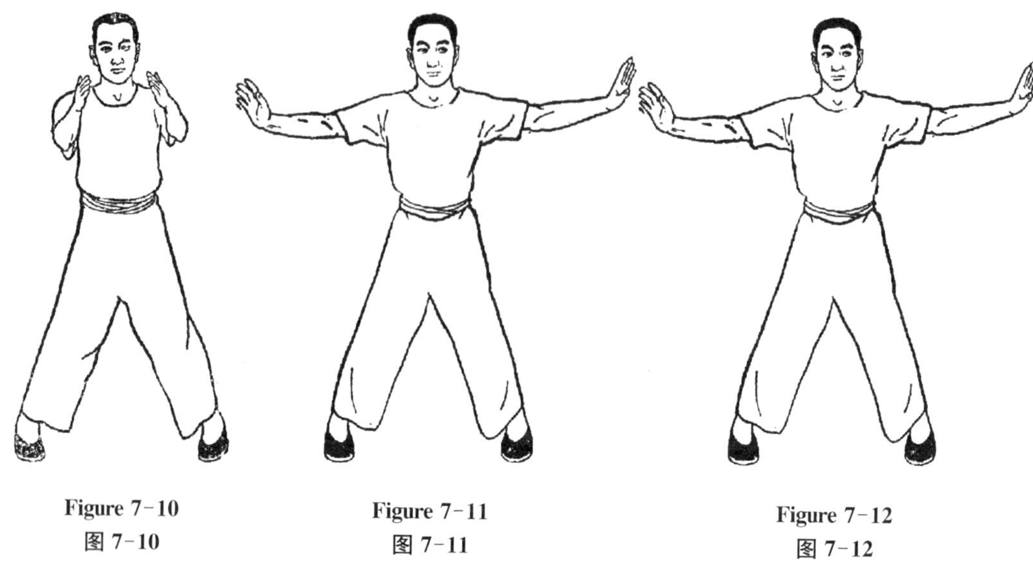

Figure 7-10
图 7-10

Figure 7-11
图 7-11

Figure 7-12
图 7-12

2.3 Phoenix spreading its wings

Training posture: Standing posture.

(1) Flex the elbows of the two arms upward, with the two hands crisscrossed in front of the chest in the standing palms.

(2) Gather the strength in the two arms, and slowly separate the two palms leftward and rightward, extend the wrists backward, close and upturn the four fingers, with the thumbs stretched outward forcefully, like stretching a bow and holding the object on the head. Look straight forward, without shrugging the shoulders, and breathe naturally (Figure 7-12)

(3) Rotate the two wrists, and flex the elbows of the two arms slowly to the center, to have the two palm centers gradually in opposition, and turn the two palms into the standing palms in front of the chest (Figure 7-13).

2.3 凤凰展翅

锻炼裆势:站裆势。

(1) 两臂屈肘上行,两手处于上胸成立掌交叉待势。

(2) 两臂运劲,两掌缓缓向左右外分,腕背伸,四指并拢上翘,拇指用力外展,犹如开弓之势,头如顶物,两目平视,不可扛肩,呼吸自然(图 7-12)。

(3) 两掌旋腕,两臂屈肘徐徐向中间收拢,使掌心逐渐相对,至两掌处于胸前交叉立掌(图 7-13)。

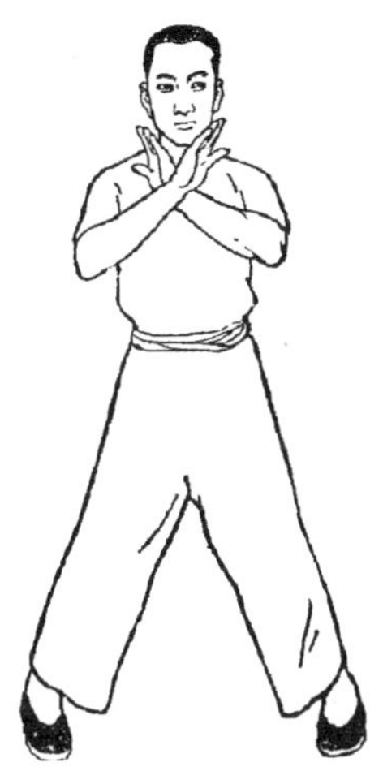

Figure 7-13
图 7-13

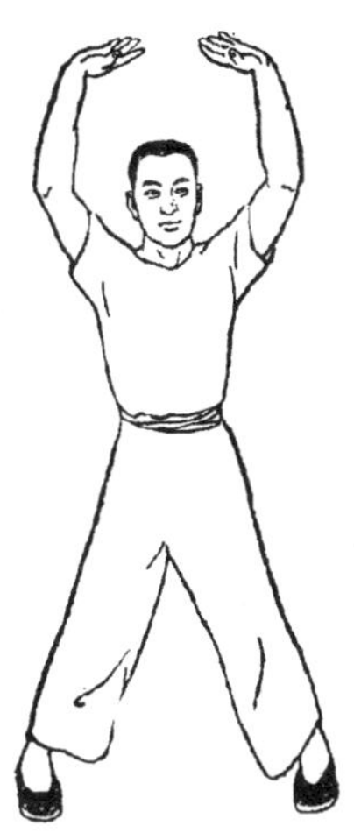

Figure 7-14
图 7-14

(4) Change the standing palms in front of the chest into the prone palms to press downward, and extend the two arms backward, as the standing posture.

(4) 由胸前之立掌化俯掌下按，两臂后伸，同站裆势。

2.4 Overload upholding a tripod

Training posture: Standing posture.

(1) Flex the elbows of the two arms into the supine palms at the body sides.

(2) Gather the strength in the fingers and palms, close the four fingers, with the thumbs stretched outward, and slowly uphold the two palms, with the palm centers upward, and while upholding over the shoulders, slowly rotate the arms, with the palm roots rotated outward, and the four finger tips of the two hands rotated inward in opposition, and with the parts of the thumb and index finger in opposition, like holding a heavy object, and slowly raise till the elbows are straightened, and look straight forward (Figure 7-14).

2.4 霸王举鼎

锻炼裆势:站裆势。

(1) 两手屈肘仰掌于腰部待势。

(2) 蓄劲于指掌，四指并拢，拇指外展，两掌缓缓上托，掌心朝天，上举过肩后慢慢旋臂，掌根旋外，两手四指指端旋内相对，虎口相对，犹托重物，徐徐上举至肘部伸直，两目平视(图 7-14)。

(3) Rotate the arms and turn the palms, with the palm centers backward, and the tips of the four fingers upward, and the thumb stretched outward, and gather the strength down and gradually withdraw the supine palms back to the two sides.

（3）旋臂翻掌，掌心向后，四指指端向上，拇指外展，蓄力而下，渐渐收回仰掌于腰部。

(4) Turn the supine palms into the prone palms to press downward, and extend the two arms backward, as the standing posture.

（4）由仰掌化俯掌下按，两臂后伸，同于站裆势。

2.5 Push the boat along with the current

2.5 顺水推舟

Training posture: Horse riding posture.

锻炼裆势：马裆势。

(1) Flex the elbows of the two hands into the standing palms at the two sides, with the four fingers forward, and the thumb stretched outward and the finger tip upward (Figure 7-15).

（1）两手屈肘直掌于胁部待势，四指向前，拇指外展指端向上（图 7-15）。

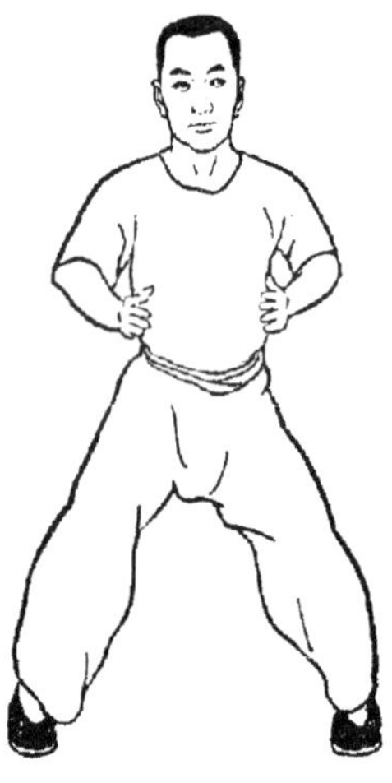

Figure 7-15
图 7-15

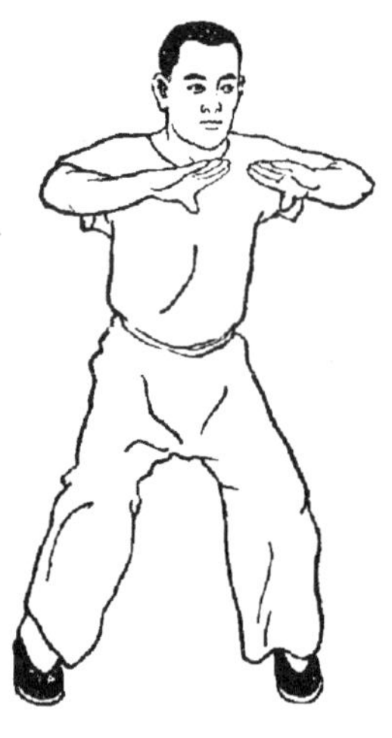

Figure 7-16
图 7-16

(2) Slowly push the two palms forward forcefully, and extend the wrist and rotate the arms as well, with the palm centers forward, the palm root rotated outward, and the parts between the thumb and index finger and the thumb tip downward, and

（2）两掌运劲徐徐向前推出，边推边伸腕旋臂，掌心向前，掌根旋外，虎口与拇指指端朝下，四指并拢，指端相对，两掌尺侧与肩肘平(图 7-16)。

close the four fingers, with the finger tips in opposition, and with the ulnar sides of the two palms at the level of the shoulder and elbow (Figure 7-16).

(3) Slowly rotate the five fingers of the two hands leftward and rightward, and flex the wrist at the level of the wrist, and turn back to the standing palms, close the four fingers, turn the thumb backward forcefully, and flex the elbow and gather the strength, and turn into the supine palms to protect the waist.

(3) 两手五指慢慢向左右外旋,并屈腕至腕平,恢复直掌,四指并拢,拇指运劲后翘,屈肘蓄力而收,成仰掌护腰。

(4) Change the supine palms into the prone palms to press downward, and extend the two arms backward, as the horse riding posture.

(4) 由仰掌化俯掌下按,两臂后伸,同马裆势。

2.6 The immortal directing the way

2.6 仙人指路

Training posture: Closed crotch posture.

锻炼裆势:并裆势。

(1) Flex the elbows of the two hands and turn into the supine palms at the waist, close the four fingers, straighten the thumbs and separate the parts between the thumb and index finger.

(1) 两手屈肘仰掌于腰部待势,四指并拢,拇指挺直,虎口分开。

(2) Uplift the right supine palm to the chest and go out as a standing palm, close the four fingers, straighten the thumbs, curve the palm into a loose palm, gather the strength from the elbow and arm to the palms, and then push the standing palm slowly forward (Figure 7-17).

(2) 右仰掌上提至胸立掌而出,四指并拢,拇指伸直,手心内凹成瓦楞掌,肘臂运劲蓄劲于掌,立掌徐徐向前推出(图 7-17)。

(3) Push out till the elbow is straightened, and then rotate the wrist and clench the fist, and gather the strength and withdraw to the waist to be the supine palm to protect the waist. At the same time, push both the left palm and right palm forward, repeatedly back and forth, in coordinative movement and natural breathing (Figure 7-18).

(3) 推出至肘直后旋腕握拳,蓄劲而收至腰部仰掌护腰。同时左掌与右掌动作相同向前推出,如此两掌一伸一收反复进行,动作协调,呼吸自然(图 7-18)。

(4) After training for the stipulated numbers and times, change the supine palms into the prone

(4) 待练好制定的次数或时间,由仰掌化俯掌下按,

palms to press downward, and extend the two arms backward, as the closed crotch posture.

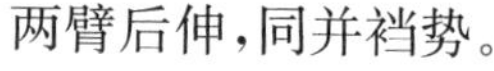
两臂后伸,同并裆势。

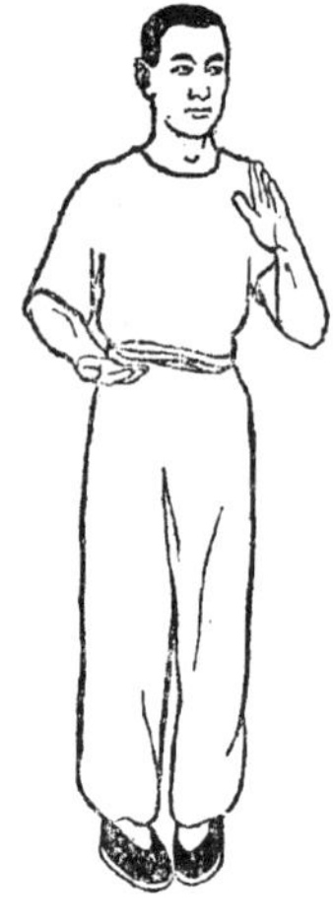
Figure 7-17
图 7-17

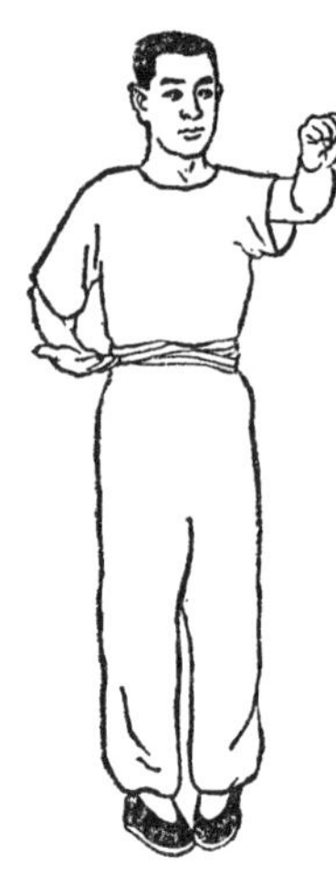
Figure 7-18
图 7-18

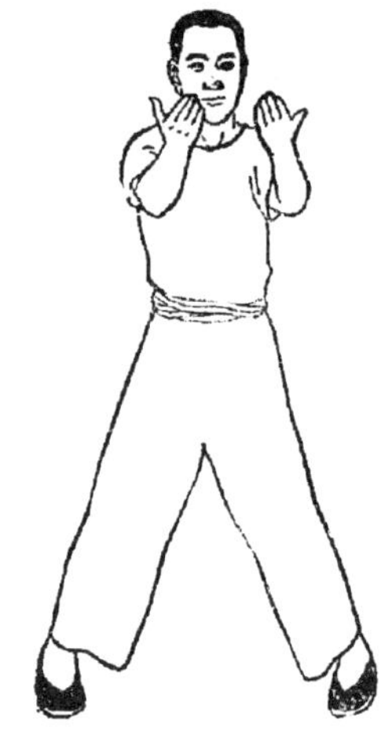
Figure 7-19
图 7-19

2.7 Uphold the pagoda with the flat hand

Training posture: Standing posture.

(1) Flex the elbows of the two hands, with the supine palms at the two sides, close the four fingers, straighten the thumbs, and separate the thumb from other four fingers.

(2) Push the two supine palms slowly forward and forcefully, and turn the thumbs leftward and rightward laterally, to maintain the flat motion of the palms, like holding object in the hand, and push continuously to the width and height of the shoulder (Figure 7-19).

(3) Turn the thumbs leftward and rightward laterally, gather the strength in the fingers and palms, and flex the elbows slowly and come back to the two sides.

(4) Change the supine palms at the two sides

2.7 平手托塔

锻炼裆势:站裆势。

(1) 两手屈肘仰掌于两胁待势,四指并拢,拇指挺直,虎口分开。

(2) 两仰掌慢慢向前运劲推出,边推边拇指向左右外侧倾斜,保持掌平运行,犹如托物在手,推足后与肩等高等宽(图 7-19)。

(3) 拇指向左右外侧倾斜,蓄劲指掌,屈肘缓缓收回至两胁。

(4) 将在两胁之仰掌化

into the prone palms to press downward, and extend the two arms backward, as the standing posture.

俯掌下按,两臂后伸,同站裆势。

2.8 Wind swinging the lotus leaves

2.8 风摆荷叶

Training posture: Standing posture.

锻炼裆势:站裆势。

(1) Flex the elbows of the two hands, with the supine palms at the two sides, close the four fingers, straighten the thumbs, and separate the thumb from other four fingers.

(1) 两手屈肘仰掌于腰部待势,四指并拢,拇指挺直,虎口分开。

(2) Gradually move the two palms upward to the chest, crisscrossed with the left palm above the right palm or right palm above the left palm, and push forward forcefully. Then, slowly separate them leftward and rightward to the body sides, with the shoulder, elbow and palm at the same height of straight line, and look straight forward and breathe naturally (Figure 7-20).

(2) 两掌渐循至上胸,左在右上或右在左上交叉,运劲前推。然后缓缓向左右外分至身体两侧,肩、肘、掌须等高成一直线,两目平视,呼吸自然(图 7-20)。

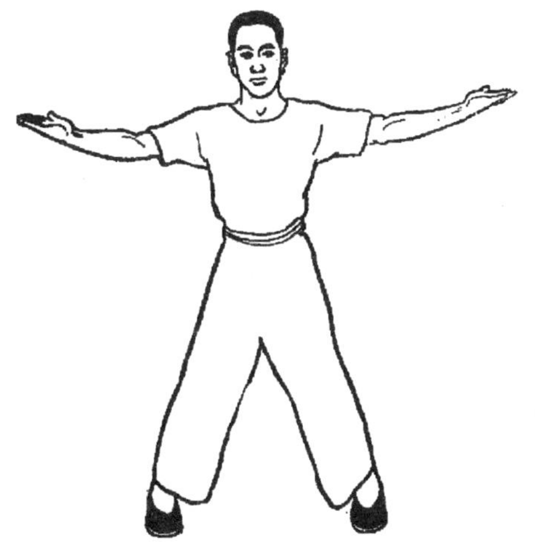

Figure 7-20
图 7-20

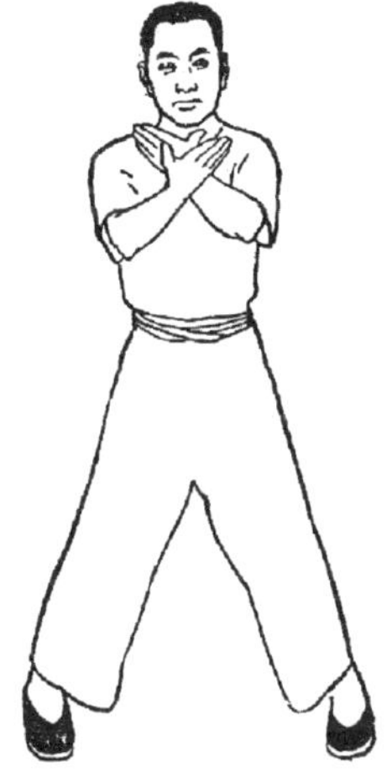

Figure 7-21
图 7-21

(3) Move the two supine palms forcefully and slowly to the front of the chest, crisscrossed with the left palm above the right palm or right palm a-

(3) 两仰掌由两侧徐徐运劲合拢至胸前,左在右上或右在左上,交叉相叠,掌心

bove the left palm, with the palms upward, and flex the elbows slightly (Figure 7-21).

(4) Withdraw the crisscrossed palms from the chest to the two sides of the waist, change into the prone palms to press downward, and extend the two arms backward, as the standing posture.

向上,两肘微屈(图 7-21)。

(4) 将胸前相叠两掌回收至腰侧,化俯掌下按,两臂后伸,同站裆势。

2.9 Pick up the moon from the bottom of a sea

Training posture: Open crotch posture.

(1) Flex the elbows of the two arms, with the supine palms at the waist.

(2) Move the two supine palms slowly upward, uplift them in front of the chest, and rotate the arms and extend the wrists simultaneously to the anterior and superior direction of the head. Then, separate them leftward and rightward slowly, with the palm centers downward, and at the same time, bend the body forward, by the straight legs, and super strength in the feet (Figure 7-22).

2.9 海底捞月

锻炼裆势:大裆势。

(1) 两手屈肘,仰掌于腰部待势。

(2) 两仰掌缓缓向上,经上胸徐徐高举,边举边旋臂伸腕至头部前上方。继而向左右两侧缓慢外分,使掌心向下,同时腰向前俯,腿不可屈,脚用霸力(图 7-22)。

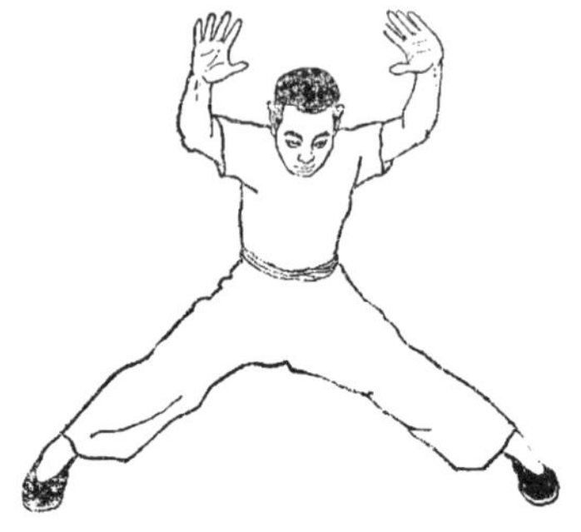

Figure 7-22
图 7-22

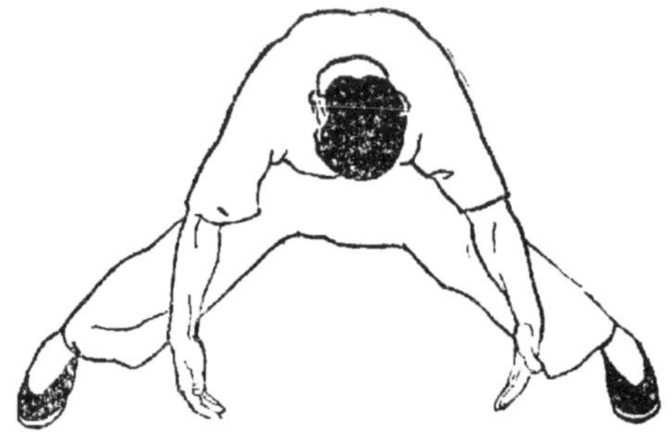

Figure 7-23
图 7-23

(3) Rotate the arms again, and move the two hands downward and pile up them inward, with the palm centers upward, like holding up object slowly, and uplift them forcefully and slowly to the front of the chest, and then withdraw the supine palms to

(3) 再旋臂,两手由上而下,由外向内相拢相叠,掌心向上似抱物慢慢抄起,用抱力缓缓提到胸前,继而收回仰掌于腰部。上身随势而

the sides of the waist. Straighten the body upright, and look straight forward (Figure 7-23).

直,两目平视(图 7-23)。

(4) Change the two supine palms into the prone palms to press downward, and extend the two arms backward, as the open crotch posture.

(4) 两仰掌化俯掌下按,两臂后伸,同大裆势。

2.10 Straighten up to the heaven and hold the ground

2.10 顶天抱地

Training posture: Closed crotch posture.

锻炼裆势:并裆势。

(1) Flex the elbows of the two hands, with the supine palms at the sides of the waist.

(1) 两手屈肘,仰掌于腰部待势。

(2) Gather the strength in the palms and fingers, uplift the supine palms to the front of the chest, extend the wrists, rotate the arms and turn the palms, with the palm center upward, the palm root turned outward, and the finger tips turned inward in opposition, and slowly raise the hands over the vertex (Figure 7-24). Up to its upmost, rotate the wrists and turn the palms, and slowly move down the two arms leftward and rightward, and at the same time bend the body forward and gradually close the two palms, with the thumbs turned outward and straightened, till the two palms are piled (with the right palm above the left palm), touching the ground with the back of the palms as much as possible (Figure 7-25).

(2) 蓄劲掌指,仰掌上托至胸前,伸腕旋臂翻掌,掌心向上,掌根外展,指端内旋相对,继续徐徐上举过头顶(图 7-24)。待推足后,旋腕翻掌,两臂缓缓向左右外分下抄,同时身向前俯,两掌逐渐合拢,拇指外展伸直,至两手掌指相叠(右掌在上左掌在下),掌背尽量碰地(图 7-25)。

(3) Then, slowly straighten up, and uplift the two palms like holding the heavy object slowly to the front of the chest, and then withdraw the supine palms to the sides of the waist (Figure 7-26).

(3) 随后腰部慢慢直起,两掌如抱重物缓慢上提至胸前,继而收回仰掌于腰部(图 7-26)。

(4) Change the two supine palms into the prone palms to press downward, and extend the two arms backward, as the closed crotch posture.

(4) 两仰掌化俯掌下按,两臂后伸,同并裆势。

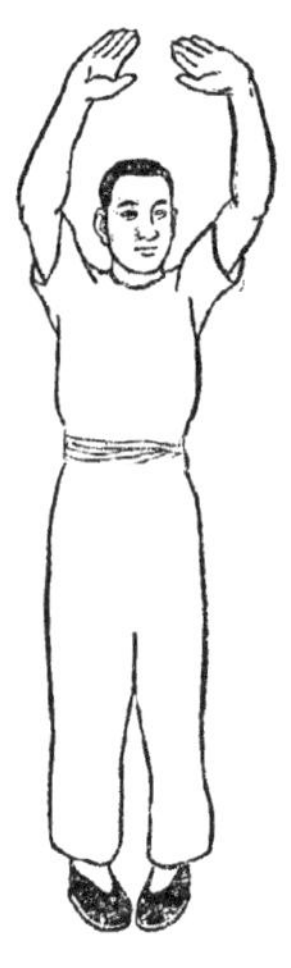

Figure 7-24
图 7-24

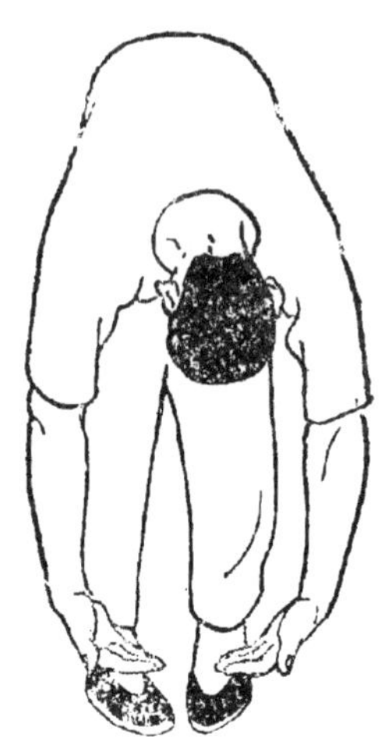

Figure 7-25
图 7-25

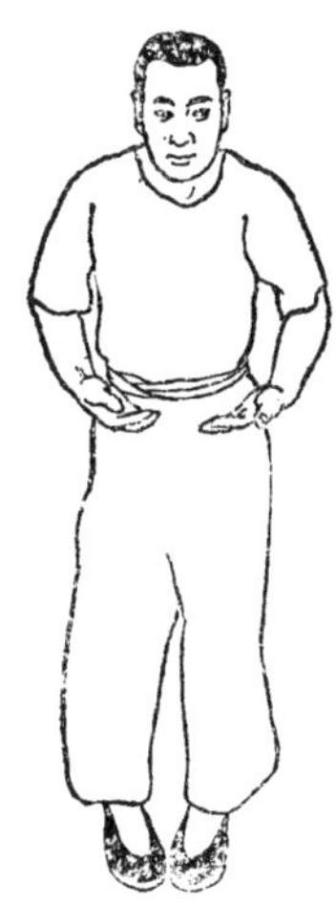

Figure 7-26
图 7-26

2.11　Rise for three times and fall for three times

Training posture: Low crotch posture.

(1) Squat down slowly, with the thighs parallel to the ground, throw out the chest and straighten up, with the two supine palms at the two sides of the waist.

(2) Rotate the arms, with the palm centers in opposition, close the four fingers, extend the thumbs backward forcefully, and push the two palms slowly forward till the elbows are straightened. Repeat this way for three times, and not to move the head with the posture, and look straight forward (Figure 7-27).

(3) In pushing the two palms for the fourth time, straighten up slowly while pushing the palms, to its utmost while the body is straightened up, and then gather the strength in the two thumbs and withdraw slowly, and finish the posture. Namely, flex the hip and flex the knee to squat down, and

2.11　三起三落

锻炼裆势:低裆势。

(1) 慢慢下蹲,大腿与地面平行,挺胸直腰,两手仰掌于腰部两侧。

(2) 旋臂,掌心相对,四指并拢,拇指运劲背伸,虎口撑开,两掌缓慢前推至肘直,如此往返三次,头勿随势俯仰摇动,两目平视(图 7-27)。

(3) 在两掌第四次推出时,身体慢慢起立,边推边起,待起来正好推足,两拇指蓄劲,缓缓收回,身体随之收势,即屈髋屈膝下蹲,待蹲下后两掌正好收回腰部,如此

withdraw the two palms exactly to the sides of the waist while squatting down. Repeat this way for three times.

往返三次。

(4) Change the supine palms at the sides of the waist into the prone palms to press downward, and extend the two arms backward, as the low crotch posture.

（4）将腰部之仰掌变俯掌下按，两臂后伸，同低裆势。

2.12 Hungry tiger pouncing on its prey

2.12 饿虎扑食

Training posture: Bow and arrow posture.

锻炼裆势：大弓箭裆势。

(1) Protect the waist with the supine palms of the two hands.

（1）两手仰掌护腰。

(2) Rotate the arms and push forward with the straight palms, and extend the wrist and rotate the arm as well, with the palm center forward, the palm root turned outward and the finger tips turned inward in opposition, and with the part between the thumb and index finger downward (Figure 7-28).

（2）旋臂直掌前推，边推边伸腕旋臂，掌心向前，掌根外展，指端内旋相对，虎口朝下（图 7-28）。

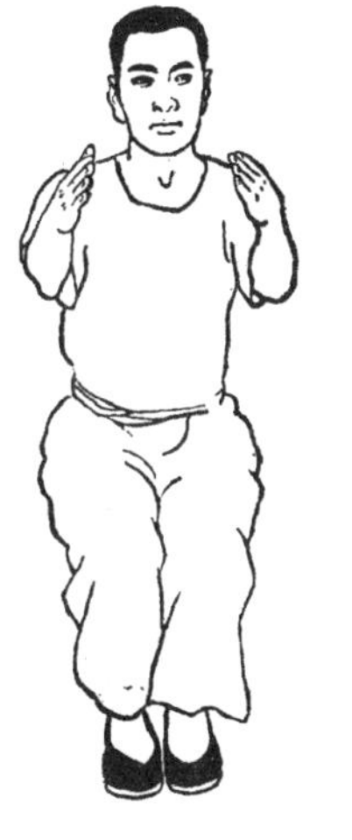

Figure 7-27
图 7-27

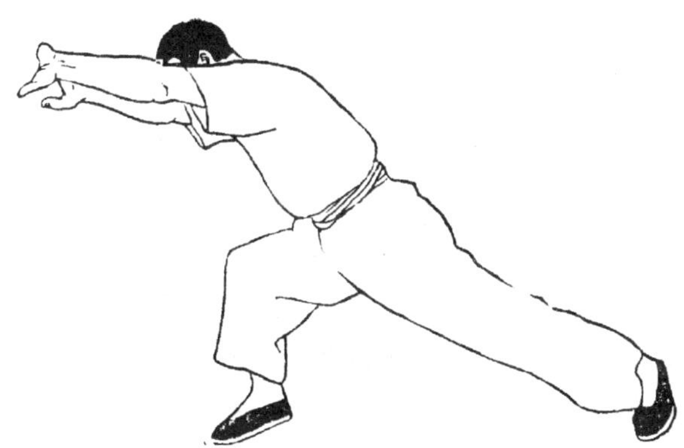

Figure 7-28
图 7-28

(3) Clench the fists with the five fingers, rotate the arms, with the fist eyes upward, and flex the elbows and gradually withdraw the supine palms

（3）五指内收握拳，旋臂，拳眼向上，屈肘渐渐收回仰掌护腰。

to protect the waist.

(4) Change the supine palms at the sides of the waist into the prone palms to press downward, and extend the two arms backward, as the bow and arrow posture.

（4）将腰部之仰掌变俯掌下按，两臂后伸，同弓箭裆势。

Section 4　Tendon-Changing Exercises (Yi Jin Jing)

第 4 节　易筋经

It is a traditional skill of long history and extensive circulation and is also an important component part in the school of one-finger massage therapy. By the specific methods, the tendon-changing exercises are supposed to train the regulation of the body, regulation of the respiration and regulation of the mind. During the training, it is requested to extend the tendons, pull the bones, contain gentleness within the firmness, contain the firmness within the gentleness, seek the motion from the tranquility, and contain the tranquility within the motion, so as to realize the goals to supplement qi, strengthen the tendons, regulate the functions of Zangfu organs, and build up the constitutional energy.

易筋经是一门历史悠久、流传广泛的中国传统功法，也是一指禅推拿流派的重要组成部分。易筋经通过特定的方法，进行自我调身、调息、调心的锻炼，锻炼过程中要求伸筋拔骨、刚中有柔、柔中有刚、静中求动、动中含静，达到气盈筋健、调整脏腑功能、培育正气的目的。

1　Wei Tuo offering the pestle

Stance: Close the two feet, like holding the object on the head, look straight forward, open the mouth slightly, touch the palate with the tongue, hold back the chest, relax the back, hold back the abdomen and buttocks, straighten the body, drop the two arms naturally to the two sides of the body, close and flex the five fingers slightly, touch the trousers seam, maintain the body upright, and tranquilize the

1　韦驮献杵势

预备姿势：两脚并拢，头如顶物，两目平视，口微开，舌抵上腭，含胸舒背，蓄腹收臀直腰，两臂自然下垂于身体两侧，五指并拢微屈，中指贴近裤缝，身体正直，心平气静（图 7-29）。

mind and have even breathing (Figure 7-29).

(1) Walk leftward for a step with the left leg, with the distance between the two feet as wide as the shoulder, relax the two knees slightly, step firm with the sole, uplift the two hands slowly, relax the shoulder, drop the elbows slightly, stretch the five fingers naturally, flex the metacarpophalangeal joints slightly, and have ball-holding posture in front of the chest. Seemly hold the object on the head, look straight forward, hold the chest, straighten the back, take in the abdomen and buttocks, open the mouth slightly, touch the palate with the tongue slightly, and concentrate the mind and regulate the respiration (Figure 7-30).

(1) 左腿向左平跨一步，两足之距约与肩宽，两膝微松，足掌踏实；双手徐徐上提，松肩，略垂肘，十指自然分开，掌指关节微屈，在胸前成抱球势。头如顶物，两目直视，含胸拔背，蓄腹收臀，口微开，舌抵上腭，凝神调息（图 7-30）。

(2) Rotate the wrist and turn the palms, with the palm centers upward, straighten the fingers, stretch the thumb and index finger, uphold the two palms over the head, slightly flex the elbows, raise the head, look at the back of the palms, and then lift the heel to support the body with the toes (Figure 7-31).

(2) 旋腕翻掌，掌心朝天，手指伸直，虎口张开，两掌上托，高过头顶。肘微屈，仰头，目观掌背，随势足跟提起，以足尖着地支撑身体（图 7-31）。

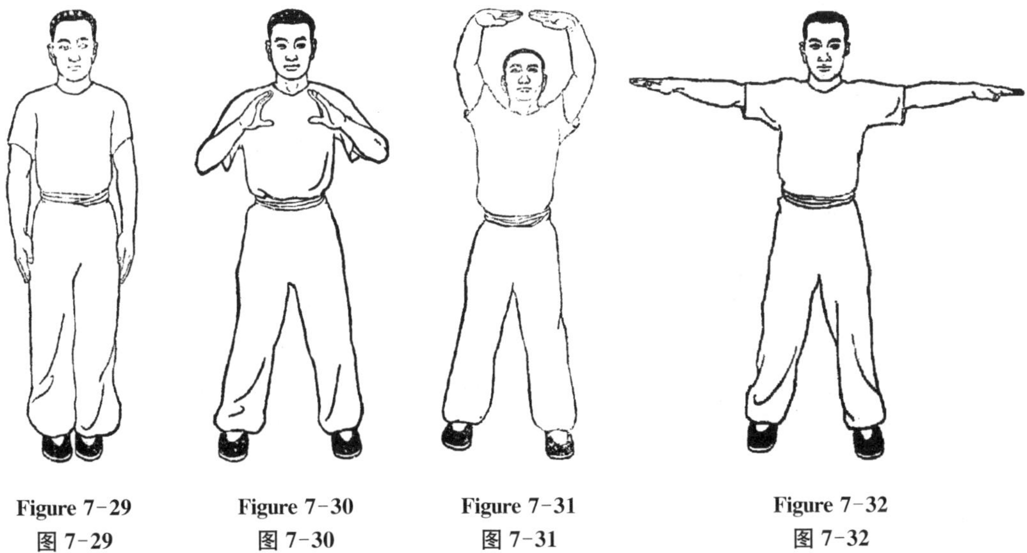

Figure 7-29 图 7-29

Figure 7-30 图 7-30

Figure 7-31 图 7-31

Figure 7-32 图 7-32

(3) Separate the two uplifted palms downward leftward and rightward, with the shoulder, elbow, wrist, and back of the palm on the same straight line, with the palm center downward, close and straighten the four fingers, and step down with the heel (Figure 7-32).

(3) 上托之两掌徐徐向左右分下，至肩、肘、腕、掌背成一直线，掌心向下，四指并拢伸直，随势足跟落地（图7-32）。

(4) Rotate the arms to turn the palm center forward, slowly close the two arms to the front and join the two palms. Flex the elbows, withdraw the two forearms and palms inward slowly, and rotate the arms simultaneously, to have the finger tip toward the chest and the middle finger pointing between Danzhong (CV 17) Tiantu (CV 22), with the shoulder, elbow and wrist flat. Stand upright, relax the shoulder, straighten the back, hold back the chest, abdomen and buttocks, keep the head upright, look forward, open the mouth slightly, and touch the palate with the tongue, and be calm in the mind and breathing.

(4) 旋臂使掌心向前，两臂缓缓向中间合拢，至两掌心相合。屈肘，两前臂与掌徐徐里收，同时旋臂，使指端向胸，中指指向膻中穴与天突穴之间，肩、肘、腕平。立身正直，松肩拔背，含胸蓄腹收臀，头端平，目前视，口微开，舌抵上腭，心静气平。

2 Reach for the stars and change the dipper

2 摘星换斗势

Stance: Same as the above.

预备姿势：同前。

(1) Move the step rightward and forward slightly with the right foot, in a T-shape with the left foot, with the right heel opposite to the left foot arch in a distance of one fist, and lean with the body slightly rightward and backward.

(1) 右足稍向右前方移步，与左足成斜丁八字步形，右足跟与左足弓相对，距约一拳，身体随势向右后侧微倾。

(2) Slightly flex the left hip and knee, uplift the right heel, and sink the upper body downward to have a loose step in the right foot. At the same time, clench a loose fist in the left hand and put it at the low back, and slightly flex the five fingers of the right hand, in a shape of hook, in front of the crotch.

(2) 微屈左侧髋膝，提右足跟，上身向下沉成右虚步；同时左手握空拳置于腰后，右手五指微屈握如钩状下垂于裆前。

(3) Uplift the right hooking hand, slightly above the shoulder, keep the forearm and upper arm almost vertically, and put the hooking hand at the right anterior direction, relax the shoulder, and flex the wrist.

(3) 右钩手上提,使肘略高于肩,前臂与上臂近乎垂直,钩手置于头之右前方,松肩屈腕。

(4) Following the above posture, rotate the forearm outward, with the hook rightward, incline with the head to one side slightly, and look at the right palm, touch the palate with the tongue, concentrate the mind and regulate the respiration, and keep the front leg loose and back leg firm (Figure 7-33).

(4) 接上势前臂旋外,钩尖向右,头微偏,目注右掌心,舍抵上腭,凝神调息。两腿前虚后实(图 7-33)。

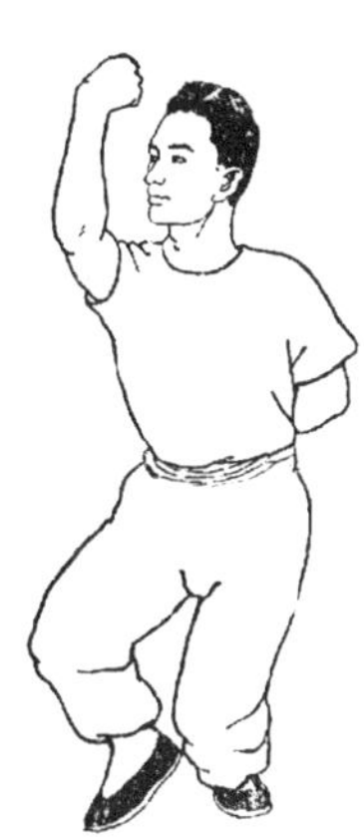

Figure 7-33
图 7-33

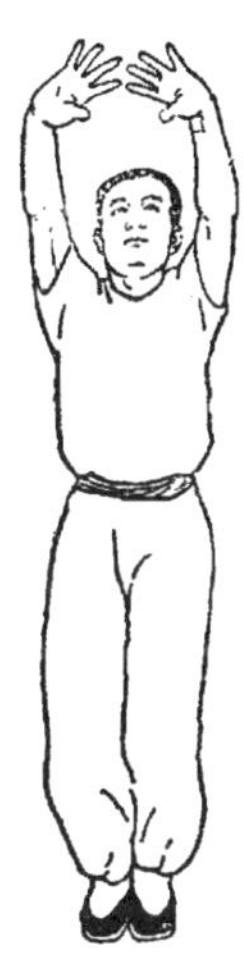

Figure 7-34
图 7-34

(5) Train alternatively the right posture and left posture, with the same movements.

(5) 左右交换,动作相同。

3 Extend the claws and show the wings

3 出爪亮翅势

Stance: Same as the above.

预备姿势:同前。

(1) Protect the two sides of the waist with the supine palms, close and straighten the four fingers. Uplift the two palms slowly in front of the chest above the head, and rotate the arm and wrist, with

(1) 两手仰掌护于腰部两侧,四指伸直并拢。两掌沿胸前徐徐上提过头顶,旋臂旋腕,掌心仍然朝天;十指

the palm upward. Separate the ten fingers forcefully, with the parts between the thumb and index finger in opposition, link with the middle and index finger of the two hands. At the same time, raise the head back, and watch the linking part of the index and middle finger, and lift the heel and support the body weight with the tiptoes. Slightly flex the elbow, straighten up and straighten the knee (Figure 7-34).

用力分开,虎口相对,两手中、食指相接;同时仰头,目观食中指交接之处,随势足跟提起,以两足尖支撑体重。肘微屈,直腰,膝不得屈(图 7-34)。

(2) Then, slowly separate the two palms downward respectively leftward and rightward, to the level of the shoulder, and stretch out the upper limbs flat (with the palm downward), and step down with the heel (Figure 7-35). Then, turn the palms upward, and separate the ten fingers forcefully (Figure 7-36).

(2) 随后两掌缓缓分向左右而下,达肩平,上肢成一字平举(掌心向下),随势足跟落地(图 7-35)。继而翻掌,掌心朝天,十指仍用力分开(图 7-36)。

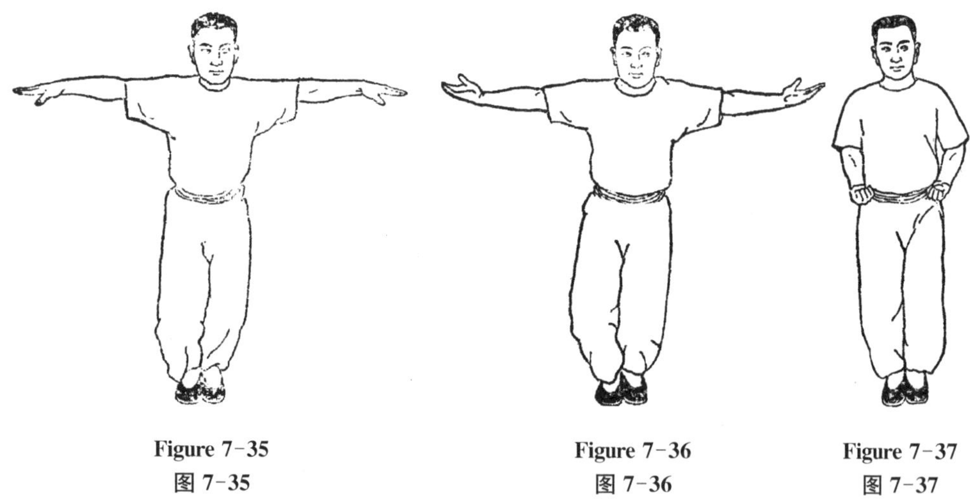

Figure 7-35
图 7-35

Figure 7-36
图 7-36

Figure 7-37
图 7-37

(3) Change the two supine palms into the fists and withdraw them slowly by flexing the elbows, to the two sides of the waist, with the palms upward (Figure 7-37).

(3) 两仰掌化拳徐徐屈肘收回,置于腰部两侧,拳心向上(图 7-37)。

(4) Change the two supine fists into the supine

(4) 两仰拳化仰掌,随即

palms, and then turn the palms into the prone palms by rotating the arms, and separate the ten fingers forcefully and push them slowly forward from the chest till the elbows are straightened, and then lift the heel from the ground (Figure 7-38, 7-39).

(5) Then, extend the two palms backward, with the palms forward and finger tips downward, and look straight forward (Figure 7-40). Afterward, flex the wrists flat, with the palm downward, and withdraw the palms to the two sides of the waist by flexing the elbows, and step down on the ground with the heel again.

旋臂成俯掌,十指用力分开,由胸前徐徐向前推至肘直,虎口相对;随势足跟提起离地(图 7-38, 7-39)。

(5) 继而两掌背伸,掌心向前,指端向上,目平视(图 7-40)。然后屈腕至腕平,掌心向下,并屈肘收回至腰部两侧,足跟随势再次落地。

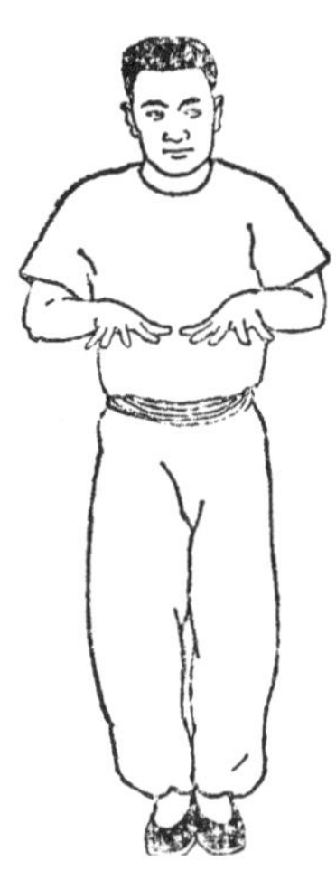

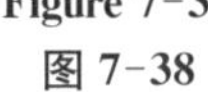

Figure 7-38
图 7-38

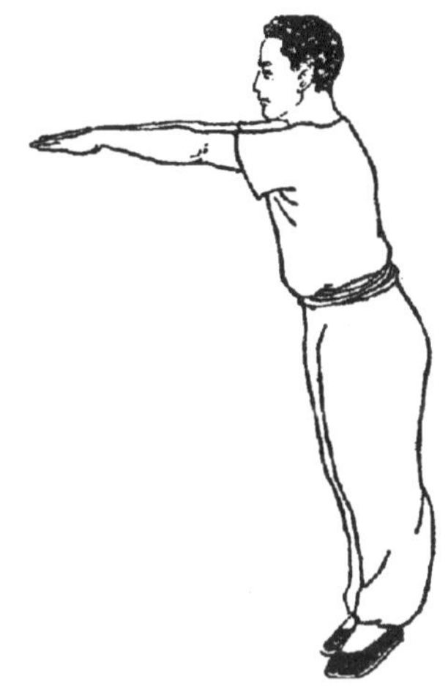

Figure 7-39
图 7-39

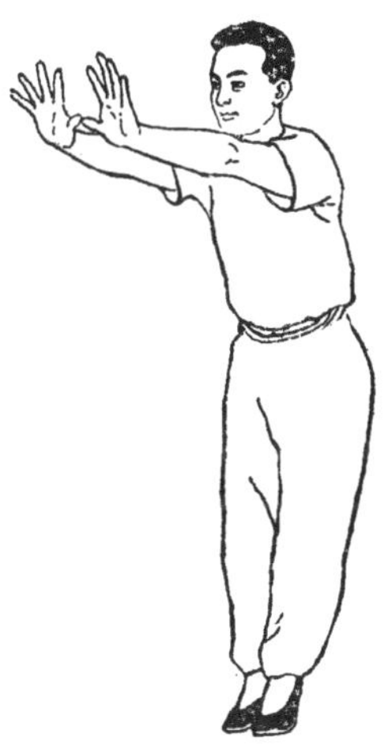

Figure 7-40
图 7-40

4 Three plates dropping on the ground

Stance: Same as the above.

(1) Walk leftward for one step with the left leg, with the distance between the two feet as wide as the shoulder, with the tiptoe turned inward, and flex the hip and knee to squat down to be a horse-riding posture, and support the waist with the two hands, throw out the chest straighten the body up-

4 三盘落地势

预备姿势:同前。

(1) 左腿向左平跨一步,两足之距比肩宽,足尖内扣,屈髋屈膝下蹲成马裆势,两手叉腰。挺胸直腰,头端平,目前视(图 7-41)。

right, keen the head upright, and look straight forward (Figure 7-41).

(2) Hold the two hands forward, with the ten fingers crisscrossed, with the back of the palm forward and the part between the thumb and index finger upward, and slightly flex the elbow, relax the shoulder, to have the upper limbs like a round plate in front of the chest (Figure 7-42).

(2) 两手由后向前抄抱，十指相互交叉而握，掌背向前，虎口朝上，肘微屈，肩松；两上肢似一圆盘处于上胸前方(图 7-42)。

(3) Rotate the wrists and turn the palms, with the two palms forward, and curve leftward and rightward and downward with the two palms, to become the supine palms in front of the lower abdomen. Then, slowly uplift them forcefully with inhalation via the lower abdomen and chest, to the eyebrows, with the distance of the two palms larger than distance between the the shoulders (Figure 7-43).

(3) 旋腕翻掌，两掌心向前，运动上肢，使两掌向左右划弧线而下，至下腹部前方呈仰掌，随吸气沿腹胸之前徐徐运劲上托，高不过眉，掌距不大于两肩之距(图 7-43)。

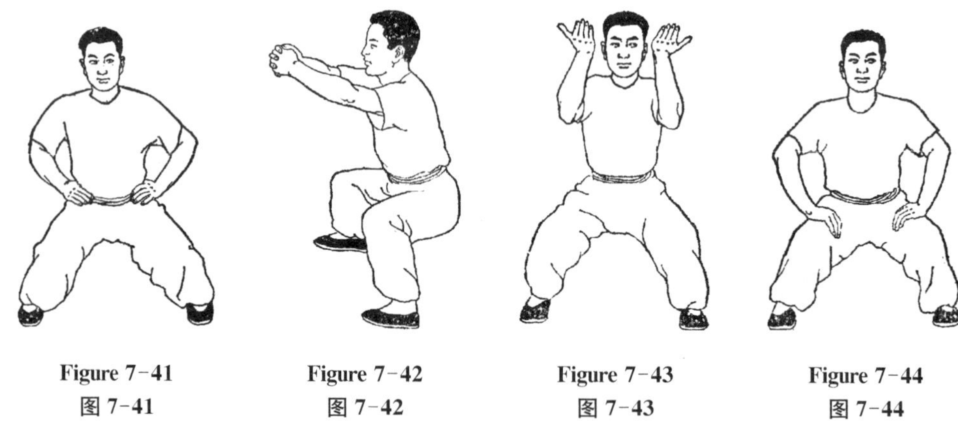

Figure 7-41 图 7-41

Figure 7-42 图 7-42

Figure 7-43 图 7-43

Figure 7-44 图 7-44

(4) Following the above posture, rotate the wrists and turn the palms, with the palms downward and the part between the thumb and index finger inward, and press downward forcefully with the two palms, and become the loose palms via the chest and abdomen in front of the upper part of the knee cap. Relax the two shoulders, flex the elbows slightly,

(4) 接上势，旋腕翻掌，掌心朝下，虎口朝内，两掌运劲下按，经胸腹之前呈虚掌置于膝盖上部，两肩放松，肘微屈曲，两臂略向内旋；前胸微挺，头如顶物，双目前视(图 7-44)。

rotate the two arms inward slightly, and throw out the chest slightly, keep the head upright and look forward (Figure 7-44).

(5) Then, stand up, put the two hands down at the body side, withdraw the left foot and return to the stance.

(5) 继而起立,两手从体侧放下,左脚收回,还原预备式。

5 Crouching tiger pouncing on its prey

Stance: Same as the above.

(1) Walk rightward for a big step with the right leg, flex the right knee and squat down to be a left crouching step, pile the two prone palms of the two hands on the right knee, straighten up and throw out the chest, and look slightly leftward (Figure 7-45).

(2) Turn the body leftward, straighten the right leg, flex the left knee and to be a posture of left bow and right arrow. Uplift the two palms from the knee via the two sides of the body to the two sides behind the ears by flexing the elbows, with the part between the thumb and index finger toward the head, the ten fingers slightly flexed and the finger tips upward. Then, push the two palms forcefully and slowly till the elbows are straightened, and look straight forward (Figure 7-46).

5 卧虎扑食势

预备姿势:同前。

(1) 右腿向右跨出一大步,屈右膝下蹲成左仆步势,两手俯掌相叠扶于右膝上,直腰挺胸,两目微向左视(图7-45)。

(2) 身体向左侧转,右腿挺直,屈左膝成左弓右箭势。扶于膝上之两掌从身体两侧屈肘上举于耳后之两旁,虎口对头部,十指微屈,指端向上。然后运劲使两掌徐徐前推至肘直,目视前方(图7-46)。

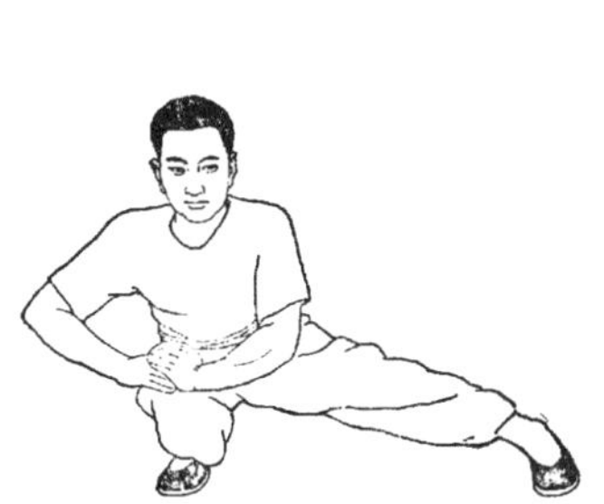

Figure 7-45
图 7-45

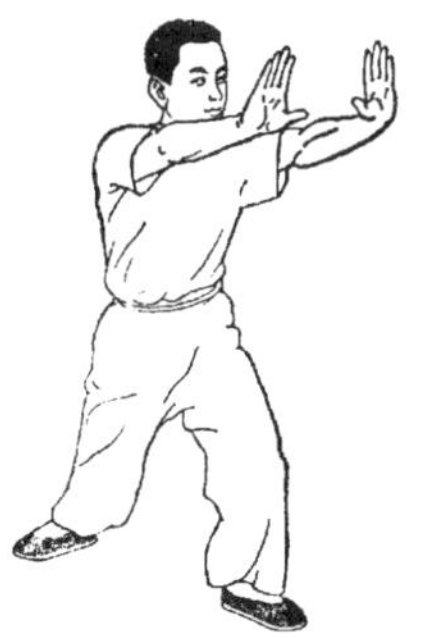

Figure 7-46
图 7-46

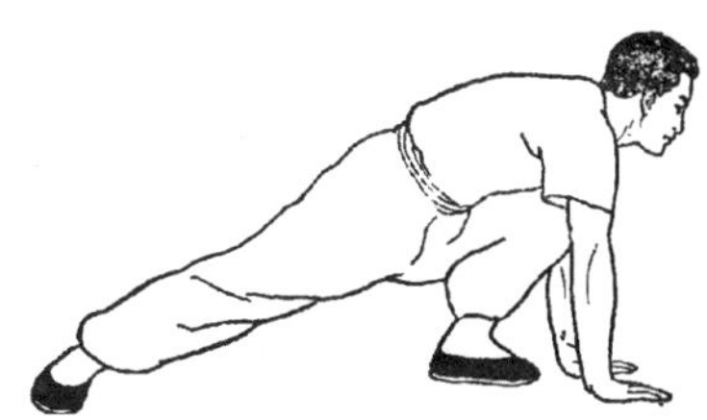

Figure 7-47
图 7-47

(3) Following the above posture, bend the body forward, press with the two palms and touch the ground with the palms or fingers, at the two sides in front of the left foot (Figure 7-47).

(3) 由上势俯腰，两掌下按，掌或指着地，按于左足前方两侧(图 7-47)。

(4) Then, lift the right heel, touch the ground with the tiptoes, and at the same time extend the left leg backward and put the left foot on the right heel, and support the body with the two palms or right foot toes. Then, flex the knee and hip (not touching the ground with the knee), and withdraw the body slowly backward, with the gravity moved backward, and keep the buttocks close to the left heel much as possible (Figure 7-48).

(4) 然后右足跟提起，足尖掂地，同时左腿后伸，做足背放于右足跟上，以两掌及右足尖支撑身体。再屈膝屈髋(膝不可接触地面)，身体缓缓向后收，重心后移，臀部尽量靠近左足跟，蓄劲待发(图 7-48)。

(5) Straighten the two knees slowly by the strength from the tiptoes, and push the body slowly forward forcefully with the two palms or fingers, and bend the body forward close to the ground as much as possible, with the gravity moved forward, like a crouching tiger pouncing on its prey. Finally, straighten the elbow, uplift the head and throw out the chest (Figure 7-49, 7-50). Thus, repeat the movements back and forth in a shape of tides.

(5) 足尖发劲，屈曲之双膝缓缓伸直；两掌或指使劲，使身体徐徐向前，上身尽量俯身贴地前探，重心前移，势如卧虎扑食；最后直肘昂头挺胸(图 7-49, 7-50)。如此后伸前探，连贯成波浪形的往返动作。

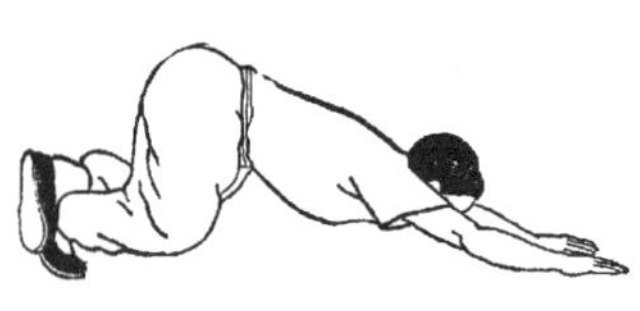

Figure 7-48
图 7-48

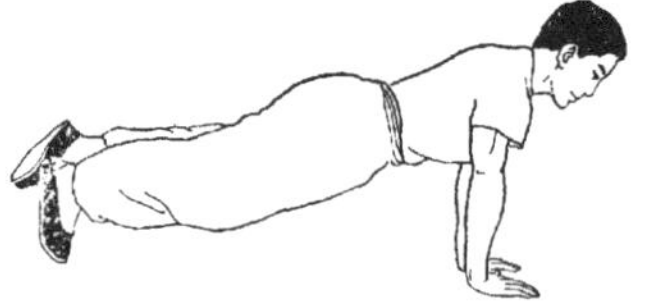

Figure 7-49
图 7-49

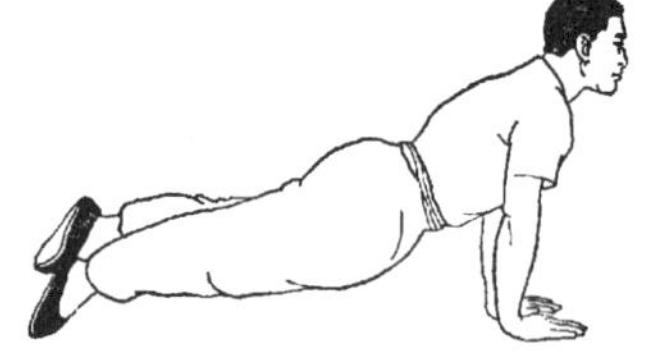

Figure 7-50
图 7-50

6　Bowing posture

Stance: Same as the above.

(1) Walk leftward for one step with the left leg, with the distance of the two feet as wide as the

6　打躬势

预备姿势：同前。

(1) 左腿向左平跨一步，两足之距比肩宽，足尖内扣。

shoulder, and the tiptoes turned inward. Uplift the two supine palms slowly from the two sides of the body to become a flat raising posture. Keep the head upright as if holding object on the head, look straight forward, relax the shoulder, and straighten the elbow, and keep the shoulder, elbow and wrist flat (Figure 7-51).

两手仰掌徐徐由身体两侧而上,成侧平举势。头如顶物,两目前视,松肩直肘,肩、肘、腕平(图 7-51)。

(2) Flex the elbow, hold the head with crossed fingers, and flex the hip and knee and squat down to be a horse-riding posture (Figure 7-52, 7-53).

(2) 屈肘,十指交叉相握抱头,并屈髋屈膝下蹲成马裆势(图 7-52, 7-53)。

(3) Following the above posture, straighten the knees and bend the body forward. Forcefully, thrust the head into the crotch, without flexing the knee and lifting the heel from the ground (Figure 7-54).

(3) 由上势直膝弯腰前俯,两手用力使头下探胯下。两膝不得屈曲,足跟不可离地(图 7-54)。

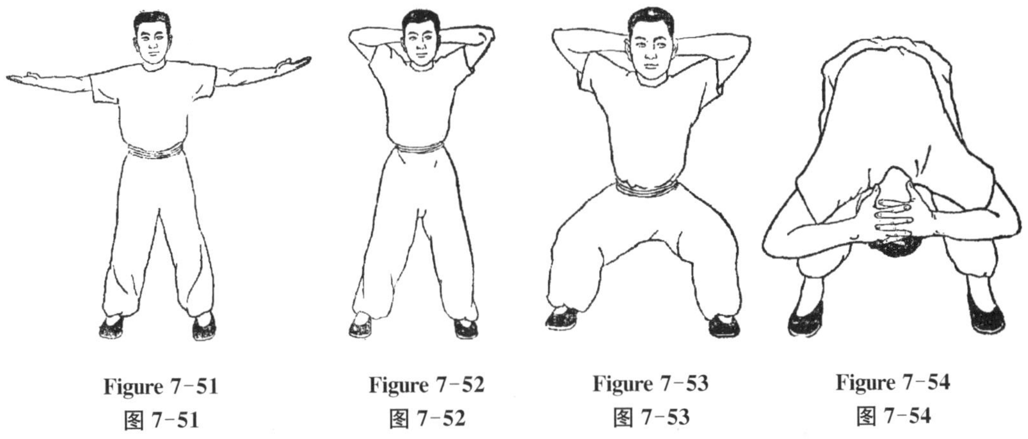

Figure 7-51 图 7-51 **Figure 7-52** 图 7-52 **Figure 7-53** 图 7-53 **Figure 7-54** 图 7-54

(4) Inhale, straighten up, flex the hip and knee and squat down to be a horse-riding posture. Then, stand up, put down the two hands along the body side, and withdraw the left foot, and return to the stance.

(4) 吸气,直腰屈髋屈膝下蹲成马裆势,继而起立,两手从体侧放下,左脚收回,还原预备式。

图书在版编目(CIP)数据

中国推拿:英汉对照/赵毅,陆萍主编. —上海: 上海浦江教育出版社有限公司,2017.9
(精编实用中医文库/陈凯先,李其忠,何星海总主编)
ISBN 978-7-81121-523-6

Ⅰ.①中… Ⅱ.①赵… ②陆… Ⅲ.①推拿—基本知识—英、汉 Ⅳ.①R244.1

中国版本图书馆 CIP 数据核字(2017)第227028号

上海浦江教育出版社出版
社址:上海海港大道 1550 号上海海事大学校内　邮政编码:201306
分社:上海蔡伦路 1200 号上海中医药大学内　邮政编码:201203
电话:(021)38284910(12)(发行)　38284923(总编室)　38284916(传真)
E-mail: cbs@shmtu. edu. cn　URL: http://www. pujiangpress. cn
上海盛通时代印刷有限公司印装　上海浦江教育出版社发行
幅面尺寸:170 mm×240 mm　印张:19. 25　字数:367 千字
2017 年 9 月第 1 版　2017 年 10 月第 1 次印刷
责任编辑:倪项根　封面设计:赵宏义
定价:80. 00 元